COMPLEX WORLDS FROM SIMPLER NERVOUS

COMPLEX WORLDS FROM SIMPLER NERVOUS SYSTEMS

edited by Frederick R. Prete

A Bradford Book
The MIT Press
Cambridge, Massachusetts
London, England

MIT Press books may be purchased at special quantity discounts for business or sales promotional use. For information, please email special_sales@mitpress.mit.edu or write to Special Sales Department, The MIT Press, 5 Cambridge Center, Cambridge, MA 02142.

This book was set in Stone sans and Stone serif by SNP Best-set Typesetter Ltd., Hong Kong. Printed and bound in the United States of America.

Library of Congress Cataloging-in-Publication Data

Complex worlds from simpler nervous systems / edited by Frederick R. Prete.
   p. cm.
"A Bradford book."
Includes bibliographical references and index.
ISBN 0-262-16223-7 (hc)—ISBN 0-262-66174-8 (pb)
1. Cognition in animals. 2. Learning in animals. 3. Animal behavior. I. Prete, Frederick R., 1948–

QL785.C545   2004
591.5'13—dc22

                                                                    2003068597

10 9 8 7 6 5 4 3 2 1

To Benjamin Andrew, Gregory Marshall, and Elizabeth Sarah

Contents

Foreword

When I started to become interested in animal behavior in the 1960s, the prevailing ideas were those of the pioneering ethologists, particularly Niko Tinbergen and Konrad Lorenz. They identified repeatable patterns of behavior, usually reliably triggered by particular stimuli. Their language was of innate releasing mechanisms and fixed action patterns, and while this approach provided a welcome framework for describing and analyzing behavior, it tended to emphasize robotlike rigidity rather than flexibility. In a well-known example, when a goose rolled an egg, the behavior would go to completion even if the egg was removed. "Not so smart," one thought.

It was the jumping spiders that lived around the University of California campus at Berkeley that started to change my thinking about arthropod behavior. The way they would turn to look at you and follow you around was endearing, as was the fact that they were furry and had big eyes. This made them look like tiny monkeys, in contrast to the inscrutable hard-faced insects that I was more familiar with. My real surprise came when I looked into the big front pair of eyes (spiders have four pairs altogether) with an ophthalmoscope. The strange boomerang-shaped retinas were moving in the image plane in a way that I soon realized was a scanning pattern. Far from waiting for some appropriate stimulus configuration to present itself, the spiders were actively interrogating images. They were seeking, as it turned out, the clues that would let them decide whether each new object was a potential prey, mate, or foe. These were not reflex machines, but inquisitive beings.

That was not all. It had been known for some years that jumping spiders could make detours to reach prey, during which time the prey was out of sight. In chapter 1, Harland and Jackson describe *Portia* making detours that last as long as 20 min. However one looks at it, a detour involves the execution of a stored plan: a motor program executed on the basis of an internal representation of the surroundings. This is sophisticated stuff, hardly to be expected of a brain the size of a pinhead. *Portia* astounds in other ways. The flexibility of its locomotor strategies in dealing with different kinds of spider prey, and the variety of cunning tactics employed for dealing with spiders in webs, would certainly fit most definitions of intelligence.

According to Nick Strausfeld, houseflies have 337,856 neurons in their brains. Bees have just short of a million. The exact numbers for the human brain are not available, but the old saying used to be (after Szentagothai's study of the cerebellum) that the brain contains 10^{10} neurons, of which 10^{11} are in the cerebellum. A factor of 10^4 to 10^5 between bee and man seems probable. And yet, qualitatively at least, there are few things a bee cannot do that higher vertebrates can (chapter 2). As "central-place foragers," bees learn the location of their nest or hive and of a variety of food sources. They use time-compensated compass cues and unfolding arrays of landmarks to get from one to the other. They communicate distance and direction of food sources to each other using the dance language discovered by Karl von Frisch. Visually they can learn colors and shapes, and can generalize abstract features, such as figure orientation and symmetry type, from the concrete examples that they have seen. They can learn to fly through mazes, and can use previously stored information to help them learn. They also readily learn cross-modal associations, for example, between the scent and color of flowers. In addition to all this, they perform a variety of very different jobs over the course of their brief lifetime.

In spite of these impressive feats of intellect, small brains must have their limitations. One assumes that there is a need to restrict the amount of information that they must process to just those features that are of greatest importance in survival and reproduction. In chapter 4 Ewert argues that by keeping its eyes still, a toad eliminates all of the biologically unimportant information about stationary objects. (If our eyes are kept artificially still for as few as 10 s, the perceived image disappears for us, too). This leaves the toad just with things that move, and these are nearly all animate: food, mates, or predators. The toad deals with these classes of objects in a sophisticated way, weighing up many of their various stimulus parameters to determine what the appropriate response should be. It is interesting that mantids (chapter 3) do very much the same thing, even employing a remarkably similar algorithm for identifying prey amid the complex background of vegetation in which it is found. Of course, when a toad moves, the stationary world reappears, and as Tom Collett demonstrated some 20 years ago, toads plan sensible routes to reach their prey. If a fence has a sufficiently wide gap in it, they go through it. Otherwise they detour around the end. Again, the praying mantis is similar. By peering back and forth or side to side, it makes the stationary objects in its world move relative to its retinae. The mantis can use this information, much as vertebrates do, to identify the location and distance of objects in its three-dimensional world.

Other examples of simplification, or stimulus filtering, include the wavelength-specific behaviors of butterflies, in which certain activities—escape, egg-laying, feeding—are linked to colors that correspond closely with the peak spectral sensitivities of individual classes of receptors (chapter 6). Effectively, the butterfly is using dedicated "labeled lines" to drive particular behaviors. It is interesting that butterflies, like bees, also have true color vision. That is to say, they can be trained to intermediate colors that do not correspond to particular sensitivity peaks. Presumably, butterflies rely on the simpler system for routine vision and keep true color vision for occasions when it is needed—distinguishing the colors of flowers, for example.

One of the common features of the sensory systems of small-brained animals is that much of the processing occurs at the periphery, presumably to simplify the brain's work. The amazing color vision system of mantis shrimps is a good example. Here, receptors with twelve different spectral sensitivities span the spectrum from 300 to 700 nm (chapter 8). One possibility is that instead of doing what we (or bees) do, which is to estimate wavelength from the ratios of activity in two or three receptor types, all a mantis shrimp's brain needs to do is to note that receptor type three, for instance, is most active. So the color must be yellow.

My favorite example of sensory simplification is the technique that fiddler crabs use to distinguish predators (requiring escape) from conspecifics (which can be fought, mated, or ignored). Instead of identifying predators (usually birds) by their form (beak, legs, etc.), all the fiddler crab has to ask is "Does this moving object intersect the horizon?" Since a line joining the crab's eye to the horizon is at crab height, anything above this is bigger than the crab, and so is probably bad news. Anything below the line is, at least, not life threatening. Simple though this is, it does require the crab to keep its elongated eye accurately aligned with the horizon, and for this it uses both visual and statocyst reflexes. Like the mantis shrimp example, a sophistication of the peripheral apparatus simplifies the central task.

Several authors have made the point, when writing, for example, about the impressive abilities of jumping spiders, bees, or mantids, that if these animals were vertebrates one might be ascribing to them abstract reasoning, even insight and intelligence. However, there is an understandable reluctance to attribute too much of an inner world to an insect. This is no doubt partly because their inflexible exoskeleton prevents their expressing anything we might regard as an emotion. However, this is certainly not true of the other group of invertebrate intellectuals, the cephalopod mollusks. Anyone who has watched cuttlefish will know that if there was ever an animal that wears its heart on its sleeve, it is *Sepia*. The changing chromatophore patterns that come and go across the skin of its mantle advertise its moods and intentions, and it is hard not to see these changes as manifestations of something akin to emotions.

Where does this leave us? Basically, with the same questions that we would address if considering "higher" vertebrates. If bees and jumping spiders have internal representations of their environment and the objects in it, as they seem to, then we have to study them in the same ways that we would if they were rats or dogs. There seem to be no reasons to consider invertebrates more robotlike than vertebrates but, equally, they are no better than rats or cats for studying consciousness and the subjective world of qualia.

This is where Jakob von Uexküll's century-old word *Umwelt* (self-world) is so useful. It implies the complex relation between the environment and an animal's internal representation of it, without suggesting that an animal's brain is just a collection of circuits on the one hand, or that it is the substrate for elaborate mentalistic imagery on the other. The nervous systems discussed in this book are possibly simpler than some, and certainly smaller, but as we have come to learn in the past few decades, the worlds they represent can be astonishingly rich, complex, and varied.

Michael F. Land
2004

Preface

In the preface to the book *The Praying Mantids* (Prete et al., 1999) I explained how, through serendipity, I came to work with these insects. In brief, on a bright, early autumn morning on the University of Chicago campus, I saw my first praying mantis at the foot of the steps to the science library. As I passed, the large, elegant insect made a characteristic defensive display, described by the famous entomologist, Jean-Henri Fabre, like this: "The wing-covers open, and are thrust obliquely aside.... [They are like] parallel screens of transparent gauze, forming a pyramidal prominence which dominates the back; the end of the abdomen curls upwards.... The murderous forelimbs ... open to their full extent, forming a cross with the body ... the Mantis wishes to terrorize its powerful prey, to paralyze it with fright" (Fabre, 1912, pp. 74–75). Although I was not quite "demoralized with fear," I was taken aback by this animal's courageous demeanor and graceful elegance. I carefully put it into my brief-case and literally ran back to my office to look more closely at this marvelous little creature.

What I had found was a female *Tenodera aridifolia sinensis*. However, before I knew its scientific name, before I had seen any scholarly papers about mantids, before I turned an analytical eye to its behavior, it was simply thrilling to watch, and after a day with my mantid, my future research agenda was set. Over the next 2 years I raised a colony of *T. a. sinensis* and *Sphodromantis lineola*, and managed to collect enough data on the psychophysics of prey recognition and the kinematics of their predatory strike to assemble a dissertation, which I finished in August of 1990. That, really, was the easy part of my research.

The difficult part of my work was convincing other people about what I had found. Fundamentally, this difficulty stemmed from the fact that prior to beginning my research, neither I nor my mantids had read any of the scientific literature written about them. I did not know that insects were "supposed" to act like simple "reflex machines" (Prete and Wolf, 1992). Likewise, the mantids did not know that they were "supposed" to be strictly limited in their visual, motor, and information-processing abilities. Hence, because of our collective ignorance, I asked my mantids complex questions (experimentally speaking), and they were generous enough to provide me with very complex answers. Neither of us knew we were in uncharted territory. And it took time before we could convince others that mantids are indeed quite different than the "simple" insects that they had been made out to be.

Similar, exciting revelations have been experienced by all of the contributors to this book. They each work with animals thought at one time to live in stark, restricted perceptual worlds. We now know that they do not. The little animals described here, and many others like them, live in extremely complex perceptual worlds; worlds that match in many ways those of the large vertebrates, even humans.

When I teach students about these little animals in courses such as Animal Behavior, I always tell them something like this: "If, when you see a praying mantis, a butterfly, a honeybee, you are not in awe, amazed by the complexity of an animal whose brain could sit comfortably on the head of a pin, you will never truly understand the wonder that is nature. Try to appreciate that wonder." I invite the reader to do the same.

Acknowledgments

A project such as this requires the goodwill and collegial cooperation of a large number of people. And indeed this book is a product of their efforts more than mine. Those to whom I am most deeply indebted are of course the many scientists who have taken their valuable time to contribute to this volume. Their friendships have been rewarding, their expertise has been invaluable, and I have learned much from each of them. I also owe a unique, personal debt of gratitude to Jörg-Peter Ewert. It was his groundbreaking work on the psychophysics of prey recognition in toads that inspired and shaped my experimental approach to prey recognition in praying mantids. I also acknowledge the efforts of Thomas Stone and Katherine Almeida, senior editors at the MIT Press, who accepted my prospectus for this book and supervised its production, respectively. Their patience, support, and guidance were invaluable. In addition, I am grateful to the referees, reviewers, editors, and production people who invested their time and talents in this project. The book was substantially improved by their efforts. It goes without saying that any errors remaining are solely mine. Finally, I thank Annie Guter, who helped me with childcare during the final stages of manuscript preparation.

Contributors

Kentaro Arikawa
Professor, Graduate School of Integrated
Science
Yokohama City University
Yokohama, Japan

Lars Chittka
Senior Lecturer, School of Biological
Sciences
Queen Mary, University of London
London, England

Vanessa C. K. Couldridge
Postdoctoral Research Associate, H. P.
Scott Center for Neuroscience, Mind and
Behavior, Department of Biological
Sciences
Bowling Green State University
Bowling Green, Ohio

Christopher Comer
Professor, Laboratory of Integrative
Neuroscience and Department of
Biological Sciences
University of Illinois at Chicago
Chicago, Illinois

Thomas W. Cronin
Professor, University of Maryland
Baltimore County
Baltimore, Maryland

Jörg-Peter Ewert
Professor, Department of Neurobiology
FB Natural Sciences
University of Kassel
Kassel, Germany

Ian G. Gleadall
Frontier Research Fellow, Institute of
Physical and Chemical Research (RIKEN)
Photodynamics Research Centre
Sendai, Japan

Takahiko Hariyama
Associate Professor, Department of
Biology
Hamamatsu University School of
Medicine
Hamamatsu, Japan

Duane P. Harland
Wool Research Organisation of New
Zealand
Christchurch, New Zealand

Robert R. Jackson
Associate Professor, Department of
Zoology
University of Canterbury
Christchurch, New Zealand

Michiyo Kinoshita
Postdoctoral Associate, Graduate School
of Integrated Science
Yokohama City University
Yokohama, Japan

Karl Kral
Associate Professor for Zoology, Institute
of Zoology
Karl-Franzens-University Graz
Graz, Austria

Michael F. Land
Professor, Sussex Centre for Neuroscience,
School of Life Sciences
University of Sussex
Brighton, England

Vicky Leung
Graduate Fellow, Laboratory of
Integrative Neuroscience and
Department of Biological Sciences
University of Illinois at Chicago
Chicago, Illinois

Justin Marshall
Queen's Fellow, Physiology and
Pharmacology
University of Queensland
Brisbane, Australia

Frederick R. Prete
President, Visuo Technologies, LLC
Morton Grove, Illinois

Heiner Römer
Professor, Institute for Zoology
Karl-Franzens-University Graz
Graz, Austria

Nadav Shashar
Assistant Professor, The Interuniversity
Institute of Eilat
Eilat, Israel

D. G. Stavenga
Professor, Department of
Neurobiophysics
University of Groningen
Groningen, Netherlands

Mandyam V. Srinivasan
Professor, Research School of Biological
Sciences
Australian National University
Canberra, Australia

Moira J. van Staaden
Associate Professor, J. P. Scott Center for
Neuroscience, Mind and Behavior
Department of Biological Sciences
Bowling Green State University
Bowling Green, Ohio

Harrington Wells
Professor, Faculty of Biological Sciences
University of Tulsa
Tulsa, Oklahoma

Shaowu Zhang
Fellow, Research School of Biological
Sciences
Australian National University
Canberra, Australia

Introduction

Sensory systems are not the transparent windows to the world that Aristotle imagined them to be. They are actually strong filters. They have evolved to extract biologically meaningful information from the world while filtering out extraneous or redundant information, and to process that meaningful information in particular, species-specific ways. Over the course of their evolution, sensory systems, even those of very small animals, have become quite complex. In fact, they have evolved so that they usually include a number of integrated, sometimes overlapping, nested subsystems that together make up the broader sensory modality in terms of which they are named. For instance, the diminutive visual system of an invertebrate may include functionally and anatomically distinct scotopic (low light), photopic (high light), wavelength-sensitive, wavelength-specific, and polarization-sensitive subsystems. In addition, it may include one or more feature-selective subsystems that are capable of assessing the configurational and/or spatiotemporal characteristics of stationary or moving objects, respectively. Each such subsystem could be thought of as an information-processing network designed to identify specific types or "classes" of biologically meaningful stimuli. Hence the modality's name, "vision," for instance, is itself a convenient label that we use to identify the complex assemblage of nested information-processing subsystems that transduce a particular range of a particular type of energy, in this example, electromagnetic energy. This is a very different conceptualization of a sensory system than that which most of us were taught as students. However, it is a conceptualization that allows a fuller, richer appreciation of the complexity of the perceptual worlds created by animals with central nervous systems that are much "simpler" than ours.

Of course, all of us—vertebrates and invertebrates, large and small—share the same planet. Hence we all face analogous, if not fundamentally similar, environmental challenges. Consequently, sensory systems can show remarkable functional and/or organizational similarities even if the organisms that possess them are phylogenetically disparate, such as humans and insects, for instance. One example of such a similarity is the organization of the retina into a central, high-acuity/low-sensitivity acute zone (or fovea) surrounded by a low-acuity/high-sensitivity peripheral area, each with functionally and anatomically distinct behavioral interfaces. Such convergent solutions to common challenges provide a window onto the general principles by which central nervous systems organize.

Conversely, organisms can face specific or unique environmental challenges that necessitate equally specific or unique solutions. For instance, stomatopod crustaceans have evolved a remarkably complex and unusual visual system that they use to analyze unique informational combinations provided by the spatial, spectral, and polarizational distributions of light in their underwater habitats. Such unique cases provide us with two types of insights. First, they teach us about the otherwise unrecognized possibilities and boundaries of neural systems. Second, by comparing a neural subsystem manifesting a unique information-processing solution with the subsystem from which it evolved, we can learn the more subtle, nuanced rules governing how the components of neural networks can alter their computational relationships to meet specific information-processing challenges.

This, then, is what this book is about. It tells a number of unique and interesting stories about the mechanisms, anatomical structures, and organizational principles that underpin some of the sensory subsystems in a handful of so-called "simpler" animals. The stories also try to give the reader a sense of the complexity and richness of the perceptual worlds to which the sensory subsystems contribute. Each story is fascinating both for what it reveals and for what it leaves out. The former teaches us how much these "simpler" animals have been underestimated. The latter tantalizes us by suggesting mysteries that are still left to be resolved.

Frederick R. Prete
June 2004

I CREATING VISUAL WORLDS: USING ABSTRACT REPRESENTATIONS AND ALGORITHMS

INTRODUCTION

Frederick R. Prete

One could argue that the central role of visual systems is to process information about various types of movement. If nothing in the world moved, it is hard to imagine why vision would have evolved. However, the visual world in which we and all other animals live is a confusing place. Not only do various objects in it move on their own, in different ways, and at different speeds, but when we move, everything in our visual field (even stationary objects) shifts its location. It would be impossible for us, even with our large human brain, to keep track of all of this information. Imagine how difficult it must be for little animals, some of which have brains no larger than the head of a pin.

All animals—people, spiders, bees, mantises, toads—can manage this dizzying array of information because their sensory systems are actually filtering systems that let in only the information that is potentially biologically meaningful; redundant or unnecessary information is filtered out. Now, what is particularly interesting is that there are fundamentally just two ways that a sensory system such as vision, for example, could do this filtering task. One way is to ignore all but some very limited, specific types of visual information. For instance, a jumping spider, a praying mantis, or a toad could be designed to recognize only a small, moving, fly-sized spot just a few millimeters away as a potential meal and ignore all other moving objects. Or a foraging bee could recognize and fly toward only yellow flowers of a certain size that appear directly in front of it. This type of filtering would ensure that a response was made to a precise and always appropriate stimulus. And, in fact, this is in many ways how small animals were once thought to operate. There is, of course, an obvious problem with this type of filtering. If the potential meal is bigger than a fly-sized spot or the flower is red, the animal goes hungry.

There is a better way to filter sensory information: that is, the way that people do. We filter sensory information by recognizing and assessing certain key characteristics of the events and objects around us, and we use that information to identify an event or object as an example of a general class of events or objects. For instance, you would not reject a meal that you had never seen before because it did not look like a specific, idealized plate of food. You would assess its characteristics (odor, color, texture, temperature), and if they all met certain criteria, you would take a bite. In this case, the novel meal is an example of the category, "acceptable meal." Likewise, we can learn that a particular task—mending a ripped curtain, for instance—is an example of the category "sewing material together." So, when attempting to mend a curtain for the first time, we apply the rules that we learned are successful in other, analogous mending tasks. In other words, we have acquired and employ an algorithm, or "rule of thumb" for solving specific problems of this general type.

In this section, you will read how several animals with comparatively very small brains filter visual information the same way that people do. They use categories to classify moving objects; they learn and use complex algorithms to solve difficult problems; and they process visual information in ways remarkably like those of humans. Such capacities are particularly interesting because they give us insights, not only into the minds of the little animals, but also into the ways that we, as people, operate. In these little animals, we can see the beginnings of the complex intellectual processes that define us as human.

1 *Portia* Perceptions: The *Umwelt* of an Araneophagic Jumping Spider

Duane P. Harland and Robert R. Jackson

The Personality of *Portia*

Spiders are traditionally portrayed as simple, instinct-driven animals (Savory, 1928; Drees, 1952; Bristowe, 1958). Small brain size is perhaps the most compelling reason for expecting so little flexibility from our eight-legged neighbors. Fitting comfortably on the head of a pin, a spider brain seems to vanish into insignificance. Common sense tells us that compared with large-brained mammals, spiders have so little to work with that they must be restricted to a circumscribed set of rigid behaviors, flexibility being a luxury afforded only to those with much larger central nervous systems.

In this chapter we review recent findings on an unusual group of spiders that seem to be arachnid enigmas. In a number of ways the behavior of the araneophagic jumping spiders is more comparable to that of birds and mammals than conventional wisdom would lead us to expect of an arthropod.

The term *araneophagic* refers to these spiders' preference for other spiders as prey, and jumping spider is the common English name for members of the family Salticidae. Although both their common and the scientific Latin names acknowledge their jumping behavior, it is really their unique, complex eyes that set this family of spiders apart from all others. Among spiders (many of which have very poor vision), salticids have eyes that are by far the most specialized for resolving fine spatial detail. We focus here on the most extensively studied genus, *Portia*.

Before we discuss the interrelationship between the salticids' uniquely acute vision, their predatory strategies, and their apparent cognitive abilities, we need to offer some sense of what kind of animal a jumping spider is; to do this, we attempt to offer some insight into what we might call *Portia's* personality. We are able to offer such a perspective because we have been immersed in the natural history of this animal over the course of many years of research. We will try to share our perspective by offering three "stories" from the life of *Portia*.

Portia is a genus containing about twenty species of primarily tropical salticids that are restricted to Africa, Asia, and Australasia (Wanless, 1978). Rain forest is the typical habitat for most of these species, and our stories take place in the rain forest of northeast Queensland, Australia. *Portia's* microhabitat within the forest is unusual. Salticids are traditionally envisaged as hunters who have little use for webs (Richman and Jackson, 1992). However, *Portia* frequents webs, both self-built and those of other species (Jackson and Blest, 1982a). *Portia* is also unusual in its appearance, both when quiescent and especially when walking.

When seen out of context, for instance on a laboratory table, *Portia's* walking gait appears overacted, even comical. With its eight legs waving about in a slow, jerky manner, *Portia* is reminiscent of a robot in a 1950s science fiction movie. Under natural circumstances, however, its gait makes sense. *Portia* is a convincing mimic of the detritus found on the forest floor and in webs. Its body is covered with a fine, low-contrast patchwork of browns, softened by fringes of hair. When walking, its exaggerated, hesitating stepping motion preserves its concealment. It appears to be no more than a piece of detritus flickering as dapples of sunlight filter through the canopy (figure 1.1A).

Stalking a Jumping Spider

Our first story begins with *Portia* slowly walking down the trunk of a tree, perhaps looking for the webs of potential prey. As do all salticids, *Portia* trails a line of silk, called a dragline, behind it as it walks (Richman and Jackson, 1992).

Many animals frequent tree trunks in the forest and before long *Portia* steps onto the draglines of another salticid. In this case they are the draglines of *Jacksonoides queenslandicus* (figure 1.1B), the most abundant salticid in the Queensland rain forest (Jackson, 1988), and among *Portia*'s favorite prey (Clark and Jackson, 2000).

Portia is sensitive to the chemical and odor cues from the other spider's draglines (Jackson et al., 2002). These cues prime *Portia* to expect to find *J. queenslandicus* in the vicinity, and the priming actually makes *Portia* more effective at visually locating the prey. When quiescent on a tree trunk, however, *J. queenslandicus*'s markings make it hard to see, and this time its camouflage is too good. However, *Portia* has a solution, something called "hunting by speculation" (Clark et al., 2001; see Curio, 1976).

Portia makes a sudden leap straight up into the air. *J. queenslandicus*, resting quietly some 15 cm away, turns to look at what moved, but *Portia* is already back on the ground, sitting still. *J. queenslandicus* does not see *Portia*, but *Portia* detected *J. queenslandicus* as it turned. Very slowly, *Portia* orients toward *J. queenslandicus* and, once *J. queenslandicus* turns away, *Portia* begins to stalk it.

When stalking other kinds of spiders, *Portia* moves slowly, with its palps hanging loosely in front of its face. When stalking a salticid, however, *Portia* moves even more slowly, exaggerating its choppy, robotlike gait, and pulls its palps back so they are hidden from the prey's view (Jackson and Blest, 1982a; Harland and Jackson, 2001).

Being a salticid, *J. queenslandicus* can see well, and this time it detects a flicker of movement as *Portia* comes up from behind, and it turns toward *Portia*. *Portia* freezes the instant its prey's large eyes come into view (Harland and Jackson, 2000a). *J. queenslandicus* looks straight at *Portia*, but sees nothing to indicate danger. Eventually *J. queenslandicus* turns and walks away. With *J. queenslandicus*'s eyes no longer in sight, *Portia* resumes its slow advance.

Portia draws steadily closer to its prey, continuously maneuvering to stay behind the *J. queenslandicus*. Eventually, from a few millimeters away, *Portia* lunges, and its fangs pierce the integument just above the brain of the *J. queenslandicus*. The victim is soon paralyzed; *Portia* feeds, and our first story comes to an end.

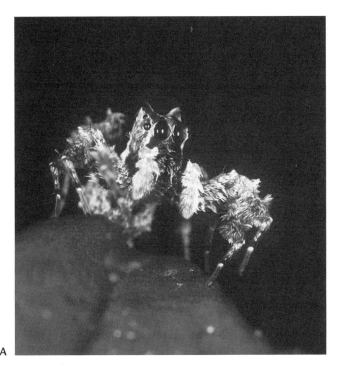

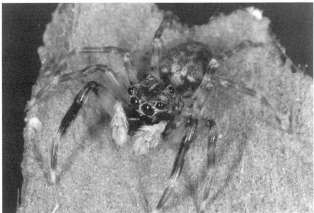

Figure 1.1
(*A*) *Portia fimbriata* subadult male from Queensland, Australia, and (*B*) primary salticid prey of the Queensland *Portia*, the insectivorous *Jacksonoides queenslandicus*. (Photo of *P. fimbriata* by D. Harland; photo of *J. queenslandicus* by R. R. Jackson.)

Deceiving an Orb Weaver

Portia sits near the edge of an orb web, looking across the sticky spirals toward the web's architect, *Gasteracantha* sp., sitting at the hub. *Gasteracantha* is a distinctive spider. It is large, powerful, and has long horny spines on its abdomen that make it difficult for *Portia* to hold on to.

Gasteracantha's eyesight is too poor to recognize *Portia* as a predator. However, *Gasteracantha* has an acute ability to detect and interpret web signals—displacements, even very small displacements, of its web's silk lines (Witt, 1975). *Portia's* task is to get within attacking distance without eliciting the wrong response from *Gasteracantha*. This large spider is fully capable of preying on *Portia* should it get the upper hand. Just walking across the web will not work for *Portia*. The resulting web signals will give it away.

So *Portia* moves slowly onto the edge of the web, reaches out with its forelegs, and begins to pluck on the silk; but *Gasteracantha* does not move. *Portia* continues to make signals, but varies them. It plucks with different legs, plucks with its palps, varies the speed and the amplitude at which its appendages move, and it shakes the web by vibrating its abdomen up and down. Complex patterns are made by simultaneously moving different sets of appendages, with different appendages moving in different ways. By using any combination of its eight legs, two palps, and abdomen, *Portia* is capable of generating an almost unlimited repertoire of web signals.

Eventually a signal may cause a reaction in *Gasteracantha*, and it may approach *Portia*. If the approach is not too fast, *Portia* will continue to signal, slowly drawing the prey spider closer (Jackson and Wilcox, 1993a). *Portia* avoids making web signals that elicit a fast approach because, when moving quickly, *Gasteracantha* is dangerous and more likely to become predator than prey.

Luring *Gasteracantha* is a slow process, and close to an hour has already passed. Then something happens to speed things up. A light tropical breeze gently rocks the web. The wind-induced web movements mask any fainter movements caused by *Portia* and the spider takes advantage of the smoke screen (Wilcox et al., 1996) by stepping rapidly across the web toward *Gasteracantha*. This time, however, when the breeze dies down, *Portia* is still several centimeters from its prey.

Now *Portia* creates a smoke screen of its own (Tarsitano et al., 2000). By violently and repeatedly flexing all of its legs at the same time, the spider shakes the web much as the breeze did. Cloaked by a succession of such diversions, *Portia* closes the remaining distance. However, when it is about 3 mm from *Gasteracantha*, something goes amiss. *Gasteracantha* suddenly turns on *Portia*, lunging forward and grabbing one of *Portia's* legs with its chelicerae. *Portia* leaps off the web, leaving the leg behind.

After landing on the forest floor half a meter below, *Portia* looks up at the web and then climbs back to it. Once there, it repeats the entire process and this time succeeds in lunging at *Gasteracantha*. *Portia* quickly punctures *Gasteracantha's* cuticle with its fangs and then lets go. *Gasteracantha* runs to the edge of the web and drops to the ground in an attempt to escape, but paralysis soon sets in. *Portia* drops to the ground on a dragline, walks in the direction of *Gasteracantha*, and scans the forest floor for the specific kind of spider it just attacked (R. R. Jackson, unpublished results). *Portia* will bypass other potential prey placed in its path, continuing to search for the expected prey, in this case, *Gasteracantha*.

Plotting a Detour

Portia walks across the forest floor until its attention is drawn to the distinctive cross-shaped stablimenta adorning the orb web of *Argiope appensa* about a meter away (Seah and Li, 2001). *Portia* moves so that the web is in clear view and approaches the tree to which it is attached. However, the web soon is out of view because of the uneven clutter on the forest floor. The journey to the tree is anything but direct. *Portia* has to continuously change direction along a route that twists around leaves, tree roots, and lumps of dirt. Intermittent visual feedback from the tree and occasionally from the web, combined with an internal sense of direction (see D. E. Hill, 1979), keeps *Portia* on course.

   Portia begins climbing the tree toward *Argiope*'s web, but *Argiope* is no ordinary spider. When it detects an intruder on its web, it rocks up and down, shaking the web violently (Jackson et al., 1993). So moving directly onto this spider's web is problematical. One misstep and *Argiope* may shake *Portia* off of the web.

   Portia stops just short of the web and slowly looks around. Eventually its line of gaze traces a path (Tarsitano and Andrew, 1999) from the top of the web to a nearby vine and down the vine and into a mass of tangled vegetation adjacent to the tree trunk. *Portia* then turns and walks away, but it is not giving up. Instead, the spider takes a long, convoluted detour, during the course of which it will temporarily lose sight of the web. After about 20 min, *Portia* arrives on the vine it saw above the web. Sitting on a leaf connected to the vine, *Portia* looks down at the resting *Argiope* and lowers itself on a dragline alongside the web without touching it. When it is level with *Argiope*, *Portia* swings in and grabs the unsuspecting prey (see Jackson, 1992a).

The Flexibility of *Portia's* Behavior

Our three stories illustrate a number of examples of behavior which, had they been described in a vertebrate predator, would probably be discussed in the context of animal cognition, animal intelligence, or problem solving. In each of the three cases, the behaviors appear to have a high level of flexibility (or plasticity) for a spider.

   Within each story, *Portia* displayed a number of sophisticated behaviors. We focus on three examples, each of which provides some insight into the remarkable sensory capacities of this spider. The behaviors are trial-and-error signal derivation, detouring, and selective attention.

Trial and Error

Although *Portia* is called a specialist because it prefers and is efficient at capturing spiders, the name can be somewhat misleading. That is, *Portia* is actually a generalist on spiders. And, if one considers the variation just in web-building spiders (Jackson and Hallas, 1986a,b), it becomes clear why *Portia*'s behavior needs to be so flexible.

Web-building spiders have only rudimentary eyesight (M. F. Land, 1985a), and so use the information provided by web signals as a primary source of sensory information (Masters et al., 1986; Foelix, 1996). Hence the web itself can be thought of as an integral part of a typical web-builder's sensory system (Witt, 1975).

After entering another spider's web, *Portia* does not approach its victim straightaway. Instead, in an attempt to gain control over its victim's behavior, *Portia* displays a number of aggressive mimicry signals (Jackson and Wilcox, 1998) that the web spider can sense. In the case of its more commonly encountered prey, *Portia* uses specific, inflexible, preprogrammed signals, as one might expect an arthropod predator to do. However, as noted earlier, *Portia* can also create an almost limitless repertoire of web signals by varying the activity of its legs, palps, and abdomen (Jackson and Blest, 1982a; Jackson and Hallas, 1986a). This allows the spider to adjust its web signals in response to feedback from the intended victim (Jackson and Wilcox, 1993a; Jackson and Carter, 2001).

When hunting commonly encountered prey, *Portia* often uses trial-and-error learning to complete a predatory sequence begun with preprogrammed signals (Jackson and Wilcox, 1998). It begins a trial-and-error sequence by presenting the intended prey with a variety of different signals. When a signal elicits an appropriate response, *Portia* stops varying its signals and repeats the successful sequence. If the prey spider stops responding appropriately, *Portia* again generates a variety of signals until one triggers a favorable response from the web's resident, and so on. This appears to be an example of flexible problem solving and represents a rudimentary cognitive ability (see Terrace, 1985; Toates, 1988, 1996).

Altering its web signals through trial-and-error learning enables *Portia* to prey effectively on a wide range of web-building spiders. In the laboratory, this includes species that *Portia* has never encountered in nature and would never have encountered in its evolutionary history.

The convergence of behavioral ecology and cognitive psychology has generated considerable interest in how the cognitive capacities of animals influence their behavior (Yoerg, 1991; Belisle and Cresswell, 1997; Dukas, 1998; Kamil, 1998). When examining this relationship, one key consideration must be the extent to which an animal's cognitive abilities are merely single-purpose adaptations tailored for specific functions rather than broader cognitive capacities (Stephens, 1991; McFarland and Boser, 1993). We are only beginning to understand how often and under what circumstances the evolution of cognitive skills has pushed animals across a threshold, so to speak, enabling them to respond flexibly and adaptively to problems outside of the context in which these skills originally evolved (see Dennett, 1996).

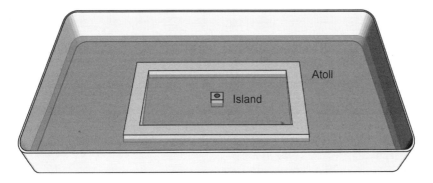

Figure 1.2
Apparatus that was used for ascertaining whether *Portia fimbriata* uses trial and error to solve a confinement problem. The spider is put on a block (island) surrounded by a frame (atoll) in a water-filled tray. It must choose to either leap or swim to reach the atoll and then again choose how it should reach the tray's edge. The successful choice was predetermined randomly. If it was successful, the spider was moved to the atoll; if unsuccessful, it was returned to the island. (Adapted from Jackson et al., 2002.)

Portia may be at this threshold. For instance, we tested *Portia* in a situation in which it had to discover a method of escape through trial and error (Jackson et al., 2001). In the experiments, *Portia* was confined to an artificial island surrounded by water (figure 1.2). This particular problem was chosen because it is unlikely to be similar to anything this spider is likely to encounter in the wild. *Portia* was forced to choose between two potential escape tactics (leap or swim), one of which would fail (it would bring the spider no closer to the edge of the tray) and the other of which would result in partial success (it would bring the spider closer to the edge of the tray). *Portia* consistently repeated choices that brought partial success and avoided choices that brought failure.

Detouring
Although detouring has been most extensively studied in vertebrates (O. von Frisch, 1962; Curio, 1976; Collett, 1982; Chapuis, 1987; Rashotte, 1987; Regolin et al., 1994, 1995a,b), more than 67 years ago Heil (1936) suggested that salticids can make deliberate detours. This was subsequently confirmed experimentally by D. E. Hill (1979) using a North American species of *Phidippus*. The detours required in Heil's and Hill's experiments were simple and short, and Hill (1979) concluded that detouring required no insight because, in the absence of a straight path to the prey, all the salticid did was to head toward an object ("secondary goal") that would bring it closer to the prey (the "primary goal"), and it continued doing this until the prey was reached. Hill's (1979) conclusion, however, does not appear to apply to *Portia*.

Portia reaches its prey by taking indirect routes (detours) when direct routes are unavailable (Tarsitano and Jackson, 1992; Tarsitano and Andrew, 1999), including detours that can be completed only by initially moving away from, and losing sight of, the prey (reverse-route detours) (Tarsitano and Jackson, 1994, 1997). In encounters with certain types of prey, such as spitting spiders, which are particularly dangerous (D. Li et al., 1999), *Portia* takes detours even when shorter, direct routes are available (Jackson and Wilcox, 1993b; Jackson et al., 1998). Solving path-finding problems by selecting a route ahead of time (Tarsitano and Jackson, 1997) implies planning ahead (i.e., a type of offline processing; see Toates, 1996), a putative cognitive ability when it is manifested by vertebrates.

Selective Attention

Chemical cues from *J. queenslandicus* have been shown experimentally to facilitate the speed with which *P. fimbriata* attend to visual cues from *J. queenslandicus*. These findings appear to be an example of attentional priming (see Roitblat, 1987). This is noteworthy in that chemosensory stimuli are priming responses to visual stimuli and because this appears to be an instance in which the priming mechanism appears to be preprogrammed.

Attentional priming, in conjunction with *Portia's* apparent use of search images (as noted earlier; L. Tinbergen, 1960; Bond, 1983; Langley et al., 1996), suggests that this spider can access a mental representation of an unseen but expected prey item. However, what "representation" might mean for *Portia* is unclear (see Roitblat, 1982; Epstein, 1982). In perhaps the simplest case, attentional priming might be explained by a direct chemosensory-induced increase in the sensitivity of a single hypothetical feature-detecting neuron in *Portia's* visual system. Further research on the mechanisms behind *Portia's* visual perception is needed.

Integrating Tactics

During much of the twentieth century, the prevailing assumption was that arthropod behavior is rigid, and researchers often expressed surprise at how varied a salticid's responses could be. For instance, Homann (1928) noted that individual spiders with the same eye experimentally occluded occasionally acted differently from one another. Crane (1949) tried to account for her spiders' behavioral variability by hypothesizing the existence of "epigamic rhythms" and short-term cyclical fluctuations of internal state. In a series of careful experiments on color discrimination, Kästner (1950) tested the salticid, *Evarcha fulcata* (Clerck), and found it preferred a striped over a uniformly colored target of identical brightness. However, during retests, many spiders switched preferences (despite the fact that neither target offered a reward or escape option). This behavior was so unexpected that Kästner admitted simply that it was impossible for him to explain these facts.

Variability is a dominant theme in *Portia's* behavior, seeming to highlight the flexibility of its prey-capture strategy. During predatory encounters, *Portia* rarely relies exclusively on any one tactic. Instead, it switches between or combines tactics, often appearing to derive a unique solution for how to capture a particular prey spider under a particular set of circumstances.

The Evolution of Behavioral Flexibility in *Portia*

Theoretical accounts of the evolution of *Portia's* problem-solving ability have emphasized the close relationship between this spider's behavior and its prey's sensory systems, the high level of risk involved in attempting to gain control over another predator's behavior, and the potential for co-evolution between predator and prey (Jackson, 1992a).

Limits of scale must place a ceiling on how flexible an animal's behavior can become, but how and where size constraints become important remain unresolved questions. Smaller animals tend to have fewer, not smaller, neurons (Alloway, 1972; Menzel et al., 1984), which means fewer components are available for brains, sensory organs, problem-solving mechanisms, and cognitive and behavioral flexibility. There is considerable evidence that even over a small size range and among closely related species, brain size influences cognitive capacities (Lashley, 1949; Rensch, 1956; Jerison, 1973, 1985; Eisenberg and Wilson, 1978; Clutton-Brock and Harvey, 1980; Mace et al., 1981; Lefebre et al., 1997). Hence, small brain size seems to present a fundamental engineering problem that potentially limits how complex or flexible an arthropod's behavior can become (Harland and Jackson, 2000b). On the other hand, *Portia's* behavior suggests that the chasm between small-brained and large-brained animals may not be quite as enormous as has been conventionally thought (see Bitterman, 1986). The key to understanding *Portia's* remarkable behavior may lie in its unusually complex sensory systems, especially its vision.

Salticid Sensory Systems

Nonvisual Senses

Vision has been considered to be essential to the behavior of salticids (Drees, 1952; M. F. Land, 1969a,b). Hence, research on salticid sensory systems has focused almost exclusively on their unique eyes. Thus what is known about their other sensory capacities is limited. However, behavioral observations indicate that salticids may rely heavily on modalities other than vision. For instance, when they are in complete darkness, some salticids readily use substrate-borne vibratory signals during mating (Taylor and Jackson, 1999). Most salticids can capture prey in total darkness (Taylor et al., 1998), and *Portia* can invade webs and use web signals in the dark (R. R. Jackson and D. P. Harland, unpublished results).

Chemoreception is also important to *Portia* (Peckham and Peckham, 1887; Heil, 1936); pheromones left by conspecifics influence courtship (Pollard et al., 1987). Furthermore, *Portia* can discriminate between itself and conspecifics, identify conspecifics as familiar, and determine the sex of conspecifics based on chemical cues imbedded in their silk (Willey and Jackson, 1993; R. J. Clark and Jackson, 1994a,b, 1995a,b). Air- and substrate-borne chemical cues are also used to detect commonly encountered prey (Jackson et al., 2002).

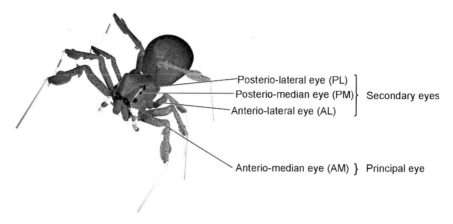

Posterio-lateral eye (PL) ⎤
Posterio-median eye (PM) ⎬ Secondary eyes
Anterio-lateral eye (AL) ⎦

Anterio-median eye (AM) } Principal eye

Figure 1.3
Drawing of *Portia fimbriata* showing the external arrangement of salticid eyes. The principal (AM) eyes function in high-acuity and color vision. The secondary eyes (PL, PM, AL) function in motion detection.

Although detailed studies of salticid mechanical senses are lacking, this modality is well described for other spider families (see Foelix, 1996). In other spiders, various mechanosensors (primarily in the form of sensory hairs and slits in the integument) mediate detection of air movement (Barth et al., 1993), deformation of the exoskeleton (Barth, 1985), temperature and humidity (Ehn and Tichy, 1994), and position of the appendages relative to the body (Seyfarth, 1985). It can be presumed that these sensory structures are also present in salticids, but more research is clearly needed.

Vision
In contrast to an insect's pair of multifaceted, compound eyes, salticids have eight camera-type eyes spaced around the cephalothorax (i.e., the frontmost segment of the body) (M. F. Land, 1985a). Acting together, these eyes (figure 1.3) serve much the same role as do the two eyes of a predatory mammal such as a lion. As in mammals, when small-field movement is detected, *Portia* will orient toward it. Once located, the object may be visually tracked, and its identity, size, range, orientation and behavior assessed (M. F. Land, 1974). However, there are important differences in how mammalian and salticid eyes perform these tasks.

In salticids there are two types of eyes, secondary and primary, or principal, eyes. The six secondary eyes, spaced along the sides of the carapace, detect movement in the periphery and enable the spider to orient toward its source. Hence the secondary eyes are functionally analogous to the peripheral retina in vertebrates. The salticid's two principal, forward-facing eyes are larger than its secondary eyes and provide detailed information about the objects toward which the spider is oriented (e.g., the object's shape, texture, and color). This is functionally similar to the mammalian fovea; that is, spatial acuity (the ability to resolve detail) is especially good in the mammalian fovea and, in the salticid, in the central region of the retina of the principal eye.

This division of functions (detection of peripheral movement and assessment of detail) into two types of eyes appears to be an evolutionary response to the limitations of size. For example, transposing the equivalent of a spherical vertebrate eye into a salticid's body would not be a workable option because an eye's optical performance is critically tied to the ratio between the diameter of the lens (aperture) and its ability to magnify (focal length) (M. F. Land, 1974, 1981; Land and Nilsson, 2002). The degree of magnification provided by a lens determines how far behind the lens an image will form, and increasing the magnification means increasing the distance between the lens and an image. If we were to design a spherical eye with a corneal lens, and an aperture and magnifying power (focal length) equal to that of the salticid's principal eye, it would have a diameter equal to the length of one of the salticid's principal eyes. The additional volume of the eye (approximately 27 times more) would mean that the single spherical, mammalian-type eye would entirely fill the salticid's cephalothorax (figure 1.4). The salticid's solution to this size-constraint problem has been to divide visual tasks between two types of eyes.

In terms of simple visual resolution, *Portia* has no rival among insects (figure 1.5). For instance, the dragonfly, *Sympetrum striolatus*, has the highest known acuity among insects (i.e., a resolving power of 0.4 deg) (Labhart and Nielsson, 1995; M. F. Land, 1997). In contrast, the acuity of *Portia*'s principal eyes is 0.04 deg, exceeding that of the dragonfly by tenfold despite the fact that dragonfly compound eyes are about the size of *Portia*'s entire cephalothorax (D. S. Williams and McIntyre, 1980)! It is interesting that the human eye, with an acuity of 0.007 deg, is only five times better than *Portia*'s (e.g., M. F. Land, 1981; M. F. Land and Nilsson, 2002).

The Secondary Eyes

The salticid's six secondary eyes are smaller than the two principal eyes (figures 1.3 and 1.4A), but each secondary eye covers a much wider field of view than the principal eyes (figure 1.6). The posterior median (PM) eyes of most salticids are regarded as vestigial because they have degenerated retinas incapable of detecting movement (Eakin and Brandenburger, 1971; M. F. Land, 1985a) (figure 1.6A). Degenerated PM eyes are thought to be a derived condition (Wanless, 1984). For instance, a number of genera in the "primitive" salticid subfamilies Lyssomaninae and Spartaeinae have large functioning PM eyes. (*Portia*, for example, is a spartaeine genus with functional PM eyes; figures 1.4A and 6B). In species with degenerated PM eyes, the fields of view of the remaining secondary eyes have apparently widened (figure 6A) so that they encompass the fields that would be covered by functional PM eyes (M. F. Land, 1985b).

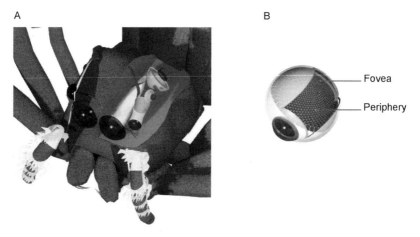

Figure 1.4
Drawing of *Portia fimbriata* showing internal arrangement of salticid eyes. (*A*) Cutaway carapace showing long eye tube of the large, forward facing principal anterior median (AM) eye and compact eye cups of secondary anterior lateral (AL) posterior median (PM), and posterior lateral (PL) eyes (see figure 1.3). Structural tissue (e.g., eye tubes) is shown in gray, retinae in red, and muscles in blue (only the principal eye has muscles). (*B*) A mammalian-type spherical eye (at the same scale and the same viewing angle as in (*A*) that would be needed to incorporate the four salticid eyes into a single eye. To retain a focal length equivalent to that of an anterior median eye, the spherical eye's diameter would have to be the same as the length of the anterior median eye tube. Additional space would be required for muscles (not shown). *P. fimbriata*'s cephalothorax would be filled with a single eye of these dimensions.

Internally, each secondary eye has a regular mosaic of well-separated receptors that form a bowl-like retina. The retina is made up primarily of three cell types: sensory cells, nonpigmented supportive cells, and pigmented supportive cells (Eakin and Brandenburger, 1971). Rhodopsins, embedded in the plasma membranes of sensory cells, detect light. Membranes containing the rhodopsin are highly folded and situated in arrays of slender microvilli (rhabdomeres) held perpendicular to the surface of the retina and the path of incoming light. The section of the sensory cell containing the rhabdomeres is called a rhabdom. Each receptor (an independent functional unit of reception) in the secondary eye is made up of two contiguous rhabdoms surrounded by accessory cells (Blest, 1985a).

The focal lengths for secondary eyes are small compared with the principal eyes, but small focal lengths help provide the secondary eyes with wide fields of view and large depths of field (i.e., there is a large distance over which an image remains in focus).

The role of the secondary eyes as motion detectors is clearly suggested by the heavily pigmented accessory cells between the receptors, which protect and

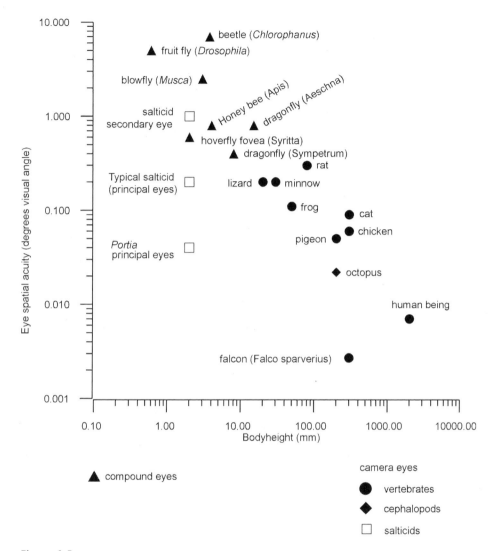

Figure 1.5

The spatial acuity of *Portia*'s eyes compared with that of other animals. The log of spatial acuity (expressed as a minimum interreceptor angle) is plotted against the log of body height. Data from Kirschfeld (1976), M. F. Land (1985a, 1997), and A. W. Snyder and Miller (1978). (Adapted from Kirschfeld, 1976.)

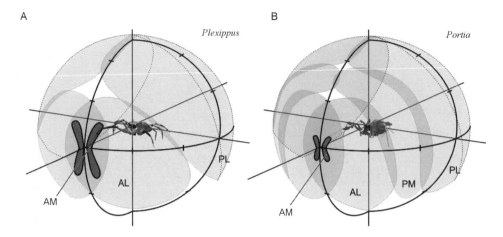

Figure 1.6
Fields of view of the eyes of (*A*) *Plexippus* sp., an advanced salticid (subfamily Salticinae) with vestigial posterior median eyes, and of (*B*) *Portia fimbriata*, a spartaeine (primitive subfamily) salticid that has large functional positerior median eyes. Overlapping visual fields indicate binocular visual fields. The orthographic view is taken from 30 deg longitude and 15 deg latitude. AM, anterior median; AL, anterior lateral; PM, posterior median; and PL, posterior lateral eye. (Adapted from M. F. Land, 1985b.)

help to isolate them optically (i.e., from the effects of stray photons) (Eakin and Brandenburger, 1971; Blest, 1985a). Furthermore, compared with receptors in the principal eyes, those of the secondary eyes tend to be larger, surrounded by supportive cells (Blest, 1983), and widely spaced.

Interreceptor spacing and receptor width are critical factors defining the degree of an eye's spatial acuity. As an image falls on the retina, it is sampled by the receptors, each receptor sampling a specific small area. Put simply, the denser the array of visual sampling units, the higher the degree of spatial detail that can be resolved. Gaps between receptors (as seen in the secondary eyes) also influence acuity by corresponding to gaps in the sampling space. An eye's spatial acuity, expressed as "visual angle" (defined as the degrees apart objects in a scene must be before they are seen as separate), is calculated from the image's quality and spread, which are determined by the aperture and focal length of the lens, plus interreceptor spacing. With visual angles varying between 0.4 and 2 deg, the spatial acuity of salticid secondary eyes tends to be comparable to that of the compound eyes of insects (M. F. Land, 1985a, 1997).

Salticids detect movement when sequential changes in image intensity stimulate adjacent receptors in the secondary eyes (M. F. Land, 1971). A stimulus change between just two adjacent receptors is enough to elicit an orientation response. For example, a small spider walking along the ground to the side of *Portia* might project an image on the posterior lateral (PL) retina that covers a single receptor. As the spider moves, its image will move from one receptor to the next on the PL retina, alerting *Portia* to the presence of a moving object.

The readiness with which a single receptor in the secondary eyes can detect an object is influenced by the size of the object's retinal image, which is a product of the object's absolute size and distance (the nearer the object, the larger its retinal image). For example, Land (1971) found that individual receptors from the PL eyes of *Metaphidippus aeneolus*, with receptive fields of 1 deg, responded to objects with retinal images wider than 0.4 deg (i.e., just less than half a receptor might be covered by the image). The probability of a response increased with the width and height of the stimulus, leveling out for stimuli larger than ~1.1 deg.

The salticid secondary eyes are monochromatic; they contain just one type of rhodopsin, with a maximum sensitivity at 535 nm (our green) (Yamashita and Tateda, 1976; Hardie and Duelli, 1978). In practical terms, this means that a salticid can detect movement of an object when there is a strong contrast in green: either a green object against a background of other colors or an object that is not green moving against a green background. For example, a green dot moving on a black background (or vice versa) provides a high level of contrast and is easily seen by a salticid. However, a red dot moving on a black background is unlikely to be detected.

When movement is detected, a salticid may orient toward the object, bringing it into its principal eyes' field of vision. Information from the secondary eyes governs orienting, which appears to depend on translating the position of stimulation on one of the secondary eye retinas into a particular number of steps by the legs, with legs on opposite sides of the body moving in opposite directions, which turns the spider a specific number of degrees to the left or right (M. F. Land, 1972).

When discussing algorithms that control orientation by animals, a distinction is commonly made between closed- and open-loop turns (Mittelstaedt, 1962; M. F. Land, 1971). Closed-loop turns require that the animal receive visual feedback from its own movement (i.e., the animal continually monitors the object's position). For this, the movement source must remain visible throughout the execution of the turn. In contrast, an open-loop turn is not governed by feedback (i.e., open-loop turns work on a single instruction). For example, movement detected 80 deg to the animal's left can be envisaged as initiating an open-loop algorithm that reads, "turns 80 deg to the left, then stop." A closed-loop algorithm, in contrast, can be envisaged as reading something like "turn a little in the direction of the movement source, after which, if the movement source is in front, stop; otherwise, repeat from the beginning."

An open-loop movement means that if the movement source is removed during the act of orientation, the animal will nevertheless be pointing toward the object's last position at the completion of its turn. Salticids generally orient toward a target in a single turn, suggesting that they rely primarily on an open-loop algorithm. However, turning is occasionally performed as a series of smaller turns, which may mean that they sometimes use a mixture of closed- and open-loop algorithms (M. F. Land, 1971).

Control of orientation toward moving objects is the best known, but not the only, function of the secondary eyes. The interplay of object size, velocity, and movement pattern may be important cues governing different responses. For example, objects that loom up (i.e., suddenly make bigger retinal images) may trigger a "panic" response (Heil, 1936). Furthermore, the speed at which an object moves influences the salticid's reaction. A slowly moving object (e.g., less than 1 deg/s for *M. aeneolus*), generally elicits no response. However, rapidly moving objects (e.g., greater than 100 deg/s for *M. aeneolus*) can provoke a "panic" response if they are large, or a chasing response if they are small (Heil, 1936; Drees, 1952; M. F. Land, 1971; Forster, 1985).

During a "panic" response, a salticid may hide quickly, make a wild leap and then freeze, or simply flee. When fleeing from a predator, salticids appear to use information from the PL eyes to keep a pursuer directly behind them (M. F. Land, 1971).

In contrast, when chasing prey, salticids appear to use information from the anterior lateral (AL) eyes to keep the prey directly in front of them (Drees, 1952; Forster, 1979). Unlike the other secondary eyes, each AL eye contains a forward-facing foveal region with higher spatial acuity (Eakin and Brandenburger, 1971; M. F. Land, 1974). The function of the AL fovea has not been studied, but perhaps it has a role in range-finding or in guiding the principal eyes' saccades.

Range-finding, or distance estimation, is the determination of the distance to an object in the visual field. This ability is important when a salticid is hunting and when it is planning detours. The AL eyes have a forward-facing region of binocular overlap (figure 1.6), which also overlaps the fields of view of each principal anterior median (AM) eye (M. F. Land, 1985b). Experiments in which various eyes were covered with opaque wax or paint suggest that the binocular overlap of the AL eye, in conjunction with the AM-AL overlap, plays a role in range-finding (Homann, 1928; Heil, 1936; Forster, 1979), but the specific contributions of each eye are not well understood.

If distance estimation is restricted to the region of binocular overlap, this may impose a significant constraint on the spider. That is, an object (e.g., an insect) in the lateral visual field may be detected by the secondary eyes, but its distance may undeterminable until it is in the frontal visual field. Suppose, for instance, that a large object (subtending 10 deg) is moving behind the salticid. From the spider's perspective, this could be a small, near object (e.g., insect prey), or a large, distant object (e.g., a predatory bird). An orienting turn might provide an answer, because it would allow the principal eyes to assess the details of the object, but with the risk of scaring off potential prey or falling victim to a predator. Larger turns probably increase the risk of both these outcomes. This may explain why *Portia* and other salticids appear willing to make short turns but reluctant to make larger turns (see M. F. Land, 1971).

The Principal Eyes

For a salticid, as for many vertebrates, orienting toward an object brings a specialized part of the visual system to bear on the target, in the spider's case the retinae of the large anterior median, or principal, eyes (figure 1.3). As indicated earlier, because of their structure, these eyes can provide information that is different from, and more detailed than, that provided by the secondary eyes. Using their AM eyes, salticids can discriminate between at least five broad classes of objects: mates, rivals, prey, predators, and features of the environment (Homann, 1928; Heil, 1936; Crane, 1949; Drees, 1952; Forster, 1979, 1982b). Some of the most basic decisions made by salticids in their day-to-day lives depend on this information. For example, *Portia* plans and executes detours based primarily on optical features of the environment acquired by the AM eyes (Tarsitano and Andrew, 1999). Its choice of signals during an encounter with a web-building spider depends on visually acquired feedback about the identity and behavior of the prey; and *Portia fimbriata* can visually discriminate between prey and conspecifics at distances of up to 46 body lengths (Jackson and Blest, 1982b; Harland et al., 1999).

The AM eyes also make it possible for salticids to identify environmental features in order to navigate detours, and this can be done at distances as far as 85 body lengths (Tarsitano and Jackson, 1997).

The Structure of the AM Eyes   On the outside of the salticid's anterior carapace are the large corneal lenses of the principal eyes. In salticids the cornea is formed by the carapace and it is both immobile and nonmalleable. Beyond the surface of the cornea there is a gradient in lens density that corrects the spherical aberration caused by the corneal surface (Blest and M. F. Land, 1977; D. S. Williams and McIntyre, 1980; Forster, 1985; see M. F. Land and Nilsson, 2002).

Despite their large size, the combined fields of view provided by the corneal lenses of the AM eyes are eclipsed by those of the flanking AL eyes (M. F. Land, 1969b, 1985b). This is because the focal length of the AM lens is greater than that of the AL lens. A greater focal length means higher magnification. However, magnification comes at a price. Magnifying an image can be envisaged as spreading the light more thinly over a larger area. Hence, to magnify an image and retain the same brightness, more light is required. The only way to get more light is to make the corneal lens wider. The other consequence of magnifying an image is that the more it is enlarged, the less of it will be in view. In short, by having a longer focal length, the AM eyes have smaller fields of view than the secondary eyes and yet they require larger lenses. Only larger lenses can provide enough light to maintain an acceptable quality for the magnified images.

Behind the AM corneal lens is a long, slightly tapering eye tube (figure 1.7). Transparent glass cells fill all except the rearmost part of the eye tube. After passing through the glass cells, light enters the matrix of cells supporting the retina (Eakin and Brandenburger, 1971). Along the optical axis, the anterior interface of this supportive matrix forms a concave pit just in front of the retina. This pit functions as a diverging lens that magnifies the image from the corneal lens (figure 1.8), boosting the eye's overall focal length. In *P. fimbriata*, the focal length of the corneal lens alone is 1701 µm. With the pit magnifying the image from the corneal lens, the eye acts as a telephoto lens system with a focal length of 1980 µm (D. S. Williams and McIntyre, 1980).

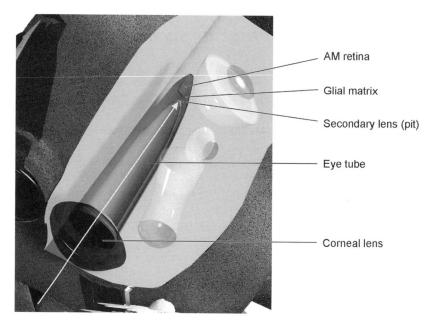

Figure 1.7
Morphology of the anterior median eye of *Portia*. Light (yellow line) enters the eye through the corneal lens and passes down the eye tube (cut along its sagittal plane), which is filled with (low optical density) glass cells. It is then magnified by the secondary lens (pit) formed by the interface with the (high optical density) glial matrix. The images focus within the retina.

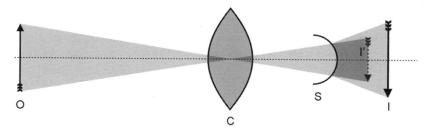

Figure 1.8
Telephoto optics of the salticid principal anterior median eye. The image (I) of an object (O) is projected by the corneal lens (C) onto the retina after being magnified by a secondary (diverging) lens (S) to make an image of size I. I' shows the approximate size and position of the image without the secondary lens. (Adapted from D. S. Williams and McIntyre, 1980.)

Salticids are not alone in using a diverging lens as a space-saving method of increasing image magnification. The eyes of falconiform birds also have foveal pits that operate as telephoto components, providing these birds with the highest spatial acuity known for any animal (up to 2.6 times greater than our own) (A. W. Snyder and Miller, 1978).

After being magnified by the secondary lens, the image is brought into focus on a complex retina. Unlike our own retina, the photoreceptors in the salticid AM retina are stacked in four successive tiers, or layers, along the light path (figure 1.9; plate 1). To reach the rearmost tier, layer I, light must pass through layers IV, III, and II (M. F. Land, 1969a; Eakin and Brandenburger, 1971; Blest et al., 1981).

Color Vision

The tiered arrangement of the AM retina plays a critical role in color vision. Light is split into a spectrum by the telephoto optics, with different wavelengths coming into focus at different distances. This is known as chromatic aberration (M. F. Land and Nilsson, 2002). Short wavelengths come into focus in layer IV, and longer wavelengths come into focus in layer I. Color vision based on chromatic aberration is effective because the photoreceptors in each layer contain different rhodopsins, each of which is sensitive to the wavelength that comes into focus on that layer (figure 1.10A) (M. F. Land, 1969a; Blest et al., 1981).

Although receptors sensitive to ultraviolet (UV), blue, green, and yellow have been found in the AM retinas of a few salticid species (DeVoe, 1975; Yamashita and Tateda, 1976), receptor location has been determined for just one species. Blest et al. (1981) found that the receptors in layer IV of *Plexippus validus* (Urquhart) have a peak absorbency in the UV range (~360 nm), and that receptors in layers I and II have a peak absorbency at 520 nm (green) (figure 1.10B). Although Blest and colleagues did not succeed in sampling receptors from layer III, optical calculations based on the position of the green and ultraviolet receptors suggest that peak absorbency in blue would enable layer III receptors to receive maximally sharp images. Wavelengths longer than green (e.g., red, ~700 nm) may also be absorbed at low efficiency by the green receptors in layers I and II (Peaslee and Wilson, 1989).

Whether salticids can discriminate light in the green region of the spectrum from light in the red region remains more controversial. Although physiological and optical studies have failed to find convincing evidence of separate green and red receptors, there are reasons to expect that discrimination is possible. In many salticid species, males have distinct red patches in their body patterns that are usually associated with courtship (figure 1.10C; plate 7), and the results of one study (Nakamura and Yamashita, 2000) suggest that salticids can learn to avoid red or green colored paper when that color is associated with heat punishment.

The tiered arrangement of the AM retina makes it tempting to suggest that salticid color vision operates by combining images from the different receptor layers into a single colored picture. However, this is probably not done, given the fact that none of the receptor mosaics match because receptors in different layers along any

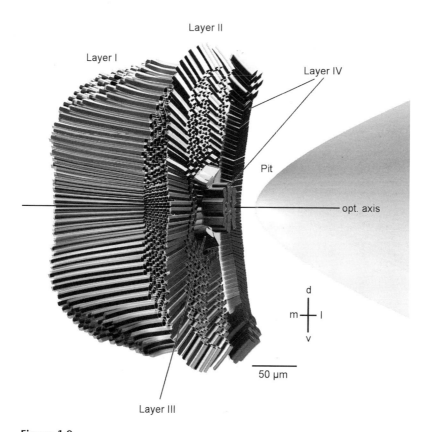

Figure 1.9
Structurally complex retina of *Portia fimbriata*'s principal eye. Behind the pit (secondary lens) are four layers of receptors (I, II, III, and IV) stacked along the optical axis. Layers II, III, and IV contain more than one receptor type. Most receptors are short, with irregular transverse cross-sectional profiles. Layer I is highly ordered with well-separated receptive segments. Separation reduces interreceptor interference. Spatial acuities as low as 2.4 min arc are supported by the central fovea of layer I. The orthographic view is taken 55 deg from the inner side of the optical axis (opt. axis) of the secondary lens. Orientation: d, dorsal; m, medial; l, lateral; v, ventral. Electron micrographs and structural descriptions were used to construct the drawing taken from D. S. Williams and McIntyre (1980), Blest et al. (1981), Blest and Price (1984), and Blest (1987a,b). (See plate 1 for color version.)

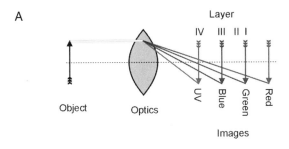

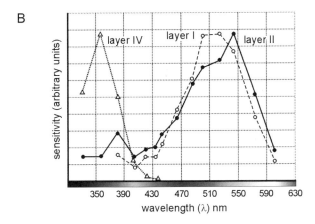

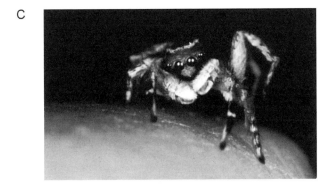

Figure 1.10

Hypothetical mechanism responsible for salticids' color vision. (*A*) Chromatic aberration of the anterior median eye optics is harnessed because green, blue, and ultraviolet (UV) components of an image come into focus on layers I, III, and IV, respectively. (*B*) Spectral sensitivity of marked cells from layers IV, II, and I within the AM eye of *Plexippus validus*. (Adapted from Blest et al., 1981.) (*C*) Undescribed adult male salticid from Sri Lanka showing colored patches associated with courtship, including red patches on the femur of each front pair of legs. (Photo by D. Harland.) (See plate 7 for color version.)

specific light path are of different sizes and shapes. Hence, the salticid cannot derive a color picture simply by combining information in a receptor-for-receptor (or point-for-point) manner. What color means to a salticid is one of the bigger unresolved questions about their vision. Obtaining an understanding of the psychological meaning of color for salticids will be an especially challenging problem for future research.

Possible Functions of the Low-Acuity Layers IV, III, and II

Structural differences in each of the layers suggests that they have functional differences that go beyond color vision. layer IV, the layer with the fewest receptors, is the first layer through which light passes in the AM retina (figure 1.9). This layer has the poorest spatial acuity but the most complex topography (figure 1.11; plate 2) (M. F. Land, 1969a; Eakin and Brandenburger, 1971; Blest et al., 1981; Blest and Price, 1984). A well-organized vertical strip of receptors lies along the outer side of the AM retina (4a), but the mosaic in the middle of the retina (4b) is poorly organized. Poorly organized regions also lie scattered peripherally (4c). The kind of information provided by layer IV is unclear. However, it has been suggested that region 4a detects the polarization plane of ultraviolet light (M. F. Land, 1969a; Eakin and Brandenburger, 1971). In other arthropods (K. von Frisch, 1949; Brines and Gould, 1982; Fent, 1986), UV polarization detectors act as a "sky compass" during navigation. Ultraviolet polarization detectors have been identified in the AM eyes of lycosid spiders (Magni et al., 1964, 1965) and the secondary eyes of certain gnaphosid and lamponid spiders (Dacke et al., 1999), but there have been no behavioral studies to determine whether salticids detect UV light polarization or use such a sky compass.

Layer III is located directly behind the central region of layer IV and is confined to a roughly circular patch in the middle of the retina (figure 1.12; plate 3) (M. F. Land, 1969a). The functions of this layer are least well understood.

In *Portia*, layer III is populated with large, irregularly arranged receptors. Unlike the secondary eye retinae, receptors in the AM eye retina are not separated by pigment. This means that the functional independence of neighboring receptors depends on them not touching. However, in layer III, rhabdoms are often contiguous, which suggests a very low spatial acuity. In some other salticids, layer III is somewhat more organized than in *Portia*, but still not to an extent that can support more than modest spatial acuity (Eakin and Brandenburger, 1971).

In most salticids, the receptor mosaic of layer II has rhabdoms that are more regularly arranged and in which the rhabdomeres are less erratically contiguous than in layer III. However, this is not the case in *Portia*. *Portia*'s layer II is only slightly more organized than layer III (figure 1.13; plate 4). The rhabdoms in layers II and III differ in appearance, depending on whether they are derived from the outer (2a and 3a) or from the inner (2b and 3b) side, but the functional significance of how they differ is not known.

In transverse section, layers I and II have a laterally compressed strip of receptors with a slight bend in the middle. The result is a boomerang-shaped (figures 1.13

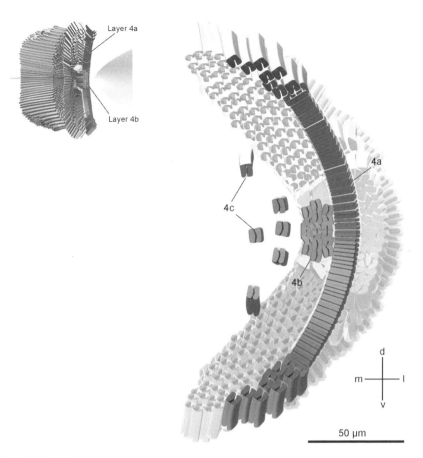

Figure 1.11
The retina of *Portia fimbriata*'s principal eye showing layer IV (shown in blue) in detail. The position of layer IV relative to other layers within the retina is shown at the top left (view angle as in figure 1.6). The transverse profile of the retina is on the right. Three types of receptors make up layer IV. Type 4a receptors form a well-organized vertical strip that may act as a simple line detector and/or be used to analyze UV polarization. Type 4b receptors form a poorly organized central patch. Type 4c receptors are scattered to the side (their positions within the figure are approximate). No function has been hypothesized for type 4b and 4c receptors. Orientation: m, medial; l, lateral; d, dorsal; v, ventral. (See plate 2 for color version.)

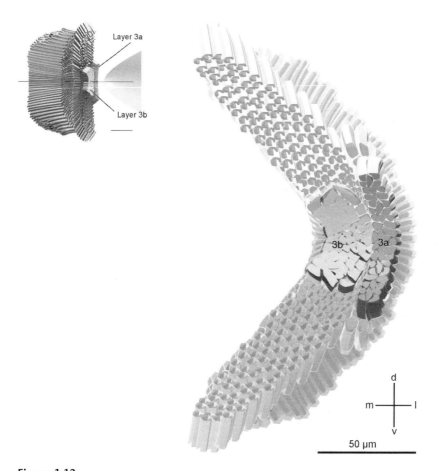

Figure 1.12
The retina of *Portia fimbriata*'s principal eye showing layer III (shown in yellow-orange) in
detail. The position of layer III relative to other retinal layers is shown at the top left (view
angle as figure 1.6). The transverse profile of the retina is on the right. Two types of receptors make up layer III: 3a and 3b receptors, which are large, short, irregularly disposed, and
have rhabdomeres that are erratically contiguous. Layer III could receive an in-focus image
in blue. The quality of any image sampled by this layer would be poor. (See plate 3 for color
version.)

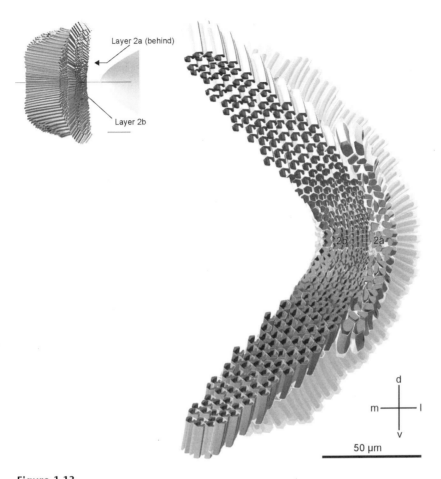

Figure 1.13
The retina of *Portia fimbriata*'s principal eye showing layer II (shown in green) in detail. The position of layer II relative to layer I is shown at the top left (view angle as in figure 1.6). The transverse profile of the retina is on the right. Two types of receptors make up boomerang-shaped layer II. At the fovea of 2b, the receptors have small interreceptor angles (although not as small as in layer I), but are arranged in a disorderly manner. The receptors increase in width toward the periphery of the boomerang arms, and the mosaic becomes more regular. Compared with layer I, the receptors in layer II are short. In *P. fimbriata*, layer II does not appear to be adapted for high-acuity vision. Orientation: d, dorsal; v, ventral; m, median; l, lateral. (See plate 4 for color version.)

and 1.14; plates 4 and 5) receptor mosaic in each of these layers, the boomerang of layer II lying over that of layer I. In *Portia*, receptor width, and therefore interreceptor spacing, in the central region of layer II (i.e., the region close to the optical axis), tends to be much greater than in the central region of layer I. This means that the central region of layer II has much lower spatial acuity. In layers I and II, receptor width and spacing tend to increase steadily toward the periphery until, at the ends of the boomerang's arms, interreceptor spacing for layers I and II roughly matches (figures 1.13 and 1.14).

Compared with the relatively high acuity of their central regions, the peripheral regions of layers I and II support only low spatial acuity. The structure of the secondary lens appears to be responsible for image quality rapidly falling off away from the fovea (Blest and Price, 1984). Close to the optical axis, the secondary lens magnifies without distortion, but the steep sides of the pit produce a distorted image away from the optical axis.

Because of its low acuity, the function of the peripheral retina probably differs from that of the central retina. For example, the periphery of layers II and I may play a role in stimulating eye tube movements (see later discussion) that line up the center of the retina on moving stimuli (Blest and Price, 1984).

The receptors in both layers II and I have almost identical absorbency spectra (figure 1.10B) (Blest et al., 1981). It is unlikely that layer II plays a role in shape perception because its image is out of focus whenever the layer I image is in focus. Perhaps layer II functions in detecting light intensity (Blest et al., 1981), has a role in pattern recognition that somehow complements the role of layer I (Blest and Price, 1984), or works with the secondary eyes to center the AM retinas on moving objects.

High-Acuity Vision: Layer I

Only layer I has the fine, regular mosaic of receptors necessary for detailed vision (figure 1.14). The internal structure of the receptors, their width and length, and their spacing in relation to other receptors are all factors that when combined define sampling performance. In the foveal region of layer I, the rhabdomeres are narrow and densely packed, which maximizes spatial sampling. In the fovea, neighboring receptors have a center-to-center spacing as low as 1.4 μm, which appears to be optimal. The rhabdomeres in layer I are also separated by cytoplasm-filled spaces, which helps isolate them optically.

Compared with other layers, layer I receptors are long, with the longest and narrowest in the fovea (figure 1.9). The additional length improves the probability that photons entering the comparatively narrow receptor will be absorbed (and hence detected).

The receptors in layer I also appear to function as light guides, which improves sampling quality in two ways. First, only light in focus on the receptor's distal tip is accepted; this reduces the probability that photons will be lost to a neighboring

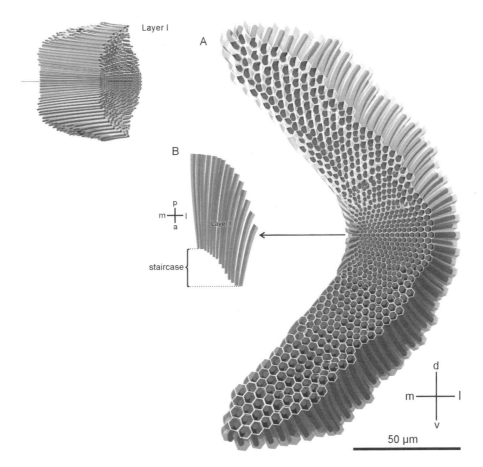

Figure 1.14
The retina of *Portia fimbriata*'s principal eye showing layer I (shown in red). The top left
shows a view 55 deg to the medial side of the optical axis (view angle as in figure 1.6). (*A*)
Transverse profile of the retina showing the detail of the layer's boomerang-shaped mosaic.
Layer I receptors are characteristically long, with a hexagonal cross-section. The mosaic is
regular, formed by rows of receptors. Receptive segments (rhabdomeres) tend to be well
separated (reducing interreceptor interference), with spacing as little as 1.4 μm at the fovea.
There is a gradual increase in receptor size (and spacing), and a gradual decrease in receptor length toward the periphery of the boomerang arms. (*B*) Longitudinal view from above
of a row of foveal receptors. These receptors are longest and arranged like a staircase. Images
of objects located from a few body lengths distant out to infinity come into focus on the
distal (anterior) tips of one or more receptors. Orientation: d, dorsal; v, ventral; m, median;
l, lateral. (See plate 5 for color version.)

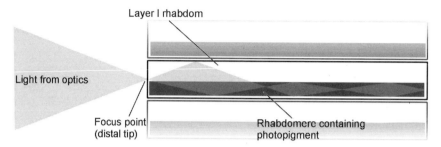

Figure 1.15
Layer I receptor acting as a light guide. Light focused on the rhabdom's anterior tip is trapped in the rhabdomere by internal reflection. Light passes back and forth through rhodopsin in the rhabdomere, enhancing its probability of being absorbed (detected).

receptor. Second, the receptors act as fiber optic cables. This effect is a consequence of the interior of the rhabdomeres being more dense than the surrounding cytoplasm. Photons entering a rhabdomere tend to get trapped by reflecting off of the optically dense rhabdomere edges. Total internal reflection enhances the likelihood that a photon will be absorbed (figure 1.15).

Layer I is specialized for resolving fine-grain spatial details, but sampling ability also depends on image quality. As noted, layers other than I have large receptors and poor sampling quality. In fact, the poor sampling quality of the more distal layers, II–IV, may be necessary for layer I to receive a maximally detailed image (D. C. Williams and McIntyre, 1980; Blest et al., 1981); that is, the interreceptor spacing and the way in which the receptors are arranged in layers II–IV diminish these layers' spatial acuity, but only minimally degrade the image received by layer I.

The minimum interreceptor angle in *Portia*'s layer I fovea is 0.04 deg (2.4 arc min) (Williams and McIntyre, 1980). In practical terms, this means that, from a distance of 200 mm, *Portia* should be able to discriminate between objects spaced 0.12 mm apart.

Compensating for Fixed-Focus Optics

The narrow receptors in the salticid's fovea can work as light guides only as long as light is focused on their distal tips. Unlike a vertebrate's eye, the salticid AM eye is a fixed lens system; i.e., it cannot accommodate. Hence, objects at different distances will come into focus at different distances behind the AM lens. For any specific receptor in layer I, when a close object is in focus on the receptor's distal tip, more distant objects tend to be out of focus (and vice versa). However, having the receptors arranged in a spatial pattern that eliminates the need for accommodation solves this potential problem.

Different parts of the foveal region of layer I are positioned on a "staircase" so that their distal tips are at different distances behind the lens (figure 1.14B). Hence, images of objects at different distances come into focus on different "stairs." The depth of the staircase (~20 μm) is sufficiently large to allow an in-focus image to form on at least one of the "stairs" from approximately two body lengths away to infinity (Blest et al., 1981). Only the layer I fovea has this structure.

The Active Principal Eye

Telephoto optics in conjunction with the unique structure of the AM retina appears to provide a solution to the problem of how a fixed-lens eye can provide both color discrimination and high spatial resolution. However, as a tradeoff, there is a drastic reduction in the AM retina's field of view. *Portia*'s layer I fovea is only fifteen receptors across, giving it a field of view little more than 0.6 deg wide, much less than the ~30–40 deg provided by the corneal lenses. What is more, most objects examined by the eye will be out of focus at some part of the "staircase," making the fovea's effective field of view even narrower. Despite these limitations, the fovea supports the remarkable feats of visual discrimination that underlie much of *Portia*'s complex, flexible behavior.

The AM eye is an "active" eye and this may be the key to understanding how the AM retina's narrow field of view works. Movement of the eye's field of view over a scene probably forms a critical part of how perception works for salticids (Kaps and Schmid, 1996). Using six muscles attached to its outside, each AM eye tube can be moved with three degrees of freedom: vertical, horizontal, and rotational (figure 1.16) (M. F. Land, 1969b). These are the same three degrees of freedom with which our own eyes move, although we are typically unconscious of the small rotational movements (McIlwain, 1996).

Small lateral eye-tube movements allow the salticid to sweep the layer I "staircase" over an object in the visual field, and larger eye movements allow this spider to sample the larger image projected by the corneal lens. The movements of the AM eyes, which can be complex, are probably a critical factor in how salticids process visual information, especially shape and form (M. F. Land, 1969b; M. F. Land and Furneaux, 1997).

Each boomerang-shaped AM retina sits in the salticid's cephalothorax with its "elbow" pointing out laterally (see figure 1.14). However the optics of the eyes invert the image both vertically and horizontally. The resulting fields of view of the two AM retinas, when held together, form an "X," with the fields of view of the two foveas not quite intersecting (see figures 1.6 and 1.17).

The X can be moved in four basic ways. The first is with wide-angle spontaneous scanning movements (figure 1.17A). At varying speeds, the center of the AM retina wanders over a large horizontal and vertical field, possibly searching for objects on which to fixate. These movements may cover the entire visual field of the AM eyes. The second is with saccades (figure 1.17B). These are rapid movements in which the centers of the retinas of both AM eyes move to fixate on some object that has just moved. Third is tracking (figure 1.17C). These are movements that keep the retinae

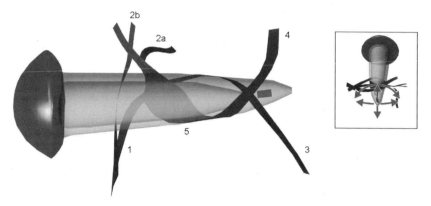

Figure 1.16
Top view of *Portia fimbriata*'s left AM eye showing probable positions of eye muscles. Five muscle bands attached to the eye tube allow the retina to be moved (inset) in the horizontal and vertical planes, and rotated about 30 deg in either direction. Although the corneal lens is wider than the eye tube (giving the eye its distinctive "mushroom" shape), the retina's field of view is never blocked because at any one time it samples only a small part of the corneal lens's field of view and because it can be moved to where the images from the sides of the corneal lens are visible. (The muscles and their numbers are taken from M. F. Land, 1969b. The eye tube is adapted from D. S. Williams and McIntyre, 1980.)

of both AM eyes fixated on a moving object. The fourth is scanning (figure 1.17D). Scanning occurs after the AM retinae fixate on a new target. During scanning, the most complex of the four movement patterns, the AM retinae move back and forth across an object at 0.5–1 Hz (approximately over the width of the layer I "staircase"), while they slowly rotate through an arc of about 50 deg.

In spite of their potential heuristic value, there are as yet no detailed studies of the movements of *Portia*'s AM eyes. However, it is known that the AM eyes of *Portia fimbriata* are more active than those of any other species that has been examined (D. S. Williams and McIntyre, 1980). In fact, they move almost continuously, even in complete darkness (D. P. Harland, unpublished results).

What the AM Eye Sees
The small window of high spatial acuity provided by layer I in the AM eye may have important implications for the kinds of fine-grained optical cues potentially available to *Portia*. Behavioral investigations of the optical cues that *Portia fimbriata* uses to discriminate between prey and nonprey has confirmed what the structural and optical investigation of the principal eye suggests. A number of critical visual cues are provided by very small, specific regions of the prey's body (Harland and Jackson, 2000a). The limited field of view provided by the AM retina means that when one region of the prey is under inspection, other regions are no longer in clear view. The

A. Spontaneous activity

B. Saccades

C. Tracking

D. Scanning

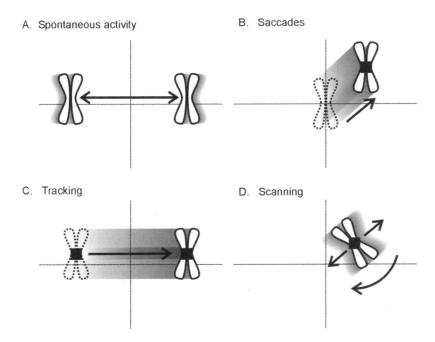

Figure 1.17
Summary of four types of eye movement made by the salticid anterior median eye. Fields of view from two boomerang-shaped retinae combine to create an X-shaped field of view. The arrows indicate retinal movement. (*A*) Spontaneous activity; retinae move unpredictably over a scene. (*B*) Saccades; fields of view are fixated on an object (the black square). (*C*) Tracking; keeps retinae fixed on a moving object. (*D*) Scanning; a newly acquired object is examined by moving fields of view back and forth while slowly rotating one way, then another. (Adapted from M. F. Land, 1969b.)

way in which the visual world is structured from such small high-resolution images appears to depend on both the pattern of the spider's eye movements and its ability to remember what cues it has seen.

Portia's Umwelt

Although salticids rely on more than one sensory modality, vision is primary. Unlike any other spider, a salticid locates, tracks, stalks, chases down, and leaps on active prey, with all phases of the predatory sequence under visual control (Forster, 1982a). Using visual cues alone, salticids discriminate between mates and rivals, predators and prey, and different types of prey, as well as other features of their environment (Crane, 1949; Drees, 1952; Heil, 1936; Jackson and Pollard, 1996; Tarsitano and Jackson, 1997; Harland et al., 1999; Harland and Jackson 2000a, 2001, 2002).

Much of human behavior, and cognition, is vision based (Dennett, 1991). Hence, we may overestimate the advantages of vision and underestimate what can be done with other sensory modalities. This potential bias notwithstanding, it seems to be the case that *Portia's* acute eyesight has a profound influence on both its behavior and its putative cognitive abilities. *Portia's* detouring behavior illustrates this point especially clearly.

Portia's ability to plan and execute long detours requires visual acuity sufficient to examine the spatial relations between objects from a distance (Tarsitano and Andrew, 1999). This visual acuity also enables it to accurately identify the location and behavior of its prey from a distance (Jackson, 1995; D. Li and Jackson, 1996; D. Li et al., 1997). All of this visual information is critical in enabling *Portia* to execute its flexible predatory tactics.

Almost a century ago, Jakob von Uexküll (1909) considered how sensory systems, styles of behavior, and cognitive profiles are interrelated. No animal, including humans, has simple, direct access to an independent physical universe. Instead, each operates inside a subjective "model" of the world (von Uexküll, 1934), or what von Uexküll (1909) called the animal's *Umwelt*. This is roughly translated as an animal's "self-world" (C. Schiller, 1957), a product of the organism's sensory intake, internal state, central processing capabilities, and motor patterns.

Natural selection sees to it that the *Umwelt* is not arbitrary (e.g., Dawkins, 1996); it has to work for the animal, enabling it to survive and propagate. However, a critical insight of von Uexküll's is that one can expect important differences among animals in the character of how they experience what is to them the outside world (Deely, 2001).

Obtaining an understanding of *Portia's Umwelt* may be a tractable problem, but it should not be confused with the notion that we might somehow come to know directly what it is like to be a *Portia* (e.g., Nagel, 1974). Although studying its sensory systems, behavior, and cognitive processes will never reveal to us precisely what it is like to be *Portia*, this is a valid approach to learning something more tangible. Although it is no trivial task, we can expect eventually to comprehend *Portia's Umwelt*. Although we are still a long way from this goal, we may be able to shed light on some of the most interesting issues with a final story.

In a Queensland rain forest, we find *Portia fimbriata* sitting on a portion of a vine that has fallen away from a tree trunk (figure 1.18A; plate 6). Based on what we know about this araneophagic predator, we think that *Portia* is prepared, in a way that we are not, to perceive webs, spider-sized animals, and potential pathways to the web via the vine and neighboring vegetation.

Of course, *Portia's Umwelt* is built from more than just visual information. In this story, for example, its feet and palps have touched silk lines on the vine's surface, triggering a number of chemoreceptors. Some of the silk is from *Jacksonoides queenslandicus*, and airborne chemical cues carry the odor of this spider. However, the source of information may not be important for *Portia*. In this example, chemosensory information from *J. queenslandicus* may prime *Portia* to detect visual cues associated with this familiar prey.

One way of interpreting such a priming effect is to suggest that chemical cues elicit some kind of representation of *J. queenslandicus* somewhere in *Portia*'s central nervous system, although what this representation might be is not clear. Certainly, it need not be anything like a picture of or the idea of the prey (Gardenfors, 1996). A more plausible explanation might be that the chemosensory information lowers the thresholds for responses by central nervous system modules (or feature detectors) associated with the visual system. What we do know is that chemosensory and visual information work together to underpin predatory behaviors appropriate for capturing *J. queenslandicus*. We are still a long way from understanding precisely how this is done, however.

The question of whether *Portia*'s *Umwelt* includes anything like the visual images (or "pictures") that we see remains unresolved, but the extraordinary eyesight of these spiders encourages us to explore this possibility. Acute vision may indeed be a central pillar of an *Umwelt* that requires recognizing distinct objects distributed at precise locations in space. This is, of course, what humans experience, and it may be reasonable to assume that *Portia*'s experiences are similar. On the other hand, given that the structural details of *Portia*'s eyes are so different from ours, we should also expect important differences in the subjective world that they help to create.

Movement of objects in the outside world must be a highly relevant part of *Portia*'s *Umwelt*. The anterior lateral eyes provide input about movement within a range of 45 deg to either side of the spider (figure 1.18C); the remaining secondary eyes gather movement information beyond that, and even behind *Portia*'s body.

Portia's *Umwelt* probably includes objects positioned at more or less precise distances, and the AL eyes probably play a major role in providing that information. The AL eyes' fields of view overlap directly in front of *Portia*, and toward the center of the visual field, the visual angle between receptors decreases from approximately 1 deg to just 0.4 deg. A disparity between the images in the AL retinae probably provides information about an object's distance. Information about additional features of the visual world, such as an object's shape, size, and color, are probably provided by the anterior medial eyes.

In this final story, for example, information from the AL eyes has directed the AM eye tubes to move their tiny field across the scene provided by the AM corneal lenses (figure 1.18D). Its AM eyes are now examining a moving object that is slightly off center. As explained earlier, the AM eye tubes are highly active, and our hypothesis is that this "scanning" activity serves to abstract relevant information from the retinal images. Input from particularly salient cues may in turn trigger patterns of scanning designed to search for certain additional visual cues that the initial cues have primed the spider to recognize. Perhaps through this type of sequential scanning for particular cues, a central nervous system-based representation of the object is constructed (figure 1.18F). The salticid eye may be surprisingly good at assessing the details of objects. However, as a consequence of doing its analysis via eye-tube movements and using a retina with only a small number of receptors, it probably takes much more time than analogous processing by a vertebrate.

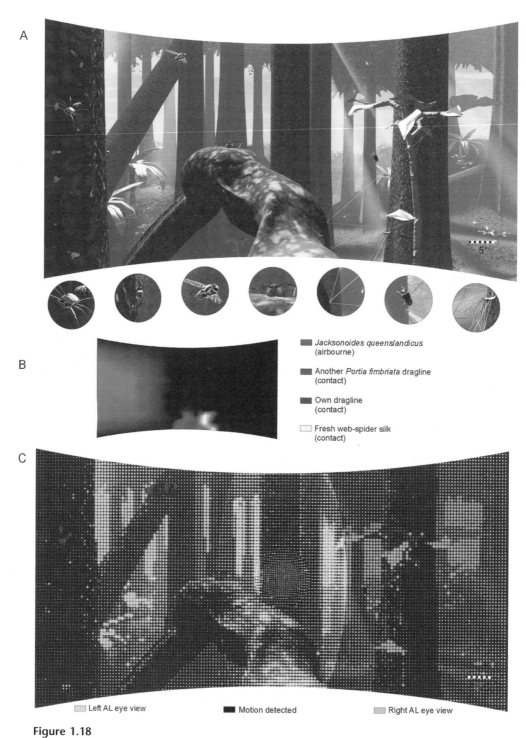

Figure 1.18

Portia fimbriata's view of the world. (*A*) *Portia*'s forest habitat (approximately 90 deg wide). The circles show some key points of interest for *Portia*. (*B*) Representation of *Portia*'s

Jacksonoides queenslandicus
(airbourne)

Another *Portia fimbriata* dragline
(contact)

Own dragline
(contact)

Fresh web-spider silk
(contact)

5°

Left AL eye view   Motion detected   Right AL eye view

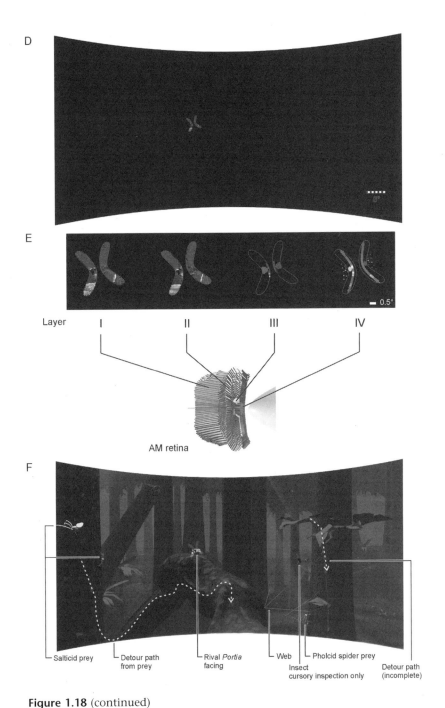

D

E

Layer   I   II   III   IV

AM retina

F

Salticid prey   Detour path from prey   Rival *Portia* facing   Web   Insect cursory inspection only   Pholcid spider prey   Detour path (incomplete)

Figure 1.18 (continued)
chemoreceptive environment. (*C*) Representation of the view seen by anterior lateral eyes. Note the region of binocular overlap used in range-finding and foveal regions. (*D*) Field of view provided by anterior median eyes. (*E*) View seen by the four layers of the AM eyes during inspection of other *Portia*. (*F*) View showing elements that *Portia* has abstracted from the scene using its AM eyes during several minutes of looking around. (See plate 6 for color version.)

Watching *Portia* pursue prey tends to be a drawn-out exercise; this spider moves through its predatory sequence at a speed that is tedious for a human observer. It may be the case that a unique (or at least a nonhuman) sense of time is a key part of *Portia's Umwelt*. The slowness of scanning-based construction of an object suggests interesting ways in which the perception of time by *Portia* might differ from our own notion of time.

Although this limited attempt to characterize *Portia's Umwelt* does not put us directly in this spider's shoes, it is a necessary, initial step toward its reverse engineering (Dennett, 1995). That in turn can be a step toward building a robot that can solve problems and behave as *Portia* does. Knowing what it is like to be *Portia* may amount to much the same thing.

2 Exploration of Cognitive Capacity in Honeybees: Higher Functions Emerge from a Small Brain

Shaowu Zhang and Mandyam Srinivasan

Despite the obvious optical differences between the human's camera-type eye and the bee's compound eye, research over the past two decades has shown that the fundamental principles of early visual processing in the two nervous systems are quite similar, at least in a qualitative sense.

The worker honeybee has a tiny brain. Its volume is only about a cubic millimeter; it weighs only 1 mg; and it contains fewer than a million neurons. However, like humans, the bee possesses excellent trichromatic color vision, motion vision, and spatial vision (K. von Frisch, 1971; Wehner, 1981). Also, like humans, the bee is capable of abstracting general features of visual patterns. Astonishingly, bees even experience some of the visual illusions that humans do (Srinivasan, 1994, 1998).

Such similarities in perceptual ability lead us to ask a number of fascinating questions about the bee's other capacities. For instance, what is the learning capacity of such a tiny brain? How complex a task can a honeybee learn? What do bees acquire, process, and memorize when they learn how to solve complex tasks? How do honeybees generalize what they have acquired in the learning process? What neural mechanisms underlie their complex behaviors?

Finding the answers to these questions is important for two reasons. First, they elucidate a number of fundamental questions in neuroscience, among which is the way in which intelligence has emerged evolutionarily from animals with tiny brains. Second, they will give engineers insight into the functional architecture and level of performance that can be attained by a computer chip as small as a bee's brain; perhaps even a chip that could be built into a learning machine capable of performing complex behaviors like a bee.

Over the past decade we have pursued the answers to many of these questions, such as the degree to which bees are able to generalize the abstract features of objects, perform "top-down" processing, learn skills and rules, group stimuli associatively, form concepts, and so on. In this chapter we review the progress we have achieved. Our review is not intended to be exhaustive. Rather, it highlights the important advances in our understanding of the processes underlying pattern recognition, perception, and the learning of complex tasks by the honeybee.

Bees Can Abstract General Properties of Patterns

Honeybees are able to learn the concrete features of objects, such as their color, shape, scent, and so on (Menzel and Bitterman, 1983; Gould and Gould, 1988; Menzel, 1990; Chittka, 1993; Lehrer et al., 1995). However, important insights into the workings of visual perception can be gleaned by examining whether honeybees are capable of recognizing and abstracting the general properties of objects. There can be little doubt that bees use some kind of neural "snapshot" to remember and recognize patterns and landmarks (Collett and Cartwright, 1983; Judd and Collett, 1998). However, it is hard to imagine that this is all there is to pattern recognition. In their daily lives, bees must remember a number of different patterns and their properties. Some examples are the shape of their nest or hive, the shapes representing nectar-bearing flowers, and the shapes of important landmarks seen on the way to and from a food source.

However, if snapshots were the only mechanisms for remembering shapes, bees would require a very large memory to store all of the images. Given that a bee's brain contains far fewer neurons than ours does, it seems unlikely that they can afford the luxury of a large memory store. One would imagine, then, that bees possess other, more economical means of representing patterns. Perhaps they can extract and remember the general properties of form.

Learning to Abstract Pattern Orientation

We first asked whether honeybees can learn to abstract a particular attribute of a pattern, such as its orientation, without having to memorize the pattern in its entirety. An early paper by Wehner (1971) hinted that bees could indeed abstract pattern orientation in this way. This issue was pursued by van Hateren et al. (1990), who used a Y-maze (figure 2.1a) in conjunction with visual cues that were random grating patterns at different orientations (figure 2.1b). In the experiments, two stimuli were presented in the vertical plane, each at the end wall of one of the arms of the maze. The stimulus representing one of the orientations was associated with a reward of sugar water; in another orientation it was not. During training, the positions of the stimuli were interchanged regularly, and the reward was moved along with the positive stimuli, to prevent the bees from simply learning to fly to a specific arm.

Two features of the apparatus and training paradigm prevented the bees from acquiring a template of the positive stimulus. First, the bees had to choose between the two stimuli from a distance too far for them to fixate on the stimulus. Second, reward trials were separated frequently by trials in which arms were marked by other random gratings that were similarly oriented, but which had different spatial structures (figure 2.1b). So to identify the positive stimulus correctly, the bees had to abstract the grating's orientation, not merely memorize (or recognize) the pattern in a photographic way.

Van Hateren et al. (1990) found that bees could be trained in this way to distinguish among vertical, horizontal, and diagonal orientations (figure 2.1c–e). Furthermore, bees trained to distinguish between two mutually perpendicular orientations were able to discriminate between similarly oriented novel patterns (figure 2.2). Hence, bees are able to extract orientation information from patterns on which they are trained and use this information to evaluate new patterns.

Learning to Detect Radial and Circular Symmetry

Horridge and Zhang (1995) showed that honeybees are also capable of extracting center-symmetric attributes of patterns. For example, they can learn to distinguish

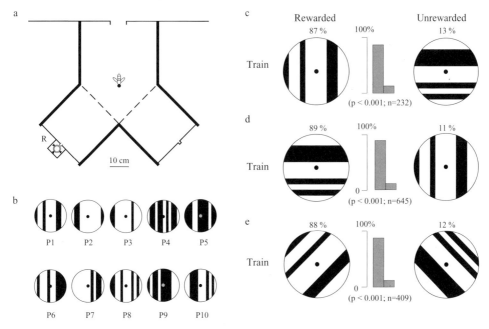

Figure 2.1
Discrimination of pattern orientation. In this and other figures, the vertical bars depict choice frequencies for the two stimuli in training or transfer tests, and n is the number of choices analyzed. The p value is associated with the t-test for examining whether the bees' preferences are significantly different from random choice. (Adapted from van Hateren et al., 1990.)

between radial symmetry and circular symmetry; that is, between a pattern composed of radial sectors and one composed of concentric rings. In these experiments, flying bees entered a Y-maze that contained a choice chamber from which they could see two patterns at the same time. During training, the positive stimulus was always a radially symmetric pattern and the negative stimulus was a circularly symmetric pattern. However, each of the two patterns used was drawn from a pool of four as shown in figure 2.3a. This tested whether the bees could learn the concepts of radial symmetry versus circular symmetry in a general sense without memorizing a specific example of each.

When trained bees were subsequently tested on various pairs of stimuli—some of which were familiar and others novel—they preferred radially symmetric patterns over circularly symmetric patterns (figure 2.3b), even when the patterns were novel patterns of bars (figure 2.3c). They also preferred a radially sectored pattern over a novel checkered pattern (figure 2.3f), but preferred the checkered pattern over a radially symmetric pattern of rings, indicating that they had learned to avoid the unrewarded pattern types (figure 2.3g).

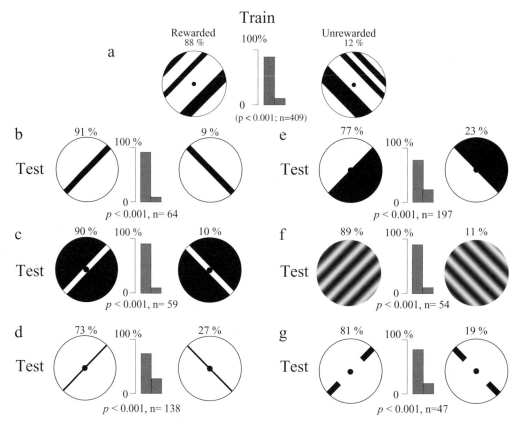

Figure 2.2
Bees trained to distinguish between random gratings oriented at plus and minus 45 deg as in (*a*), are able to extract the orientation information in these patterns and use it to discriminate the orientations of other patterns not previously encountered (*b*)–(*g*). The patterns in (*f*) represent sinusoidal gratings. (Adapted from van Hateren et al., 1990.)

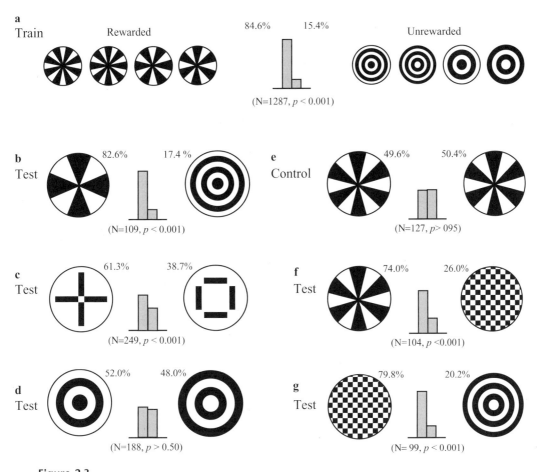

Figure 2.3
Bees can make a generalized discrimination between radially sectored and ring patterns.
(Adapted from Horridge and Zhang, 1995.)

The bees showed no preference if the stimuli were identical (figure 2.3e) or if they were both composed of concentric rings, differing merely in the proportion of black (figure 2.3d).

Learning to Detect Bilateral Symmetry

Perception of symmetry has been demonstrated in humans, birds, dolphins, and apes. Horridge (1996) found that honeybees, too, can recognize bilateral symmetry and discriminate the axis of symmetry. In his experiments, bees were trained on seven different pairs of four-bar patterns that were presented successively to prevent the bees from learning any one pattern. In each trial, one of each pair of patterns presented always had the attribute of bilateral symmetry. The bees learned to choose the pattern with bilateral symmetry, irrespective of the orientation of the axis of symmetry. They also were able to discriminate between a pattern with one axis of bilateral symmetry and the same pattern rotated by 90 deg, irrespective of the actual pattern (figure 2.4a–g).

The bees were then tested with the pairs of positive and negative stimuli rotated 180 deg; nevertheless, the positive stimulus had a horizontal axis of symmetry and the negative stimulus had a vertical axis. The bees continued to discriminate and make choices consistent with their original training (figure 2.4h–n).

Giurfa et al. (1996) also demonstrated that bees can learn to discriminate bilaterally symmetric from nonsymmetric patterns and then transfer this knowledge to novel stimuli, suggesting that they can learn to recognize the difference between symmetric and nonsymmetric forms.

In all of these studies, bees have clearly demonstrated that they can detect and learn certain abstract characteristics of objects. In addition, they can learn the average angular orientation of parallel bars, irrespective of their exact locations in a pattern (van Hateren et al., 1990). They can discriminate between radial and tangential edges, irrespective of the pattern (Horridge and Zhang, 1995), and between patterns with different axes of bilateral symmetry, also irrespective of the pattern (Horridge, 1996). Furthermore, they can generalize what they have learned during training and apply their knowledge to novel discrimination tasks. Bees can also learn other abstract properties of objects, such as their color and size, without having to memorize the objects' images literally (e.g., Ronacher, 1992; Horridge et al., 1992b).

It is important to emphasize that in all of the experiments we have described, the bees' ability to generalize what they have learned has been demonstrated by training them to not one, but a number of stimuli that differ in detail but share the key property that is to be generalized. For example, the patterns associated with reward might all have the same orientation or the same kind of symmetry (e.g., left-right symmetry). However, during training the stimuli would be shuffled randomly to ensure that the bees would in fact learn the stimulus characteristic associated with the reward and not just recognize one particular pattern (Horridge, 1999).

How might the bee's visual system extract the orientation of a pattern independent of its structure and without simply memorizing it? Srinivasan et al. (1993)

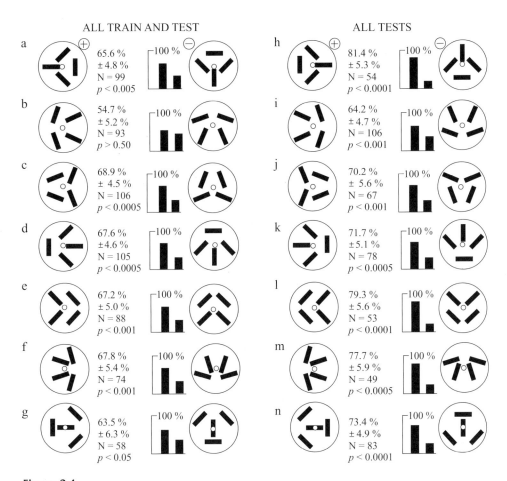

Figure 2.4
Bees detect bilateral symmetry and discriminate its axis. (Adapted from Horridge, 1996.)

provided evidence that in bees pattern discrimination is based on the geometric cues that are intrinsic to the pattern and not on any cues derived from the direction of apparent image motion. Furthermore, E. C. Yang and Maddes (1997) found large-field, orientation-sensitive neurons in the bee's lobula (in the optic lobe). Horridge (1999) suggested that bees possess large-field filters that respond selectively to abstract stimulus properties such as symmetry, relative proportion of radial and tangential edges, angular size, orientation, and so on. The existence of such filters is suggested by the fact that bees can respond to a generalized cue extracted from a group of patterns that they have encountered.

Honeybees Perceive Illusory Contours

The human visual system perceives an illusory contour where there is a fault line across a regular striped pattern. In essence, our brain fills in the missing information from ·experience; this is one way that our visual system recognizes an object that is partially occluded by another, closer object. For example, in the so-called "Kanizsa illusion" (figure 2.5a), the gaps in the lines and the cutouts in the black disks create the perception of a triangle that is not there. Von der Heydt et al. (1984) discovered that certain cortical neurons that normally respond to oriented contours of objects also respond to illusory contours such as those in the Kanizsa illusion.

Van Hateren et al. (1990) explored whether such illusory contours are also experienced by honeybees. They trained bees in a Y-maze in which they had to distinguish between random gratings that were oriented at plus or minus 45 deg. Only the former choice was rewarded (figure 2.5b). When these trained bees were tested with rectangles in the same two orientations, they preferred the rectangle with the same orientation as the grating rewarded during training (figure 2.5c). The bees were able to abstract information about orientation and apply it to the novel discrimination task. When the grating-trained bees were tested with illusory rectangles oriented at plus and minus 45 deg, again they showed a significant preference for the plus 45 deg orientation (figure 2.5d). This suggests that the bees did indeed perceive the illusory rectangles as do we. Further, note that when the stimulus components were scrambled, the bees' preference and presumably, their perception, of the illusory rectangles disappeared (figure 2.5e).

Insects experience many other illusions that we do, such as the waterfall illusion, the Benham illusion, and the Mueller-Lyer illusion, among others. This suggests that insects may process many types of visual information in ways that are similar to those used by humans (Srinivasan, 1993). In fact, Horridge et al. (1992a) examined the dragonfly's perception of a type of illusory contour that in humans has been explained by the existence of an end-stopped edge, or line detectors in the striate visual cortex (von der Heydt and Peterhans, 1989). Horridge et al. found a class of neurons in the dragonfly's lobula that responded directionally to motion of the illusory contour, as if to a real edge or line.

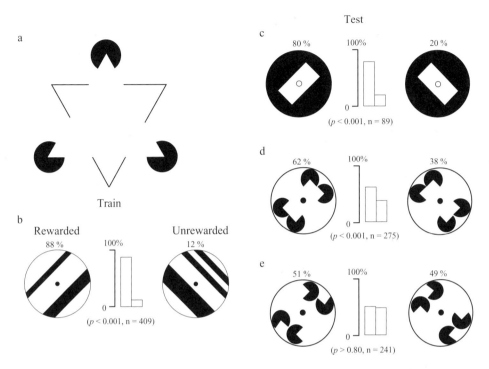

Figure 2.5
Like humans, honeybees perceive illusory contours. (Adapted from van Hateren et al., 1990.)

"Top-Down" Processing

It is well known that prior knowledge or experience aids us tremendously in recognizing objects that are poorly visible, partially hidden, or camouflaged. For instance, many of us who view the scene in figure 2.6 for the first time would not see a familiar object, especially if we have not been told what the picture contains. Once the camouflaged Dalmatian has been discovered, however, it is recognized instantly every time the picture is reencountered (Lindsay and Norman, 1977; Goldstein, 1989; Cavanagh, 1991).

Top-down processing of this kind can speed up the analysis of the retinal image when a familiar scene or object is encountered, and help fill in, or complete, details that are missing in the optic array (Cavanagh, 1991). Is this ability to enhance visual processing restricted to highly developed visual systems, such as those of humans and higher mammals, or does it extend to relatively simple visual systems, such as those of invertebrates? Zhang and Srinivasan (1994) approached this question by investigating whether bees are able to use prior experience to facilitate the detection of

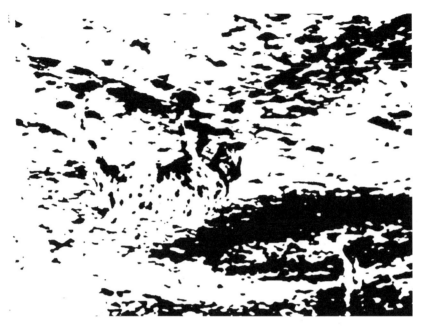

Figure 2.6
A familiar, but camouflaged object. Readers experiencing difficulty in recognizing the Dalmatian dog may wish to view the picture upside-down. (Photo courtesy of R. C. James. Modified from Lindsay and Norman, 1977.)

objects and the discrimination of their shapes. First, they attempted to train bees to distinguish between a ring and a disk when each shape was presented as a camouflaged (textured) figure positioned 6 cm in front of a similarly textured background (figure 2.7a). Although the figures are well camouflaged, they can be detected by the relative motion between the figure and the more distant background as the bee flies toward them. It turned out that the bees were unable to learn this discrimination, despite training that lasted for more than 100 rewarded trials per bee.

Next, Zhang and Srinivasan examined whether bees could learn to distinguish the camouflaged patterns if they were first trained on a related but simpler task: distinguishing between a black ring and a black disk, each presented 6 cm in front of a white background. The ring and the disk were the same size and shape as their textured counterparts, and their spatial configuration in relation to the background was identical to that in the previous experiment. The bees were able to learn this new task (figure 2.7c). Then, when the pretrained bees were tested on the original task, they distinguished between the camouflaged patterns almost immediately (figure 2.7d). Evidently the bees were able to learn to use the motion parallax provided by the figure

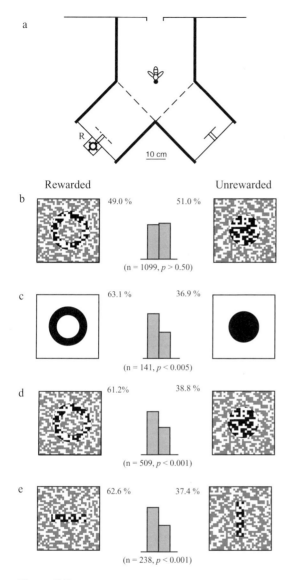

Figure 2.7
Investigation of top-down processing in honeybees. (Adapted from Zhang and Srinivasan, 1994.)

and background as a cue to break the camouflage, but only after they had been pre-trained on uncamouflaged versions of the same shapes.

In this experiment, bees used knowledge acquired from the simpler discrimination task to solve the more difficult task of recognizing the camouflaged figures. Moreover, bees trained in this step-by-step fashion could go on to learn to distinguish between other camouflaged objects that they had not previously encountered, such as two differently oriented bars (figure 2.7e), without pretraining on black-and-white versions of the new shapes. Hence, the enhancement in the bees' performance was not restricted to the specific training shapes, such as the camouflaged ring and disk. Rather, the bees were extracting a novel cue, motion parallax, from the stimulus and using it to discriminate between the novel shapes.

Learning to Negotiate Complex Mazes

The discovery of top-down processing by bees inspired us to pursue other experiments using mazes to examine whether honeybees can learn skills and rules to solve complex tasks and then apply what they have learned to novel situations.

Maze learning has been investigated extensively using a number of higher vertebrates, notably rats, mice, and pigeons (Pick and Yanai, 1983; Dale, 1988). Relatively few studies, however, have explored this capacity in invertebrates. We were initially interested in whether bees could learn to negotiate complex mazes that required several correct decisions to reach a goal.

Zhang et al. (1996) tested bees in a variety of complex mazes, each of which consisted of a 4×5 matrix of identical cubic boxes. Each wall of each box had a hole in its center so that a path through the maze could be created by leaving some holes open and blocking others. The task was to fly through a particular sequence of boxes to reach a feeder containing sugar solution (figure 2.8).

Learning a Maze by Following a Sign

In one series of experiments, bees had to find their way through the maze by learning to following a 4- × 4-cm green square on the wall below the correct exit in each box (figure 2.9a). Bees were trained to negotiate the maze by moving a feeder step by step along the correct path until it was in the third box along the path. During this training period, the bees had the opportunity to learn that the green square in each box indicated the correct exit. After the training period, the feeder was moved directly into the last box along the path, left there briefly, and then moved to its final position, the feeder compartment behind the last box. Before each test, the boxes were swapped to remove possible olfactory cues.

The bees' performance was tested immediately thereafter. During the test, only one bee at a time was allowed into the maze. Its performance was scored by assigning each of its flights to one of four categories: Category C_1 was assigned to flights in which a bee flew through the entire maze without making any mistakes. In category

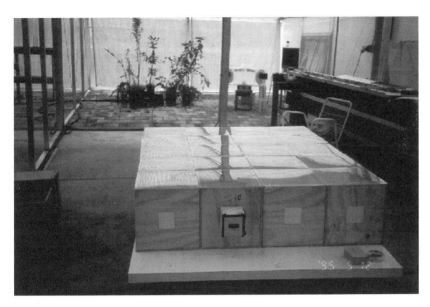

Figure 2.8
Maze apparatus in the All Weather Bee Flight Facility. (Adapted from Zhang et al., 1996.)

C_2 flights, the bee turned back and retraced its path one or more times but remained on the correct path. In category C_3, a bee made one or more wrong turn but still arrived at the goal within 5 min. Finally, category C_4 consisted of flights in which the bee did not reach the goal within 5 min, regardless of whether it was on the correct path. Also, in some tests the time needed to reach the goal was measured. The results show clearly that after their initial training in the first portions of the maze, the bees were able to find their way through the rest of the maze (test 1, figure 2.9b). Performance was also good when the bees were tested on a novel path created by rearranging the maze (test 2, figure 2.9b).

Evidently the bees had not only learned to follow cues provided by the green squares but were also able to use this strategy in a novel situation.

The control condition shown in figure 2.9 depicts the results of a test that measured how well the trained bees could follow an unfamiliar route in an unmarked maze. Their performance is a baseline against which the performance of the experimental bees can be compared. Clearly, the experimental bees learned to use the colored marker as a guide to negotiating complex mazes.

Learning a Maze by Using a Symbolic Cue
We also found that bees could use symbolic cues to negotiate mazes (Zhang et al., 1996). In these experiments, a color on the back wall of each box indicated whether the bee was to turn to the left or the right (figure 2.10a, left panel).

a

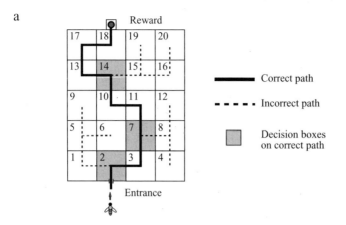

b

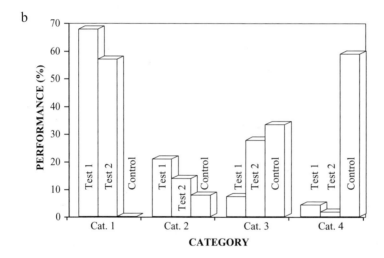

Figure 2.9
Learning to negotiate mazes by following marks. (Adapted from Zhang et al., 1996.)

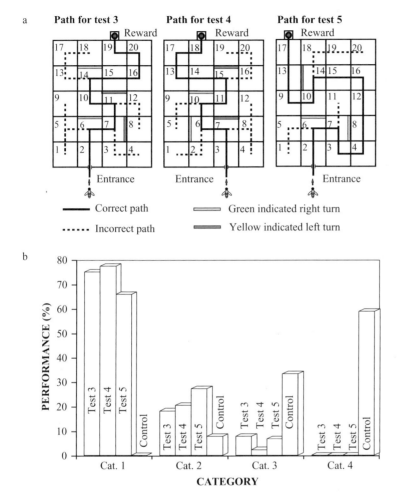

Figure 2.10
Learning to negotiate mazes by using a symbolic cue. (Adapted from Zhang et al., 1996.)

Initially, bees were trained and tested on a specific path using procedures similar to those described earlier (figure 2.10a, left-hand panel, path 3). Bees learned this task very well (test 3, figure 2.10b). In fact, their performance was just as impressive as in the previously described experiments.

Here again, the trained bees were immediately able to use the left or right cue to successfully negotiate novel mazes (figure 2.10a, middle and right-hand panels; tests 4 and 5, figure 2.10b). In all cases, the experimental bees performed better than the controls (figure 2.9b).

It is interesting that walking honeybees are also capable of using visual stimuli as navigational signposts when learning to follow a route (Zhang et al., 1998).

Negotiating Unmarked Mazes

Zhang et al. (1996) also examined the ability of bees to learn to negotiate unmarked mazes (figure 2.11a). Here bees were trained step-by-step through the entire maze, from the entrance to the reward box. After 5 days of training, the bees had indeed learned to negotiate the maze, although their performance was poorer than when they followed a colored cue. Nevertheless, their performance was better than that of a control group. Examples of the bees' performance in two mazes are shown in tests 6 and 7 of figure 2.11b. Presumably the bees learned the mazes by memorizing the sequence of turns that had to be made at specific distances (or box counts) along the route. There is evidence that bees use visual odometry to estimate the distance they have flown (Srinivasan et al. 1997, 2000), and that they are able to count landmarks en route to a goal (Chittka and Geiger, 1995).

When bees that have learned to negotiate a maze with the aid of signs or symbolic cues are later tested on the same routes without the signs or cues, their performance is significantly poorer than that of bees that have been trained on unmarked mazes (Zhang et al., 1996). Evidently when they are trained in this way, bees rely almost exclusively on visual cues for navigation and pay little "attention" to the route per se.

Negotiating Mazes by Learning Path Regularity

We have seen that bees' performance in unmarked mazes is not as good as in mazes with visual cues that indicate the appropriate turn to be made at each stage in the maze. This is because the only way that a bee can navigate an unmarked maze, in general, is to memorize the sequence of turns necessary to get through the maze successfully. It is conceivable, however, that some unmarked mazes are easier to learn than others. For example, mazes that require a regular pattern of turns might be learned more readily than those that do not; that is, if bees have the ability to recognize such patterns.

Zhang et al. (2000) tested the ability of bees to learn unmarked mazes of various configurations, some with path regularity and some without. Four different configurations were used, each in a different experimental series: constant-turn mazes in which the appropriate turn in each decision chamber is always in the same direction;

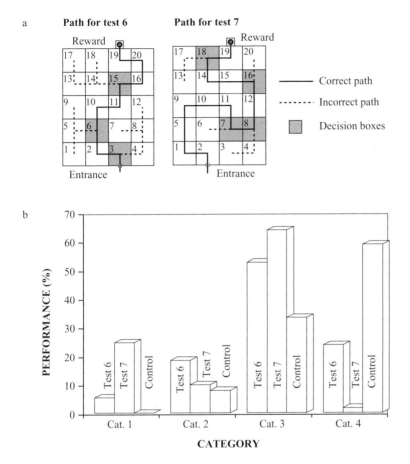

Figure 2.11
Learning to negotiate unmarked mazes. (Adapted from Zhang et al., 1996.)

zig-zag mazes in which the appropriate turn alternates left and right; irregular mazes in which there is no pattern to the appropriate turns; and variable irregular mazes in which the bees were trained to learn four irregular mazes simultaneously (figure 2.12). To facilitate comparisons of performance in these four types of mazes, the mazes were six decision chambers long, unless specified otherwise.

Vertically oriented cylinders were used as modules to construct the mazes. A bee flying a correct path through the maze entered a cylinder through one hole and could leave through one of two exit holes, positioned 45 deg to the left and right of the entrance hole. One exit hole represented the correct path and the other one led to a cylinder that was a dead end. The final cylinder on the correct path contained a feeder that provided a solution of sugar water.

Again, bees were trained step-by-step through the entire maze, from the entrance to the reward box. The baseline performance of the bees was obtained in control experiments in which bees were trained in a variable irregular maze and then tested in a novel irregular maze.

We evaluated the bees' performance using the same categories as described earlier (C1, C2, C3, and C4, and flight time through the maze). Flight durations were grouped into five categories: T1, 1–30 s; T2, 31–60 s; T3, 61–90 s; T4, 91–120 s; and T5, 121–300 s (5 min); T1 was the best performance and T5 the worst.

The Right-Turn Maze

In one series of experiments (series 1 in the tables) we used a constant-turn maze in which every correct turn was in the same direction (e.g., figure 2.12a). The performance of bees trained on a right-turn maze for 1 day and then tested in an identical maze was surprisingly accurate. During the test phase, most flights had durations of less than 30 s and contained no errors (tables 2.1, 2.2).

Bees trained in the right-turn maze were also tested in an extended right-turn maze that had an additional right-turn chamber at the end. The bees showed a clear tendency to make a right turn in the final chamber, indicating that they were continuing to apply the rule that they had just learned.

When tested in a novel irregular maze (figure 2.13a), bees originally trained in a right-turn maze succeeded in arriving at the feeder by simply using the always-turn-right rule (figure 2.13a). The rule allowed them reach the goal eventually, even if they entered some dead-end chambers en route. When tested in a number of irregular mazes, bees trained on the right-turn rule showed a strong and significant preference for making right turns no matter what maze they encountered (figure 2.13b). These bees can also negotiate left-turn and zig-zag mazes because the right-turn rule (or left-turn rule, for that matter) can, in principle, be applied to all of the mazes and will eventually yield success (Zhang et al., 2000).

The Zig-Zag Maze

A second series of experiments (noted as series 2 in the tables) examined whether bees could learn to negotiate a zig-zag maze in which the correct turns alternated right and

a. Right-turn-maze

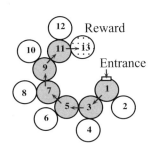

Correct path: 1 > 3 → 5 → 7
→ 9 → 11 → 13

b. Zig-zag maze

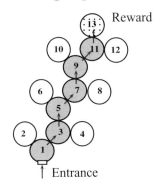

Correct path: 1 > 3 → 5 → 7
→ 9 → 11 → 13

c. Irregular maze

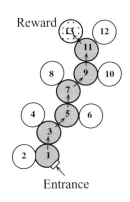

Correct path: 1 > 3 → 5 → 7
→ 9 → 11 → 13

d. Variable configuration

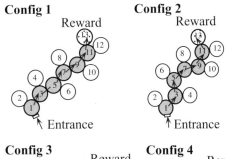

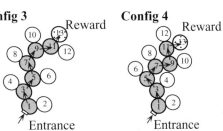

Correct path: 1 > 3 → 5 → 7
→ 9 → 11 → 13

Figure 2.12
Four types of maze configurations.

Table 2.1
Summary of maze performance as evaluated by categories

		C1	C2	C3	C4	Total
Series 1	Number of flights	87	18	161	0	266
	Percentage	32.7%	6.8%	60.6%	0	
Series 2	Number of flights	33	4	86	0	123
	Percentage	26.8	3.3%	69.9%	0	
Series 3	Number of flights	21	5	99	0	125
	Percentage	16.8%	4.0%	79.2%	0	
Series 4	Number of flights	0	1	55	0	56
	Percentage	0	1.8%	98.2%	0	
Control	Number of flights	1	0	34	7	42
	Percentage	2.4%	0	80.9%	16.7%	

For each series of experiments, performance is indicated by number and percentage of flights in each category: C1, C2, C3, and C4.

Table 2.2
Summary of maze performance as evaluated by flight time

		T1	T2	T3	T4	T5	Total
Series 1	Number of flights	138	78	30	13	7	266
	Percentage	51.8%	29.3%	11.3%	4.9%	2.6%	
Series 2	Number of flights	64	45	11	3	0	123
	Percentage	52.0%	36.6%	8.9%	2.4%	0	
Series 3	Number of flights	39	49	27	10	0	125
	Percentage	31.2%	39.8%	21.6%	8.0%	0	
Series 4	Number of flights	7	23	11	3	12	56
	Percentage	12.5%	41.1%	19.6%	5.4%	21.4%	
Control	Number of flights	3	13	10	3	13	42
	Percentage	7.1%	31.0%	23.8%	7.1%	31.0%	

For each series of experiments, performance is indicated by number and percentage of flights in each time zone: T1, T2, T3, T4, and T5.

Training in right-turn maze, transfer test in an irregular maze

a. Transfer test in an irregular maze

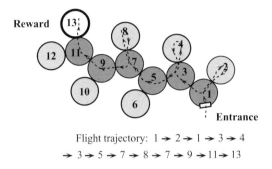

Flight trajectory: 1 → 2 → 1 → 3 → 4
→ 3 → 5 → 7 → 8 → 7 → 9 → 11→ 13

b. Performance in Transfer tests

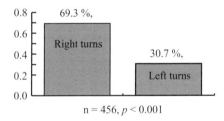

$n = 456, p < 0.001$

Figure 2.13
Training in a right-turn maze and subsequent test in an irregular maze. (Adapted from Zhang et al., 2000.)

left (figure 2.12b). Again, after just 10 hr of training, bees learned the zig-zag maze nearly as well as a constant-turn maze (tables 2.1 and 2.2) (Zhang et al., 2000).

We then tested these bees in a number of ways. First, we found that the bees negotiated an extended zig-zag maze equally well and in the final additional chamber showed a clear tendency to choose the correct exit.

In another test, bees flew in a maze similar to the zig-zag maze in figure 2.12b, but with a special chamber (chamber 5) added in the middle (figure 2.14a). The special chamber had only one exit, directly opposite the entrance, so that the bees could not choose to go left or right. The question here was how would the bees behave in the next chamber, given that they had made a left turn prior to being forced to fly straight? After leaving the special chamber, the bees showed a clear tendency to turn left, which suggests that that they treated the special chamber as if it required a right. In essence, the spatial chamber was treated as if it were a "valid" chamber along the route.

Transfer test in augmented zig-zag maze

a. Maze configuration   **b. Sequential performance histogram**

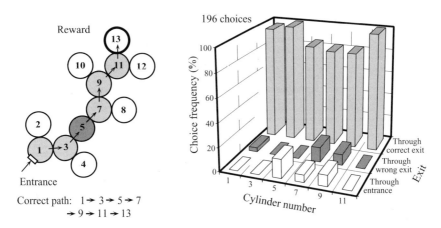

Correct path: 1 → 3 → 5 → 7
              → 9 → 11 → 13

Figure 2.14
Training in a zig-zag maze and transfer test in an augmented zig-zag maze. (Adapted from Zhang et al., 2000.)

Zhang et al. also investigated the ability of bees to negotiate an irregular maze (i.e., series 3 in the tables), and four variable irregular mazes simultaneously (i.e., series 4 in the tables). In brief, what we found was that the bees were not able to learn four irregular mazes as well as just one, demonstrating that there is a ceiling to their maze-learning abilities. In general, we found that the bees' performance was best in the constant-turn maze, slightly better in the zig-zag mazes than in the fixed irregular mazes, and better in the fixed irregular maze than in the variable irregular mazes.

These experiments show that honeybees can negotiate mazes by recognizing and learning regularities in the paths through them, if such regularities exist. Furthermore, their performance is better in mazes with path regularities than in irregular mazes. Finally, honeybees can negotiate novel mazes by using the rules that have proven to be successful in the past.

Context-Dependent Learning

Gadagkar et al. (1995) examined whether honeybees could learn to associate environmental cues with rewards in a context-dependent manner. In these experiments, they set up two different contexts, one at the hive and one at a feeder 12 m away. At both locations bees were offered a choice of two colors: blue and green. At the feeder,

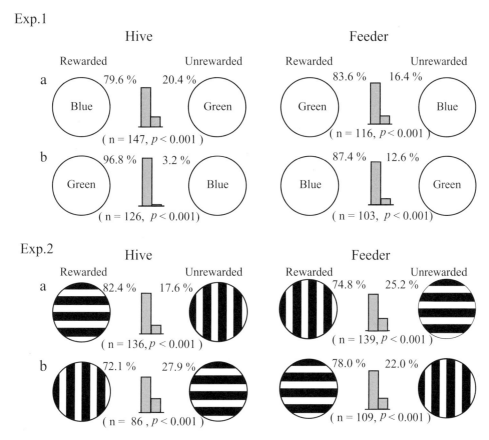

Figure 2.15
Context-dependent learning by honeybees.

green gave them access; at the hive, blue was the correct choice. The bees learned this task very well (figure 2.15, experiment 1a; for the complementary experiment, see figure 2.15, experiment 1b). Similar results were obtained using stimuli that consisted of gratings that were oriented vertically or horizontally (figure 2.15, exp. 2a and b). Not only could bees learn these context-dependent tasks, but they were able to reverse their preference in the 2 s that it took to fly from the feeder to the hive.

Colborn et al. (1999) also examined context-dependent learning, but in bumble-bees. The question was whether contextual cues can prevent interference during the acquisition of potentially competing visuomotor associations. Their findings are consistent with the hypothesis that different contextual signals are associated with either approaching the nest or approaching the feeder, and that these contextual signals facilitate learned associations between orientation detectors and motor commands.

Learning the Principles of "Symbolic Matching"

One of the more complex tasks that has been used to investigate the principles of learning and memory has been the delayed match-to-sample task (DMTS). This task has been investigated in a number of vertebrate species, such as monkeys (e.g., D'Amato et al., 1985), dolphins (e.g., Herman and Gordon, 1974), and pigeons (e.g., Roberts, 1972).

Most DMTS tasks follow the same general procedure. Each trial begins with the presentation of a sample stimulus. The sample is followed by a delay or retention interval and then by the presentation of two or more test stimuli, one of which is identical to the sample stimulus. If the animal chooses the test stimulus that corresponds to the sample, it obtains a reward. Hence the name delayed match-to-sample. Most experiments use two or three sample stimuli that are varied randomly from trial to trial.

A more complex variant is called a symbolic delayed match-to-sample task (SDMTS). Here, none of the test stimuli match the sample physically. The experimenter arbitrarily designates the correct choice. So the animal has to learn to associate each sample stimulus with the arbitrarily correct test stimulus. We wanted to know if bees could learn such tasks.

Honeybees have evolved a number of navigational skills that enable successful foraging. Collett and Wehner suggested that foraging insects travelling repeatedly to a food source and back to their homes navigate by using a series of visual images, or "snapshots," of the environment acquired en route (Collett and Kelber, 1988; Collett et al., 1993; Collett, 1996; Judd and Collett, 1998; Wehner et al., 1990, 1996). By comparing the currently viewed scene with the appropriate stored image, the insect is able to ascertain whether it is on the correct path and make any necessary corrections. Hence, successful foraging may require the bee to be able to solve tasks analogous to SDMTS tasks.

Learning Symbolic Delayed Match-to-Sample Tasks with Visual Stimuli
Zhang et al. (1999) trained honeybees to fly through a compound Y-maze consisting of a series of interconnected cylinders (figure 2.16a). The first cylinder carried the sample stimulus. The second and third cylinders each had two exits. Each exit was marked with a visual stimulus and the bees had to choose between them. If a bee made a correct choice in the second as well as in the third cylinder, it arrived in a fourth cylinder where it found a feeder with sugar solution. Hence, the second and the third cylinders acted as decision stages. In each of these cylinders the bee had to choose between two stimuli, and the initial, single sample stimulus (seen in the first cylinder) determined the choice that had to made in the two decision stages.

During training, the sample stimulus was a black-and-white grating oriented either horizontally (stimulus A) or vertically (stimulus A'). The second cylinder (first decision stage) offered a choice between a blue square (stimulus B) and a green one (stimulus B'), and the third cylinder a choice between a pattern consisting of a

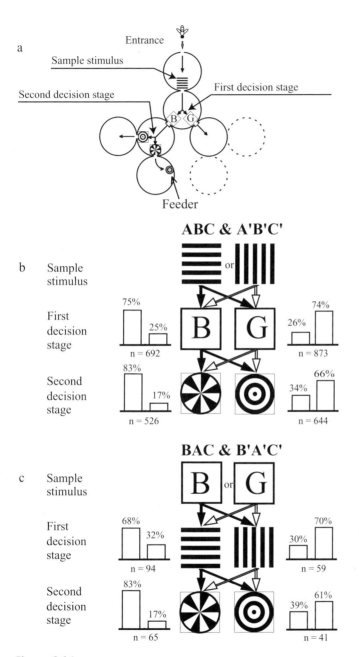

Figure 2.16
Learning a symbolic delayed match-to-sample task using vision. (Adapted from Zhang et al., 1999.)

sectored disk (C) or concentric rings (C') (figure 2.16b). When the sample stimulus was the horizontal grating, the feeder could only be reached if the bee chose blue in the second cylinder and the sectored disk in the third. However, when the sample was the vertical grating, the bee could reach the reward only if it chose green in the second cylinder and the ring pattern in the third.

After training, the bees were tested not only on the training sequences ABC and A'B'C' (learning tests) (figure 2.16b), but also in transfer tests that presented five other permutations of the training sequences. The results of tests on one of the permuted sequences (BAC and B'A'C') are illustrated in figure 2.16c.

The bees were indeed capable of learning SDMTS tasks. This suggests that when the bees viewed the sample stimulus, it triggered recall of the stimulus that should be chosen in the subsequent choice points (figure 2.16b). In general terms, exposure to any one of the stimuli that were encountered in training (A,B,C, A',B',C') was sufficient to trigger associative recall of all of the other stimuli belonging to that set. In all of the tests, changing the sample stimulus (from A to A', B to B', or C to C') caused the bees to change (and reverse) their stimulus choice at subsequent stages of the maze.

It should be noted that in this experiment, the bees were not specifically trained to distinguish between the sample stimuli A and A'. Nevertheless, they distinguished between them in the transfer tests. It is also clear from these experiments that the bees were capable of treating the stimulus pairs (i.e., B, B' and C, C') as sample stimuli, even though these were never encountered as sample stimuli in the training.

These findings suggest that bees solve the SDMTS task by mapping the six visual stimuli encountered during training into two distinct sets—A, B, C and A', B', C'—as illustrated in figure 2.17. After training, exposure to any stimulus belonging to a member of one of these sets triggers recall of the other two members.

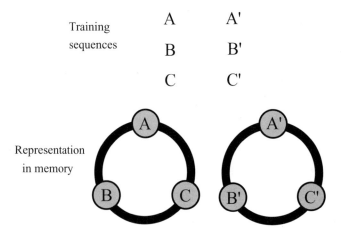

Figure 2.17
A model for associative grouping derived from the results of the symbolic delayed match-to-sample experiments.

Learning the Symbolic Delayed Match-to-Sample Task across Sensory Modalities

Can bees learn an SDMTS task when they are required to make associations that span different sensory modalities? Clearly, humans display impressive cross-modal associative recall. It is a common experience that an odor or sound can trigger a vivid recollection of a past event, with all of its rich, multimodal sensory qualities (Baddeley, 1993).

Srinivasan et al. (1998) explored this issue by asking whether bees could learn to associate specific scents with specific colors. The experimental setup consisted of a compound Y-maze with a single decision stage (figure 2.18a). The sample stimulus, presented in the first cylinder, was either a lemon or mango scent. The decision stage offered a choice of two colors, blue or yellow. When the bees encountered a lemon scent at the entrance, they had to learn to choose blue in the decision stage; when they encountered a mango scent, they had to choose yellow. The bees learned this task (figure 2.18b, experiment 1) and its converse (figure 2.18b, experiment 2) very well. They could also learn to associate a color at the entrance with a scent at the decision stage (figure 2.18c,d, experiments 1 and 2).

Learning an SDMTS task across sensory modalities requires that the bee be able to recall stimuli of a modality different from that of the triggering stimulus. For a foraging honeybee, cross-modal associative recall can facilitate the search for a food source. For example, detecting the scent of lavender could initiate a search for purple flowers.

Learning the Concepts "Sameness" and "Difference"

In vertebrates, the capacity to learn the concepts of sameness and difference has been studied using two experimental procedures, the delayed match-to-sample task, and the delayed nonmatch-to-sample task (DNMTS) (e.g., Holmes, 1979; Zentall and Hogan, 1978). The DNMTS task is similar to the match-to-sample task except that the animal is required to respond to the stimulus that is different from the sample. It should be pointed out, however, that the ability to learn the concept of sameness or difference is demonstrated only if the animal can transfer the learning to a novel set of stimuli. Otherwise the task demonstrates only the simple association of two stimuli.

Giurfa et al. (2001) trained bees to choose a sectored or ring pattern in the decision chamber of a Y-maze, depending on whether the sample stimulus seen at the maze entrance was a sectored or a ring pattern (figure 2.19a and 2.19c, left-hand panel). The trained bees were then given a transfer test in which the stimuli were simply blue and yellow rather than black-and-white patterns. The bees immediately transferred their ability to use the matching rule to the new task (figure 2.19c, right-hand panel). They were also able to transfer the matching rule to other novel stimuli, such as gratings oriented at plus or minus 45 deg.

Bees can also be trained to match odors (figure 2.20a and 2.20c, left panel), and then transfer the matching rule to colors (figure 2.20b and 2.20c, right panel). Hence the concept of sameness, once learned, is easily transferred across sensory modalities.

Finally, bees can also learn the concept of difference. That is, they can be trained to choose the nonmatching stimulus, rather than the matching one. Figure 2.21a

a Training and test odor to color

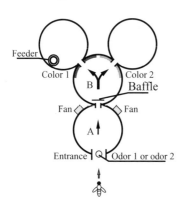

b Scent-to-color association

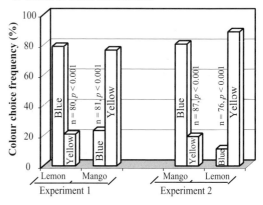

c Training and test color to odor

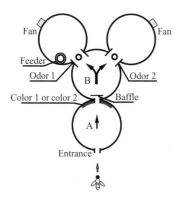

d Color-to-scent association

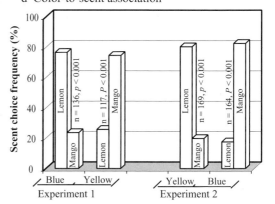

Figure 2.18
Learning a symbolic delayed match-to-sample task across the sensory modalities. (Adapted from Srinivasan et al., 1998.)

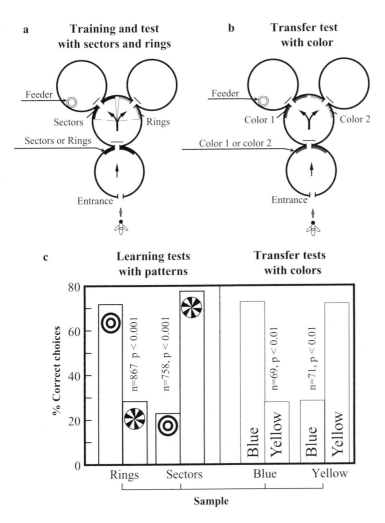

Figure 2.19
Learning the concept of "sameness" in the visual modality. (Adapted from Giurfa et al., 2001.)

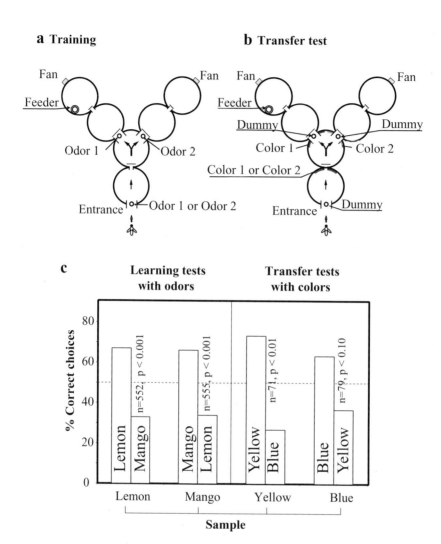

Figure 2.20
Learning the concept of "sameness" across sensory modalities. (Adapted from Giurfa et al., 2001.)

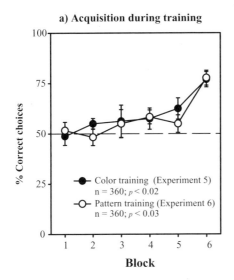

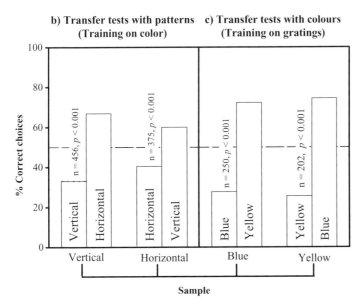

Figure 2.21
Learning the concept of "difference." (Adapted from Giurfa et al., 2001.)

shows learning curves obtained in two experiments investigating this capability. In one experiment, the training stimuli were colors (blue and yellow). Here, bees had to learn to choose yellow in the decision chamber when they encountered blue at the entrance and vice versa. In another experiment, the training stimuli were horizontally and vertically oriented linear gratings. In this case, the bees had to learn to choose the vertical grating in the decision chamber when they encountered a horizontal grating at the entrance, and vice versa. Once bees learned these tasks, they were immediately able to transfer the nonmatching rule to novel stimuli (figure 2.21b,c).

Biological Relevance of Cognitive Processes in Honeybees

Why is it that honeybees can perform some of the same complex cognitive tasks that mammals, including humans, can perform? In other words, why are honeybees so smart? In this section we would like to discuss the biological relevance of, and the possible evolutionary reasons why honeybees possess such cognitive capacities.

It is well known that the honeybee is a social insect that can survive only as a member of a colony. In order to maintain their nest and care for their brood, worker bees regularly leave and return to their nest site to feed, to protect and nurse the larvae, to store food, and to hide from adverse environmental conditions. Since they forage for flower nectar and pollen at unpredictable sites, they have to learn the celestial and terrestrial cues that can guide their foraging trips and return flights over long distances (Seeley, 1985; K. von Frisch, 1967).

Through the course of evolution, honeybees have developed a variety of sensory systems for foraging. Although they rely heavily on their visual system for navigation and object recognition, they have also evolved a well-developed olfactory system and auditory, magnetic, tactile, and gustatory systems.

Honeybees have also evolved the ability to learn. They learn to relate the sun's position and the sky's pattern of polarized light to the time of day within the framework of the time-compensated sun compass (Lindauer, 1959), as well as landmarks associated with their nest site. Hence, their success at foraging is a product of the evolution of cognitive capacities that allow them to exploit their sensory systems to the maximum.

The honeybee brain is tiny, about one millionth of the weight of a human brain. But, like the brains of humans and other mammals, it has evolved into an organ with specialized functional and morphological divisions. A large part of the research on the honeybee brain has focused on the visual and olfactory pathways, and on the so-called mushroom bodies in the protocerebrum, which are believed to be the structures of the insect brain most closely associated with higher-order sensory integration, learning, and memory (Withers et al., 1993). About half of the total neurons within the bee's brain belong to the optic lobes, which are made up of three distinct neuropilar masses: the lamina, medulla, and lobula. In addition, the antennal lobes receive their principal sensory input from olfactory receptors on the antennae (Winston, 1991;

Hertel and Maronde, 1987). Output neurons in the antennal lobe project to the mushroom bodies, which also receive visual input (Menzel and Muller, 1996).

Visual information is acquired through a pair of compound eyes that take up a substantial part of the bee's head and are capable of a wide range of photoreceptive functions. Their color vision is mediated by UV, blue, and green photoreceptors whose spectral sensitivities are well suited to flower discrimination (Chittka et al., 1993; Vorobyev and Menzel, 1999). The evolution of shape perception allows bees to respond innately to some features of natural flowers, resulting in a spontaneous preference for flowerlike patterns (Wehner, 1981; Lehrer, 1995), and the ability to abstract key features of flowers and to memorize them efficiently is critical to successful foraging. Srinivasan et al. (1993, 1994) have suggested that the existence of feature-extracting mechanisms in the insect visual system might be comparable, functionally, to those known to exist in the mammalian cortex.

Associative learning is an essential component of the bee's central-place foraging behavior and dance communication (Hammer and Menzel, 1995). To forage successfully, a worker bee has to remember not only the color and shape of nutrient-rich flowers, but also how to locate them. A foraging bee is able to ascertain whether it is on the correct path and make any necessary corrections by comparing the currently viewed scene with the appropriate stored image. If a bee happens to forage at more than one site, then it needs not only to memorize a separate set of images for each route that it has learned, but also to retrieve the set of images that is appropriate to each route. Associative grouping and recall of visual stimuli provide an effective means of retrieving the appropriate navigational information from memory.

Antennal chemoreceptors give the honeybee an excellent sense of smell. The combination of visual and olfactory attractants allows the bee to find food sources accurately and efficiently.

Like mammals, including humans, honeybees accumulate experience and remember what they learn, especially after they start their orientation flights and become foragers. Withers et al. (1993) found that age-based division of labor in adult worker honeybees (*Apis mellifera*) is associated with substantial changes in certain brain regions, notably the mushroom bodies. Moreover, these striking structural changes are dependent, not on the bee's age, but on its foraging experience. This demonstrates a robust anatomical plasticity associated with the complex behavior of the adult insects.

Although the mushroom bodies of honeybees and the hippocampi of birds and mammals are very different anatomically, they appear to subserve similar cognitive functions. There is considerable evidence that one function of the avian and mammalian hippocampus is to create and maintain a mental map of space. For instance, food-storing passerine birds that are able to remember a large number of cache locations have a much larger hippocampus than do nonstoring passerines of comparable brain size. Even within families of food-storing birds, the size of the hippocampus is correlated with reliance on stored food (Sherry, 1998).

As social insects, bees are able to communicate with each other, particularly to inform nest mates about available resources outside the nest (K. von Frisch, 1967). The navigation and communication of honeybees requires them to have sophisticated cognitive processes; for example, the use of a time-compensated sun compass. As the sun moves in the sky during the day, bees are able to take this movement into account and adjust their flight directions. Likewise, when bees are ready to start a new hive, workers search for nest sites and communicate the direction, distance, and quality of the site to their nest mates through modifications of the so-called waggle dance, which are based on environmental cues indicating the sites location (Lindauer, 1955). Hence, some consider the bee's dance communication system a semantic system that symbolically encodes various features of distant sites.

In summary, research over the past 30 years or so is beginning to suggest that learning and perception in insects is more intricate and flexible than was originally imagined. Honeybees are capable of a variety of visually guided tasks that involve cognitive processes that operate at a surprisingly high level. Bees can abstract general features of a stimulus, such as orientation or symmetry, and apply them to distinguish between novel stimuli. They can be taught to use new cues to detect camouflaged objects. They can learn to use symbolic rules for navigating through complex mazes and to apply these rules in flexible ways. Honeybees are able to form "concepts", and to group and recall stimuli associatively.

While the processes of learning and perception are undoubtedly more sophisticated in primates and some other mammals than in insects, there seems to be a continuum in these capacities across the animal kingdom, rather than a sharp distinction between vertebrates and invertebrates. The abilities of an animal seem to be governed largely by what it needs in order to pursue its lifestyle, rather than whether it possesses a backbone.

3 In the Mind of a Hunter: The Visual World of the Praying Mantis

Karl Kral and Frederick R. Prete

The praying mantids are an intriguing group of predatory insects. Their striking morphology, unusually mobile head, large compound eyes, piercing gaze, and the remarkably fast strike of their spined, raptorial forelegs have captured people's attention and imagination for millennia (Prete and Wolf, 1992).

Consistent with the scientific mindset of the time, early experimental reports depicted mantid behavior as simplistic, mechanistic, and stereotyped. However, more recent organism- (rather than theoretically) centered studies have revealed that mantids, like many other insects, are actually remarkably complex animals that respond to their environment with a variety of quite plastic behaviors, all of which are underpinned by equally complex information-processing capabilities. However, mantids are remarkable not only for what they do, they are also remarkable for who they are. That is, the mantids are most closely related to insects that are (at least on the surface) much less remarkable (but see chapter 10 in this volume). Thus they capture our attention, as does the human genius born of humbler parents. We look at them and wonder how they manage to construct and maneuver through a perceptual world seemingly unimaginable in even their closest relatives.

In this chapter we explore some of the anatomical, neurophysiological, and information-processing mechanisms by which mantids make sense of, and respond to, their complex visual world. In particular, we are interested in the ways that mantids parse their visual world, how they recognize objects in that world, and how they construct and understand the three-dimensionality of the world in which they live.

Phylogeny

Kristensen (1991) grouped ten extant insect orders to form the "basic Neoptera" or Polyneoptera, fossil members of which appear as early as the upper Carboniferous period (about 300 million years ago; Sharov, 1968; Gorochov, 1995). The Polyneoptera include the monophyletic group, Dictyoptera. The Dictyoptera include the Mantodea (mantids), Blattodea (cockroaches), and Isoptera (termites) (Eggleton, 2001). Amazingly, the Blattodea and Mantodea apparently diverged from a primitive cockroach-like Paleozoic ancestor. The fossil of what may be an early mantid dates from the Lower Permian (about 270 million years ago) (J. Kukalova-Peck, personal communication), and fossil mantids date from the Upper Cretaceous period (about 70 million years ago), and Paleocene (60 million years ago) and Oligocene epochs (30 million years ago) (Nel and Roy, 1996). So the mantids were probably well established around 60 million years ago, during the Tertiary period.

Understandably, the mantids and cockroaches display many fundamental anatomical and organizational similarities to members of the orthopteroid, proper (grasshoppers, crickets, and katydids), to which they are more distantly related. To avoid confusion, and the misperceptions created by the casual use of "orthopteroid" as an umbrella category, we will refer to the broader group (Dictyoptera plus orthopteroid, proper) as orthopteroidea (Gonka et al., 1999).

Family Characteristics

Based on morphology, the mantids have been divided into eight families. The Metallyticidae include one genus, *Metallyticus*. These are blue or green metallic-colored insects restricted to the Malayan region. The Chaeteessidae, too, contain only one genus, *Chaeteessa*. They do not have the strong hook-shaped spine on the end of their foreleg tibia as do other mantids, and their other foreleg spines are thin and delicate. Again, there is just one genus, *Mantoida*, in the family Mantoididae. These neotropical insects are the smallest mantids, similar in appearance to *Chaeteessa* except that their forelegs look like those of most other mantids.

The Amorphoscelidae are small mantids that range from the Mediterranean countries and Asia to Africa and Australia. This group is characterized by lateral tubercles (tiny, cone-shaped extensions) behind the eyes and a short pronotum. Their forelegs have a unique arrangement of foreleg spines.

The Eremiaphilidae are stout, ground-dwelling mantids that live in the desert and semidesert regions of northern Africa and Asia. They have a globe-shaped head, slightly protruding eyes, small antennae, a short trapezoidal pronotum with a bumpy surface, strong predatory forelegs armed with short spines, and meso- and metathoracic legs that are long and thin, which make them fast runners. Their wings are always reduced and nonfunctional.

The Empusidae are slender, unusual-looking mantids that are found in southern Europe, Africa, Madagascar, and western Asia up to China. They are distinguished by a number of characteristics, including comblike projections on both sides of the male's antennae, an elongated vertex (i.e., a point on top of their head), and frequently, lobes on the meso- and metathoracic legs. The Hymenopodidae are found in all tropical countries except Australia. The group includes the spectacular flower mimics such as the orchid mantid, *Pseudocreobotra ocellata*.

The remaining roughly 361 genera, including 80% of the species, are grouped in the family Mantidae. This is a very diverse group, including both the more common-looking mantids and most of the grass and bark mimics. They are a grossly paraphyletic assemblage, and a taxonomic reorganization based on a formal phylogenetic analysis is needed (G. Svenson, personal communication). Virtually all research on mantids has been done on members of this group (figure 3.1). Hence, any reference to "mantid" characteristics should be considered a convenient shorthand. There are little comparative behavioral or physiological data, and we do not as yet know the extent to which any data are generalizable across species or families.

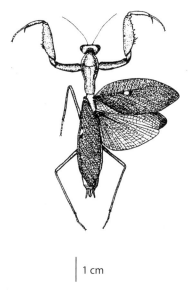

1 cm

Figure 3.1
Sphodromantis lineola. A relatively common southern European and African species on which a considerable amount of psychophysical data has been collected. (Drawing by Phil Bragg for Prete et al., 1999. Reproduced with the kind permission of Johns Hopkins University Press and Phil Bragg.)

Most recently, Svenson and Whiting (2004) completed the first formal phylogenetic analysis of mantid relationships using molecular data. Parsimony analysis of DNA sequence data of five genes (16S + 18S + 28S ribosomal DNA + cytochrome oxidase II + histone 3) using optimization alignment (POY-random additions = 600, tree length = 8913) resulted in a single most parsimonious tree (figure 3.2). Mantid relationships inferred from this analysis are well supported by nonparametric bootstrap and Bremer calculations.

The analysis supports *Mantoida schraderi* as the most basal mantid, sister to the rest of the Mantodea. The Mantidae, Hymenopodidae, Thespidae, and Iridopterygidae are all paraphyletic groups. The family Amorphoscelidae is nested within Iridopterygidae, suggesting that a short thorax is not a reliable character in identifying basal lineages (G. Svenson, personal communication). Rather, amorphoscelids are only derived members of the Iridopterygidae.

The Compound Eye

All praying mantids have two large, laterally protruding, forward-directed compound eyes, each consisting of some 9,000 individual sampling units or ommatidia. As is typical for insects, each ommatidium contains eight photoreceptor cells.

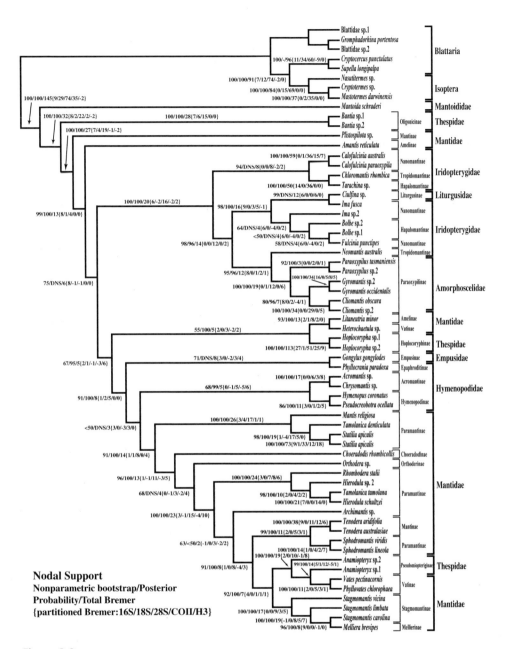

Figure 3.2

Phylogeny of Mantodea. Total evidence molecular tree based on five genes, 16S rDNA + 18S rDNA + 28S rDNA + cytochrome oxidase II + histone 3. Optimization alignment produces a single most parsimonious tree using equal character weighting (length = 8913). Nonparametric bootstrap and Bremer values were calculated in Phylogenetic Analysis Using Parsimony (PAUP) from the implied alignment (via POY) and given for each node (bootstrap/posterior probabilities/Bremer). (Adapted from Svenson and Whiting, 2004 with the authors' kind permission.)

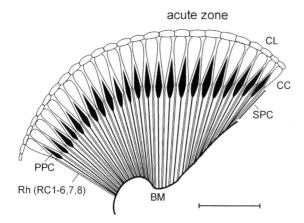

Figure 3.3
Schematic of a horizontal section through the equatorial region of the compound eye of *Tenodera sinensis*. Adjacent ommatidia are optically isolated from each other by primary pigment cells (PPC) and secondary pigment cells (SPC). Note that the forward-directed acute zone has larger lenses, longer ommatidia, and smaller interommatidial angles than elsewhere in the eye. BM, basement membrane; CC, crystalline cone; CL, corneal lens; Rh, rhabdom of receptor cells (RC). Scale bar = 200 μm. (Drawing by K. Kral.)

The compound eyes are the apposition type, in which the ommatidia are shielded optically from one another by pigment. Within ommatidia, there is a direct connection between the corneal lens and the crystalline cone (the dioptric apparatus) and the central, fused rhabdom, which is formed by the light-sensitive microvillar extensions (the rhabdomeres) of the ommatidial photoreceptors (figure 3.3). In this type of eye, the distal tip of the rhabdom lies in the focal plane of the corneal lens (Horridge, 1978, 1980; for review, see Nilsson, 1989).

The compound eyes allow the mantid to see in nearly every direction. Its visual field has a vertical extension of 245 deg and a horizontal extension of more than 230 deg. This includes a large, forward-looking binocular area, with a vertical extension of more than 240 deg and a maximum horizontal extension of 70 deg (Rossel, 1979).

The compound eyes function in a range of light intensities spanning more than four log units. In comparison, the human visual system can operate over a range of approximately thirteen log units. The amplitude of the on-transient component of the mantid's electroretinogram (ERG) varies with the log of light intensity (Walcher, 1994; Walcher and Kral, 1994), indicating that a large range of light intensities are compressed into a manageable scale. This enables the eye to respond over a tremendous dynamic range, from starlight to sunlight. It also permits the mantid to distinguish between different objects via differences in contrast.

Spatial Resolution

Spatial resolution refers to the ability to perceive neighboring points in space as separate from one another. The smaller the distance between points (i.e., the higher the spatial frequency) that can be discriminated, the higher the spatial resolution. This can be estimated anatomically by the ommatidial characteristics.

Each ommatidium or, more specifically, each rhabdom, acts as a collecting point, as it were, for incident light. This means that no further spatial resolution is possible within an ommatidium and the spatial angle viewed by an ommatidium is the limiting factor for spatial resolution. Consequently, spatial resolution is limited by ommatidial spacing, expressed in terms of the interommatidial angle, or the angle between the optical axes of neighboring ommatidia. The highest resolvable spatial frequency is determined by the smallest interommatidial angle. The smaller the interommatidial angle, the higher is the potential resolution of the eye, or what is sometimes referred to as the anatomical resolution.

In the frontal, binocular region of the mantid's eye, interommatidial angles are as small as 0.6 deg. More laterally, dorsally, and ventrally, they increase to 2.0–2.5 deg (Rossel, 1979).

Spatial Resolution versus Contrast Sensitivity

The mantid's interommatidial angles lie at the lower limit at which the eye can still function optimally. Although a decrease in facet (ommatidial lens) diameter improves resolution, it also reduces the photon capture rate per ommatidium. This reduces the eye's ability to resolve contrast and degrades image quality.

Mantids resolve this dilemma by compromising between spatial resolution and contrast sensitivity (Horridge and Duelli, 1979). The distribution of interommatidial angles in the eye is such that the smallest are in the so-called "acute zone," the forward- and slightly downward-facing region in which spatial resolution is relatively high and image quality is maximized by smaller rhabdom diameters and larger facet diameters compared with the rest of the eye (Rossel, 1979). In addition, the ommatidia are significantly longer there and have longer crystalline cones and rhabdoms, resulting in a distinctly greater radius of curvature and a corresponding flattening of the surface curvature compared with the rest of the eye (Horridge, 1980).

The eye's light sensitivity, calculated as the product of facet diameter and interommatidial angle, is higher outside of the acute zone (i.e., sensitivity is lowest in the acute zone). Hence the acute zone functions only at light intensities greater than those at which the rest of the eye can be active. In analogy to the human eye, the acute zone is photopic and the rest of the eye is scotopic.

The ommatidial aperture also affects both spatial resolution and contrast sensitivity, and it is not fixed; it fluctuates with lighting conditions, creating what is termed a physiological acceptance angle. Strictly speaking, the physiological acceptance angle is determined by the combination of the physiological acceptance angles of the lens and rhabdom. The physiological acceptance angle of the lens corresponds to the halfwidth of the intensity distribution arising from diffraction occurring at the lens of an ommatidium.

The physiological acceptance angle of the rhabdom corresponds to the halfwidth of the rhabdom acceptance function and is expressed as the projection of the rhabdom diameter into space. The total physiological acceptance angle of an ommatidium reaches its maximum in darkness and diminishes with increasing brightness. In dim light it is medium sized, and in dazzling sunlight it is at its smallest. This adaptation to light intensity is brought about by a displacement of pigment at the dioptric apparatus, by a displacement of pigment between the ommatidia, and possibly, also by a change in the rhabdom diameter and the index of refraction between the rhabdom and the surrounding cytoplasm.

In the light-adapted state, the physiological acceptance angle is of the same order of magnitude as the interommatidial angle, and there is a constant relationship between the two angles over the entire eye. The angular values measured in the daytime under light-adapted conditions range from 0.7 deg in the acute zone up to 2.5 deg at the periphery (Rossel, 1979). A smaller physiological acceptance angle in the acute zone would not be possible, owing to diffraction (see earlier discussion). In the rest of the eye, the acceptance functions of the rhabdoms constitute the limiting factor for the physiological acceptance angle (Rossel, 1979).

Of course the theoretical spatial resolution of the mantid compound eye gives no indication of whether mantids are in fact capable of spatial perception. It only demonstrates that the eyes provide optimal preconditions for this. Theoretically, the two eyes could capture about 18,000 individual pixels from the visual surroundings. In the frontal binocular visual field, the angle between pixels would be considerably less than 1 deg, while in the rest of the visual field, the angles would reach a value of about 2 deg. Such a high spatial resolution in the frontal region of the eye (although a hundred times lower than in the human fovea) is, however, only possible in the high light intensities provided by bright daylight.

The degree to which the theoretical limits of the compound eye's spatial resolution is maintained at the neuronal level is a function of the connections between the photoreceptors and the neurons in the first optic ganglion, the lamina. These connections will in turn limit the type of information processing that can take place in more central optic ganglia.

Temporal Resolution

As a rule, a direct relationship exists between spatial resolution and temporal resolution (see Srinivasan and Bernard, 1975). The high spatial resolution of the acute zone suggests a high temporal resolution and a consequent facility for motion detection.

A simple technique for studying temporal resolution is via electroretinograms recorded in flickering light. In *Tenodera aridifolia sinensis*, the maximum flicker fusion frequency (the maximum resolvable flicker rate) is 50 Hz. At 52 Hz, the ERG response misses cycles and lags behind the light stimulus (K. Kral, unpublished results). This indicates a medium-fast, but not a fast eye; the latter have flicker fusion frequencies of 200 Hz or more (Autrum, 1950; Autrum and Stöcker, 1952). It should be noted that these ERG recordings were made using a dark-adapted eye, which may have lower spatial resolution but greater sensitivity than a light-adapted eye. Furthermore, ERG responses of the acute zone could not be isolated from ERG responses of the rest of the eye, even when a different electrode was placed on the acute zone. Thus, the temporal resolution of the acute zone has yet to be determined, but could be expected to be higher than that of the rest of the eye. Nonetheless, very fast temporal responses are metabolically demanding, and a higher response rate is probably not necessary for this relatively slow-moving and, in some cases, slow-flying insect.

Motion Sensitivity

The minimum discernable time during which an object passes through the receptive field of an ommatidium is an important parameter with respect to the mantid's motion sensitivity. This time period can be defined as the integration time. It is the halfwidth of the impulse response function and is directly dependent on the physiological acceptance angle of the ommatidium. No exact measurements exist for the mantid eye; however, when the critical flicker fusion frequency is taken into account, it appears that conditions are similar to those in the apposition eyes of locusts. In locusts, in daylight, the physiological acceptance angle is 2 deg and the integration time is 19 ms; at night, after dark, these values increase to 4 deg and 54 ms, respectively (D. S. Williams, 1983; Howard, 1981). This suggests that the photoreceptor cells are faster during the daytime than at night. In daylight, the photoreceptor cells in the acute zone should be distinctly faster (with integration times less than 10 ms) than those in the rest of the eye. This organization parallels that of vertebrates, in which cones reside primarily in the fovea and rods reside in the extrafoveal and peripheral regions of the eye.

Information Transfer through the Optic Lobe

Visual Processing in the Lamina

Monopolar Cells and Intrinsic Cells   In *T. sinensis*, axons of each set of the six largest photoreceptors (R1 to R6) project directly to three large monopolar cells (LMCs), where together they form a cartridge. Hence, the 9,000 ommatidia are represented in the lamina by 9,000 cartridges, which means that the lamina is organized in a strictly retinotopic manner. Likewise, the axons of the LMCs project to the medulla retinotopically. In contrast, the axons of the two smallest photoreceptors (R7 and R8), which are probably ultraviolet sensitive, project through the lamina cartridge directly to the outer neuropil of the second optic ganglion, the medulla. In addition to these direct centripetal visual pathways, amacrine and tangential cells establish connections among the individual cartridges in the lamina. There may also be feedback neurons between lamina neurons and photoreceptor cell axons. In addition, centrifugal fibers project from the medulla and enter the cartridges via the external chiasma (figure 3.4) (Leitinger, 1994, 1997; Leitinger et al., 1999).

The retinotopic organization of the cartridges is clearly visible in horizontal, ultra-thin sections through the lamina. In the cartridges, axons of the photoreceptor cells

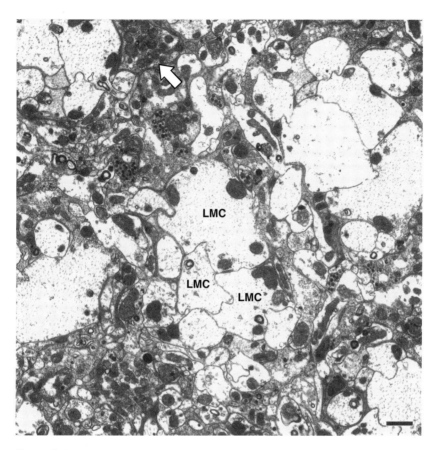

Figure 3.4
Electron micrograph of a cross-section through several lamina cartridges in an adult *Tenodera sinensis*. Each cartridge consists of at least three large (electron-lucent) monopolar cells (LMC). The LMC axons are surrounded by receptor cell axons (e.g., as indicated by the white arrow). The electron-lucent profiles located more peripherally may belong to the other monopolar cells and join profiles of intrinsic cells and centrifugal fibers. Scale bar: 1.3 μm. (From Leitinger, 1997, with the author's kind permission.)

are found at the cartridge periphery and the axons of the three LMCs are located in the center. The cartridge also contains axons that presumably belong to the two or three small monopolar cells (Leitinger, 1994, 1997; Leitinger et al., 1999). Individual cartridges are clearly delimited, as is typical in apposition eyes, which suggests that information from individual ommatidia is transmitted separately (for a review, see Kral, 1987). However, this demarcation does not seem to be present at all levels of the neuropil; some of the dendrites of the monopolar cells leave their own cartridge and presumably establish connections with neighboring cartridges (figure 3.4) (Leitinger, 1994, 1997).

What is particularly interesting is the question of how the acute zone is represented in the lamina. Specific comparisons between the lamina structure in the region that may represent the acute zone and other laminar regions have yet to be made. However, no conspicuous laminar subdivisions have been observed in *T. sinensis* (Leitinger, 1994, 1997). It may be that in the lamina, the optical information of the acute zone is treated in the same way as that of the rest of the eye. A differentiation of the neural structures corresponding to the acute zone would then be expected only at more central levels, in the medulla and/or in the lobula complex. Of course, a uniform handling of incoming information at the level of the lamina would not result in any reduction in the relatively greater spatial resolution provided by the more densely sampled acute zone; the acute zone would remain relatively more highly represented informationally.

Signal Amplification Provides Information about Illumination   As in other insects (e.g., Laughlin et al., 1987), a principal function of the mantid lamina may be signal amplification to enhance information about variations in illumination, even though this may occur at the expense of information about average brightness.

In other orthopteroidean species, the LMCs exhibit a greater response to changes in light intensity than do photoreceptors R1–R6. The synapses between R1–R6 and the LMCs are inhibitory, and the signals are inverted (depolarizations in the photoreceptors are transformed into hyperpolarizations in the LMCs). Typically, an LMC hyperpolarization is both filtered and amplified. It becomes much more phasic, and its amplitude is larger than that of the photoreceptor response (see Laughlin, 1981, 1989).

Specifically, the photoreceptor responds to a light stimulus with an initial peak depolarizing potential, followed by a sustained, smaller depolarization that lasts until the end of the stimulus. In contrast, an LMC responds to an "on"-stimulus with a large, transient hyperpolarization and responds at the end of the stimulus with a transient depolarization. During the stimulus there is almost no response, and the potential of the membrane is close to its dark resting potential. Thus the LMC always responds to changes in light intensity from the same level of membrane potential, i.e., from a potential that is close to the resting potential. This means that in the lamina, there is a loss of information about mean levels of illumination, but a considerable increase in information about changes in illumination or, in other words, responses to background illumination are filtered out, while responses to small changes in light intensity are amplified. This is, of course, analogous to the response characteristics of vertebrate retinal ganglion cells.

These response characteristics are reflected in the fact that the LMCs exhibit steeper intensity-response curves than do photoreceptors. The steeper the curves, the greater the sensitivity to small changes in light intensity. This sensitivity is associated to a certain extent with a reduction in the range of light intensities under which the visual system can function. However, it would seem that the working range of the LMCs in the praying mantis is sufficient to handle the changes in light intensity with which the insect is usually confronted.

Intensification of Contrast and Spatial Resolution   Another important function of the mantid lamina, indicated by the lateral interconnections between the LMCs of neighboring cartridges (and electrophysiological data from other orthopteroideans) is contrast intensification by lateral inhibition. This sharpens the receptive field contrast of the ommatidia and in turn allows an LMC to respond to small stimuli centered in its receptive field, but diminishes or prevents responses to stimuli a few degrees off center and/or stimuli that affect the receptive fields of several LMCs. Such signal transformations may serve to counteract the unavoidable signal degradation caused by synaptic noise at the next optic ganglia, the medulla.

Visual Processing in the Medulla

The axons of the three LMCs and of the two or three small monopolar cells project into the neuropil of the medulla. In doing so, they cross in the chiasma, connecting the posterior medulla with the anterior lamina (Leitinger, 1994, 1997; Leitinger et al., 1999). The axons terminate in corresponding columns, each of which seems to contain several classes of neuron. In other orthopteroideans (e.g., *Locusta migratoria*), ten different classes of neuron have been found in these columns (James and Osorio, 1996). In mantids, this ganglion is probably where the initial processing of movement information takes place.

Medulla Columnar Neurons   Very little is known about the electrophysiological properties of the medullary columnar neurons in mantids. However, in other orthopteroideans, these include small-field neurons with receptive fields the same size as those of photoreceptors R1–R6.

Medulla Large-Field Neurons   In *T. sinensis*, large neurons have been identified that form extensive arborizations in the medulla and the axons of which project to the ipsilateral or contralateral midbrain (Leitinger et al., 1999). Likewise, Berger (1985) identified three movement-sensitive medullary cells in *Mantis religiosa*, also with extensive arborizations. He labeled these M1, M2, and M3. Cell M1 responded preferentially to a moving dot and the vertical movement of a single stripe; M2 primarily to a stripe or dot irrespective of direction; and, M3 to a stripe or grating irrespective of direction. M1 projects only to the ipsilateral tritocerebrum. The other two cells project to the contralateral optic lobe (figure 3.5). We think that rapid processing of movement information by these large-field medullary cells plays a role in rapid

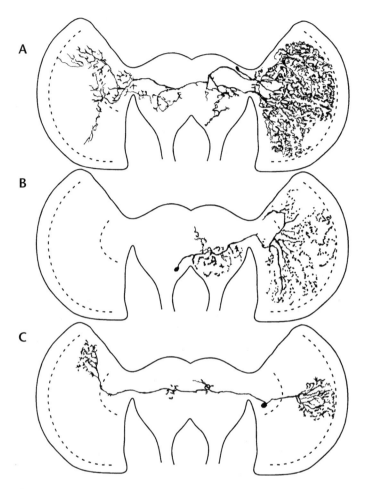

Figure 3.5
Sketches of three movement-sensitive medullary neurons in *Mantis religiosa* identified and named by Berger (1985). The outermost dashed line indicates the lateral border of the medulla. (*A*) Cell M-2 responds to the movement of spots, stripes, and gratings in the entire ipsilateral half of the visual field, with no direction preference. Its receptive field also extends slightly into the contralateral visual field center. Its punctate responses to a horizontally (but not vertically) moving grating indicate its high spatiotemporal sensitivity in this direction. (*B*) Cell M-1 has a high spontaneous firing rate on which is superimposed a preference for small-field (i.e., a dot) movement horizontally or dorsally, in or just below the visual field center (i.e., in the acute zone). It does not respond to large-field (i.e., grating) movement or a horizontally moving stripe. It does, however, respond sharply to a vertically moving stripe in the visual field center. (*C*) Cell M-3 is responsive to a moving stripe in the entire visual field, although it is most sensitive in the visual field center. It is also responsive to a moving grating, with no direction preference. (Redrawn from Berger, 1985, with the author's kind permission.)

orientation and avoidance behaviors which do not require detailed information about the eliciting stimulus, for instance, orienting to a small moving object or ducking when a looming object moves overhead. This would be analogous to the reflexive responses mediated by peripheral retina-to-midbrain pathways in vertebrates, including humans.

Local Processing of Contrast Information   The medullary columnar neurons receive amplified signals containing information on temporal and spatial variations in illumination from LMCs. However, the response properties of these neurons differ from the LMC's graded responses. In other orthopteroideans, medullary columnar neurons preferentially exhibit nongraded responses to either on-stimuli or off-stimuli. So-called P1–P4 cells respond to positive contrast steps, while the N cells (N1–N6) respond to negative contrast steps (James and Osorio, 1996). It is possible that these separate on and off afferent pathways project out of the medulla and are later combined, but these remain open questions for mantids.

Elementary Motion Detection   As a result of lateral connections, the medullary columnar neurons of orthopteroideans are motion sensitive (Osorio, 1986) and represent so-called "elementary motion detectors." Each elementary motion detector could be connected via the corresponding LMCs to the photoreceptor cells (R1–R6) of two neighboring ommatidia. In theory, in an elementary motion detector, the signal originating in one photoreceptor is delayed and is then combined with the signal from the second photoreceptor. By this means the detector correlates the signal from the first photoreceptor with a signal originating slightly later in the second photoreceptor (see Srinivasan et al., 1999). It is possible that a medullary column contains various types of elementary motion detectors, each adapted to detect a different movement direction or speed.

Spatial Integration   Another important function of the medulla may be the spatial integration of information resulting from elementary motion detection. Such integration would involve interconnections between the elementary motion detectors, possibly represented by motion-sensitive columnar neurons. These interconnections could even create preferential responses to particular spatial configurations in target neurons located in the medulla and/or lobula.

The medullary elementary motion detectors could also have connections with medullary large-field neurons, such as those identified in *T. sinensis* and *M. religiosa*. This is the case in the lepidopteran, *Papilio aegeus* (Ibbotson et al., 1991). Such spatial integration is essential to detection and interpretation of motion and motion direction.

Visual Processing in the Lobula
In the lobula complex, which in mantids consists of four distinct regions, some retinotopic organization is lost owing to convergence of afferents onto motion-sensitive

small- and large-field neurons (Leitinger, 1997; Leitinger et al., 1999). Presumably, small-field neurons receive inputs from a small number of medulla elementary motion detectors, and large-field neurons receive inputs from relatively more. The output processes of some lobula neurons are known to synapse onto descending interneurons that carry information to thoracic motor neurons (figure 3.6) (Berger, 1985).

Heide et al. (1982; also see Berger, 1985) identified a number of motion-sensitive lobula cells in *M. religiosa*. These neurons responded to horizontal and/or vertical movements with either increases or decreases in spike rate. For the most part, the centers of the regions of motion sensitivity were located near the median plane of the mantid. Specific responses to large-field stimuli were generally weak. Heide et al. found that of seventeen neurons, nine were monocular ipsilateral, two were monocular contralateral, and six were binocular.

Seeing the World through the Mantid's Eyes: How the World Is Represented on the Retinae

Local Image Motion

In general, a discontinuity in local motion (i.e., small-field movement) will result in the mantid's perception of a discrete object, which could be a moving leaf or another animal. For instance, for an *Empusa fasciata* waiting in ambush, an approaching bee would give rise to small-field movement, which would contrast clearly with any random movements in the background vegetation. If the characteristics of that local image motion meet certain criteria, it could signal prey. However, the mantid cannot rely on local image motion alone to distinguish between a small nearby object (prey, perhaps) and a large distant object (a potential predator); other characteristics of the image need to be assessed.

Figure 3.6 ▶

Sketches of four movement-sensitive lobula neurons in *Mantis religiosa* identified and named by Berger (1985). The innermost dashed line indicates the lateral border of the lobula. (*A*) L-1 is sharply responsive to small-field movement in any direction and the upward movement of a stripe in the acute zone. It has virtually no spontaneous firing rate and is insensitive to large-field movement. This cell synapses on a descending interneuron in the ipsilateral nerve cord (DIMD). (*B*) L-6 displays a moderate spontaneous firing rate and is very sharply sensitive to small-field movement in the visual field center. (*C*) L-4 has a high spontaneous firing rate on which are superimposed inhibitory responses to both a moving dot and a stripe in the visual field center. It also displays an initial, transitory inhibitory response to the movement of a grating. (*D*) L-11 has a moderate spontaneous firing rate on which is superimposed a preference for horizontally or vertically moving stripes in the visual field center. It also responds to the contralateral and vertical movement of a grating. However, its highly punctate responses to the grating suggest that it is resolving the individual stripes as they move. (Redrawn from Berger, 1985, with the author's kind permission.)

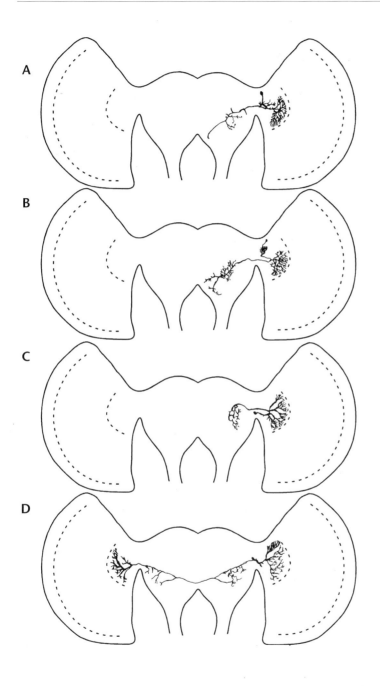

Although only a modest amount of data has been gathered on precisely what types of information signal a predator rather than prey, we do know that overall stimulus size (generally greater than about 12×12 deg) and movement pattern (e.g., erratic) will elicit defensive rather than appetitive behaviors in male *Sphodromantis lineola* (Prete et al., 2002). We also know that small-field visual stimuli that create local image motion but do not meet the specific set of criteria defining prey (as explained later), or preylike stimuli that have been preceded immediately by another visual stimulus (even another preylike stimulus) will elicit defensive rather than predatory behaviors in female *S. lineola* (Prete et al., 1993). Hence, the perception of a prey object is created by a relatively specific type of small-field movement experienced within a certain type of experiential context.

Of course, in the wild there is probably no absolute dichotomy between local image motion that elicits predatory versus that which elicits defensive (predator elicited) responses in mantids. Descriptive behavioral and experimental evidence (reviewed in Prete and Wolfe, 1992 and Prete et al., 1999) indicates that predatory versus defensive behaviors are actually opposite ends of a continuum. All else being equal, some visual stimuli (e.g., small arthropods) will always be identified as prey. Larger stimuli (e.g., large arthropods or very small vertebrates) may elicit defensive responses in smaller (e.g., male) mantids and, initially, in the larger females. Females, however, may then switch from an initially defensive behavior to a predatory behavior and capture the animal (e.g., Fabre, 1912; for other references see Prete and Wolf, 1992). Finally, some visual stimuli (e.g., large vertebrates) will always be perceived as threats and elicit defensive responses (Edmunds and Brunner, 1999; Liske, 1999; Maldonado, 1970).

Whether a predatory or a defensive response is emitted in any particular situation, and precisely what defensive response occurs (defensive striking, remaining motionless and cryptic, flight, threat posturing) will be determined by a complex interaction among a number of as-yet little-studied factors. However, we know that the characteristics of any local image motion must be integrated with other information, for instance, that pertaining to physiological state, immediate prior experience, a modest amount of learning (e.g., taste aversion; Bowdish and Bultman, 1993), and/or a mantid's species, sex, or developmental stage (Edmunds and Brunner, 1999; Liske, 1999).

Global Image Motion

Movement in the environment, for instance, a surround of swaying vegetation or the shadows of drifting clouds, will yield coherent global (i.e., panoramic) image motion in the mantid's eyes, although the overall perception of coherence may result from a combination of any number of different, individual motion signals. In some cases, global image motion may simply represent noise, while in others it may provide useful information. For a mantid waiting in ambush, swaying vegetation is probably noise. However, when performing back-and-forth peering movements to gauge the distances to stems or branches, the relative movements of the individual pieces of vegetation will provide information that can be used to determine their distances.

Optic Flow

Whenever a mantid moves within a structured environment, optic flow occurs over the retinae. Optic flow is the total pattern of velocity vectors corresponding to the objects in the visual field. The vector velocities will vary, depending on the velocity of the mantid, the direction of the mantid's line of sight relative to the direction of motion, and the distance to the objects being viewed. Optic flow resulting from movements of the mantid itself can include, for example, expansions and contractions of the panorama caused by back-and-forth peering; lateral displacements caused by side-to-side peering; and rapid, centrifugal image expansion during flight landing.

When we refer to retinal image motion or motion patterns, it should be kept in mind that these are not received directly as such by the mantid; they are merely a useful shorthand to describe the geometric projections of the visual surroundings on the retina. The precise detail and characteristics of the visual flow field will be shaped by the local optical characteristics (and resolution capacities) of the mantid's eyes. As indicated earlier, the acute zone has the highest resolution, and resolution decreases posteriorly. It is interesting that this matches in some ways the structure of the image motion.

The information contained in the time- and space-dependent luminosity values of the retinal images must be optimally filtered by the nervous system to reduce both noise and redundancy, and processed in ways that lead to appropriate behavioral responses. Admittedly, however, we can make only relatively modest speculations in this direction, since our knowledge of mantids still faces sobering limitations. One such limitation is that much of the data that we have on mantids and related species has been collected (of necessity) under comparatively austere laboratory conditions, with stimuli whose characteristics have not been explicitly matched to those of the natural world. Thus the associated behaviors and neuronal responses cannot easily be matched to those that occur under the complex dynamic stimulus conditions that occur naturally.

Visual Perception in the Natural Environment: Transforming Local Image Motion into Prey Recognition

It is a sunny day in May, and the air is growing steadily warmer. A female *Empusa fasciata* is perched motionless on a grass stem, waiting for prey. She is surrounded by flowers swaying gently in the breeze. Suddenly a bee appears and approaches a flower. By tensing her body, turning her head, and drawing up her forelegs, the mantis reveals that she has noticed the bee even though it is still half a meter or more away. She visually tracks the bee as it flies closer, turning her head and forelegs without moving the rest of her body. She strikes only when the bee is in the binocular visual field and within reach, just a few centimeters away. The strike is accurate and quick, lasting only about 60 ms (Gombocz, 1999; also see Prete and Cleal, 1996).

How was this mantis able to recognize the bee as potential prey? How did it know what it was and where it was? The answers to these questions are interesting, not only in and of themselves, but also because they reveal the extent to which mantid visual perception approaches the complexity of that of many vertebrates.

To begin with, mantids are opportunistic, generalized predators that prey primarily—but not exclusively—on arthropods and their larvae (e.g., Bartley, 1983; Fagan and Hurd, 1994; Hurd and Eisenberg, 1984a,b, 1990; Moran and Hurd, 1994). The particular mix of prey items that a mantid eats is limited only by the rate at which the prey is encountered and can be successfully captured, and could include beetles, bees and wasps, crickets, grasshoppers, caterpillars, or butterflies (e.g., Bartley, 1983). In addition, mantids may capture much larger prey, such as same-sized conspecifics, and even newts, lizards, frogs, small birds, small turtles, or mice (e.g., Edmunds, 1972; Johnson, 1976; Nickle, 1981; Ridpath, 1977; Tulk, 1844; for a review, see Prete and Wolfe, 1992).

Given the variety of retinal images created by these different prey items, it is clear that mantids do not identify prey by a simple matching to template procedure (e.g., "the object looks like a bee at 2 cm"). Certainly, beetles, butterflies, grasshoppers, other mantids, and the occasional newt do not look like bees. In fact, it is hard to imagine what they do have in common. The common thread, however, is that each of these prey items is a representative of the category "prey" that is constructed by the mantid's visual system.

To understand the idea of a perceptual category, consider again the example used in the introduction to this section. When you decide if a particular meal is fit to eat, you do not have in mind a picture of one invariant, acceptable meal (i.e., a template) to which you try to match the meal on the table in front of you. Rather, you weigh a variety of stimuli (the odor, the color, the taste, the texture) associated with the meal and if, all together, the stimuli are acceptable, you eat. In fact, in some instances, one particular stimulus might be quite unacceptable if you considered it in isolation (e.g., the smell of Roquefort cheese), but may be delectable if it is accompanied by a number of other acceptable stimuli (e.g., those of an elegant tossed salad). In this case, the entire set of stimuli associated with the tossed salad is one example of the category *acceptable meal*. The category can be understood as a theoretical, perceptual envelope that includes all of the various combinations and permutations of the original, key stimulus parameters (odor, color, taste, texture), and it may contain combinations as diverse as sushi, pizza, borscht, and goulash.

A mantid's visual system does the same thing when it decides what an acceptable meal is. It identifies an object as an example of the category "acceptable prey item" by assessing each of ten stimulus parameters. Only if a sufficient number of parameters are satisfied will the mantid attempt to capture the prey. The ten stimulus parameters are (1) the overall size of a compact stimulus, (2) the length of the leading edge of an elongated stimulus, (3) stimulus contrast with the background, (4) location of the stimulus in the visual field, (5) apparent speed of the stimulus, (6) the geometry of the stimulus in relation to its direction of movement, (7) the overall direction of the movement, (8) the distance that the retinal image of the stimulus moves, and (9 and 10) the degree of spatial and/or temporal summation of any subthreshold stimulus elements (Prete, 1992a,b, 1993, 1999; Prete and Mahaffey, 1993; Prete and McLean, 1996). Of these ten, items 1–5 are fundamental.

Psychophysical Studies
Virtually all of our psychophysical studies have been done on female *Sphodromantis lineola*. However, we have also collected some data on male *S. lineola*, and female *T. sinensis* and *Hierodula membranacea* (e.g., Prete, 1999; Prete et al., 2002; Gonka et al., 1999). In all cases, the data were concordant.

The basic experimental procedure was to present tethered mantids with either mechanically driven or computer-generated visual stimuli. The former were flat shapes of various types that were moved across an enclosed arena floor at specified speeds. The latter were computer animations. In all cases, we could assess the degree to which a stimulus was categorized as prey by calculating the overall rate at which the mantis stuck at (strike rate) and/or attempted to chase a particular stimulus (approach rate).

Geometry in Relationship to Direction   In a typical experiment using mechanically driven stimuli, we presented mantids with various squares and rectangles. In some cases the stimuli were black and moved against a white or patterned background and in others the stimuli were patterned to match the background over which they moved (cryptic). In all cases the results were the same.

A number of such experiments, including tens of thousands of trials with scores of mantids, revealed that the mantids were identifying two types of stimuli as prey: relatively small squares (compact stimuli) and narrow rectangles (elongated stimuli) that moved parallel but not perpendicular to their long axes. In the amphibian literature, elongated stimuli moving parallel to their long axis have been referred to as "worm" stimuli, those moving perpendicular as "antiworm" (e.g., Ewert, 1987; Ingle, 1983; for similar preferences in salamanders, see Roth, 1987).

From the mantid's perspective, mechanically driven stimuli subtended approximately 1 deg of visual angle per millimeter. So, for instance, *T. sinensis* preferred (i.e., categorized as prey) compact stimuli that were 6×6 deg and elongated stimuli with a leading edge no wider than 6 deg. Analogously, *S. lineola* preferred compact stimuli that were 12×12 deg and elongated stimuli with a leading edge no wider than 12 deg. As suggested by these results and confirmed by additional experiments, mantids attended preferentially to the leading edge of the moving stimuli (figure 3.7).

Here we would like to emphasize the point that the mantids were not responding to the elongated stimuli based on size per se. That is, within the dimensions specified, worm configurations were consistently preferred over same-sized antiworm configurations. In other words, the mantids were responding to stimulus geometry in relationship to direction of movement, not size by itself.

Speed   Theoretically, the speed of a moving prey item could inform a mantid about either its identity (e.g., what species it is) or its distance. However, given the mantid's eclectic tastes, the former is unlikely. Mantids will capture both slow prey and

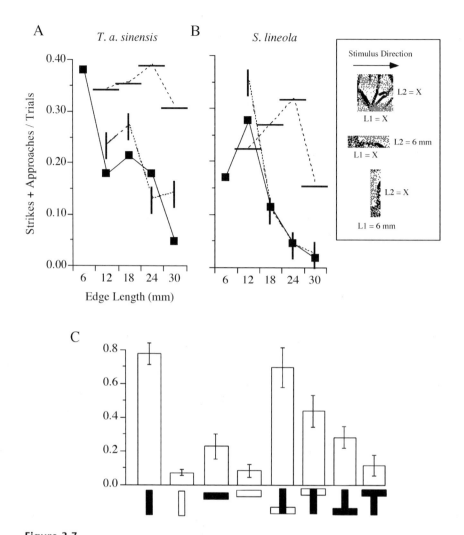

Figure 3.7

(*A*), (*B*) The average responses of two mantid species to mechanically driven, patterned rectangular stimuli moving against a similarly patterned background (inset). Note the species difference in the smallest preferred square and the overall preference for worm versus same-sized antiworm stimuli. (Redrawn from Prete and McLean, 1996, with the kind permission of S. Karger AG, Basel and Johns Hopkins University Press.) (*C*) Columns 1–4 are average response rates of *S. lineola* to mechanically driven, rectangular stimuli moving against the patterned background shown in the inset. In all graphs the error bars represent standard errors. Mantids preferentially identified worm (versus antiworm) and darker (versus lighter) worm stimuli as prey. Columns 5–8 are response rates to mechanically driven, T-shaped stimuli moving against the patterned (columns 5 and 6), or a white background (columns 7 and 8). The response rates were suppressed when the crossbar was at the leading (versus) trailing edge of the stimulus, indicating that the mantids were attending preferentially to the leading edge of the stimuli. (Redrawn from Prete, 1992b, and Prete et al., 1999, with the kind permission of S. Karger AG, Basel and Johns Hopkins University Press, respectively.)

fast-moving prey, even when the latter move slowly (e.g., a walking fly). Thus speed is always confounded with prey type. However, the speed of an object could be used as a cue to the object's distance. We know that mantids do in fact assess the distance between themselves and prey. They will stalk or chase prey that is too distant to capture, and they will adjust the distance that they lunge during a strike according to the distance to the prey (e.g., Cleal and Prete, 1996; Prete and Cleal, 1996; Prete et al., 1990, 1992).

Because mantids have immobile eyes with fixed-focus optics, the distance of an object cannot be inferred by ocular convergence (Srinivasan, 1992). So like other insects, they extract relative distances from the relative speeds of the retinal images of the objects in the environment. The retinal images of nearer objects will move faster than the images of more distant objects. Thus from the mantid's perspective, a slowly moving image that subtends a visual angle small enough to be considered prey (e.g., 10 deg) probably represents a very large distant object (such as a bird flying by). However, a quickly moving image that subtends the same 10 deg probably represents a small nearby object (and perhaps a meal).

The critical role that retinal image speed plays in recognizing prey and assessing the distance of objects is evidenced by the results of experiments using both mechanically driven and computer-generated stimuli. First, an otherwise preylike visual stimulus must be moving within a preferred velocity range to reliably elicit predatory strikes. In experiments with *S. lineola*, this ranged from approximately 35 to 85 deg/s. Second, in keeping with the explanation made in the previous paragraph, we found convincing evidence that mantids use image speed as a cue to distance. That is, slower moving preylike stimuli are perceived as more distant and elicit primarily approaching behavior (which would bring the stimulus within range of a strike). Faster moving preylike stimuli, perceived as being closer and already within the range of a strike, elicit only strikes (figure 3.8).

Location, Direction, and Distance Moved   As discussed earlier, mantids have an acute zone (sometimes referred to as the fovea), a forward- and slightly inward-looking area of high acuity in each compound eye. The acute zone creates an area of high spatial and temporal resolution in the lower center of the visual field. This means that as an image moves across the fovea, luminance changes created by its edges will be sampled at a higher rate than if the object were moving in the periphery. In other words, the fovea is particularly sensitive to the movement of an object. As might be expected, then, if all else is equal, a preylike object moving through the lower center of the visual field (i.e., the area sampled by the fovea) should be more likely to elicit predatory behavior, and this is indeed the case.

Interesting, too, is the fact that the direction of the image's movement is superimposed on this location preference. Downward-moving images are preferred and elicit the highest strike rates. Again, this makes sense in that from a mantid's perspective, for instance, when it is perched on a stem, a downward-moving retinal image would represent an object moving toward the mantid along the stem. Upward-moving images are least preferred; these would represent objects moving away from the

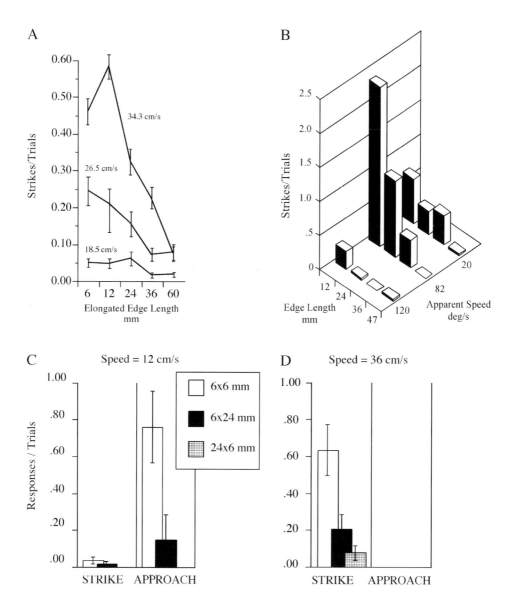

Figure 3.8
(A) Average response rate of *S. lineola* to black, mechanically driven worm stimuli moving against a white background at three speeds. The width of the leading edge of the stimuli was 6 mm; their lengths are indicated on the abscissa. Data from Prete et al. (1993). (B) Average response rate to black, computer-animated square stimuli that moved against a white background in an erratic path around the center of the mantid's visual field for 10 s per trial. Note in both (A) and (B) the dramatic effects of stimulus speed. (C) The speed of an object is used as a cue to its distance. Hence, slower moving, mechanically driven stimuli elicit primarily approaching (i.e., stalking or chasing) behavior (left graph); faster moving stimuli elicit primarily striking behavior. This is also true for computer-animated stimuli. (Redrawn from Prete et al., 1993, with the kind permission of S. Karger AG, Basel and Johns Hopkins University Press.)

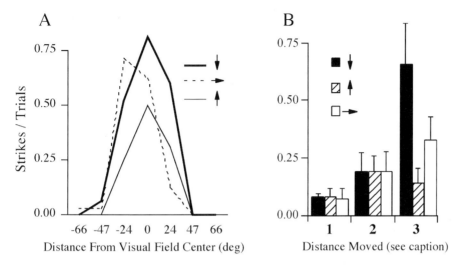

Figure 3.9
(*A*) Computer-generated, black square stimuli moving linearly elicit the highest average strike rate when they move downward through the visual field center (heavy line), or horizontally just below the visual field center (dashed line). (*B*) Average response rate to 6 × 24-deg black, computer-animated stimuli moving against a white background. In condition 1, the stimulus began 58 deg from the visual field center and disappeared when its leading edge reached the center; in 2, the stimulus began 24 deg from the visual field center and disappeared when its trailing edge was 24 deg past the center; in 3, the stimulus began when its leading edge was 58 deg from the visual field center and disappeared when its trailing edge was 24 deg past the center. (Redrawn from Prete, 1993, with the kind permission of Cambridge University Press and Johns Hopkins University Press.)

perched mantis. Horizontally moving images, which would be created by objects moving across the mantid's visual field, elicit intermediate rates of striking (figure 3.9).

The overall distance that an object's retinal image moves also affects the probability that it will elicit a strike. For instance, if a preylike worm stimulus appears 24 deg lateral to the visual field center, moves through the visual field center, and then disappears when its trailing edge is 24 deg past the center, it is unlikely that it will elicit a strike, irrespective of its direction. Likewise, the stimulus will do poorly if it appears as much as 58 deg from the visual field center (i.e., in the periphery) and disappears when its leading edge just reaches the center of the visual field. In contrast, downward and horizontally moving worm stimuli elicit the highest rates of striking when they begin in the periphery and do not disappear until their trailing edge is 24 deg past the visual field center (figure 3.9).

All told, then, an otherwise preylike object is most likely to be categorized as prey if its image moves through or just below the center of the visual field, it moves downward over the retinae, and it travels a sufficient distance over the retinae.

Relative Contrast   Although it is clear from their behavior that mantids can see moving stimuli that are brighter than the background, a stimulus must be darker than the background to be classified as prey. This makes sense for two reasons. First, in general, moving objects will be perceived as decreases in luminance; that is, as darker than the average background luminance. The second, more interesting reason is that small increases in luminance (i.e., small bright spots) actually mean something different than prey to mantids. They are in fact recognized as droplets of water (Prete et al., 1992).

The predilection to recognize relatively darker visual stimuli as prey items is consistent with data collected by Bowdish and Bultman (1993) in their investigations of the visual cues used by the mantis, *T. sinensis*, in food avoidance learning. After exposing the mantids to toxic milkweed bugs, these researchers presented *T. sinensis* with visual stimuli that were black, orange, or black and orange. Under all conditions, the mantids struck most frequently at the solid black (i.e., the relatively darkest) stimuli.

Spatial and Temporal Summation   If we see a cat walking behind a picket fence, we do not interpret what we see as several independently moving furry pieces of cat. The synchronously moving images are seen as portions of a single, larger, moving object. This perceptual penchant causes us to perceive an array of synchronously moving small shapes as a single unified object, even if the array is moving against a similarly patterned background against which it would be undetectable if it were motionless (e.g., a "Julesz pattern") (Cutting et al., 1988; Julesz, 1971; Prazdny, 1985). Mantids also have this perceptual ability, even if tiny black rectangles, each too small to elicit any response individually, are arranged into a larger prey-sized array (figure 3.10).

The fact that mantids behave as if they perceive a moving Julesz pattern as a single, unified object indicates that their visual system sums inputs over both space and time. This was demonstrated further in experiments using computer animations in which the distance between successive retinal images of a preylike stimulus was increased incrementally. A series of still images in which each image was displaced 20 deg or less from its predecessor created the illusion of a single moving object for the mantis, whereas images displaced more than 20 deg did not. This phenomenon is, of course, also experienced by people. If two stimuli are flashed in different places on a screen, one immediately after the other, it appears as if the first image "jumps" to the second position if the distance between the two images is not too great. Hence the spatial and temporal proximity of successive retinal images is also a key parameter affecting prey recognition in mantids.

The results of the two sets of experiments just described suggest that the probability that an object will be perceived as prey increases in proportion to the number of adjacent (or at least very closely spaced) sampling units (ommatidia) that experience a decrease in luminance, as long as the total affected retinal area at any given time does not exceed the preferred size or leading-edge width for preylike stimuli. We confirmed this hypothesis by presenting mantids with an array of nine 25 × 25-deg black, square, computer-generated stimuli that varied systematically along two

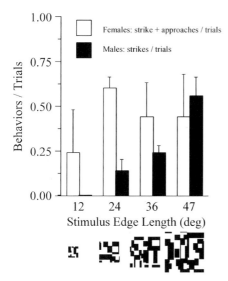

Figure 3.10
Average response rates of female and male *S. lineola* to patterned (as shown), square, computer-generated stimuli that moved against a similarly patterned background in an erratic path around the visual field center for 10 s per trial. Such stimuli are undetectable when they are stationary (even by humans). (Redrawn from Prete and Mahaffey, 1993, and Prete et al., 2002, with the kind permission of Cambridge University Press and Elsevier Science, respectively.)

dimensions: the number of black pixels that made up their border (level B, for border) and the number of black pixels that made up their internal detail (level D, for detail) (figure 3.11).

The square with the fewest pixels elicited visual tracking but no striking whatsoever. As the number of pixels increased, the strike rate increased proportionately, regardless of whether pixels were added to the border or the interior of the stimulus (figure 3.11). In other words, as the number of pixels in the 25 × 25-deg array increased, so did the number of ommatidia within the boundaries of the overall retinal image that experienced a decrease in luminance at any given time. As the number of affected ommatidia increased, so did the probability that the stimulus would be classified as prey.

Neural Underpinnings of Prey Recognition
Over the past decade or so we have been studying mantid prey recognition using a top-down approach. As explained, we have discovered that mantids rely on a computational algorithm that involves the simultaneous assessment of a number of identified stimulus parameters. Remarkably, the algorithm is much the same as that used

A

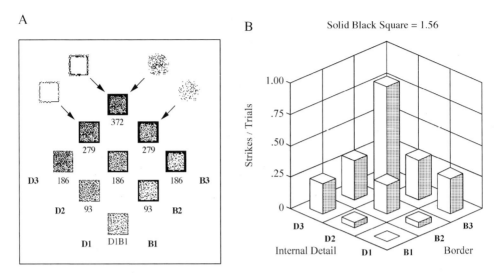

Figure 3.11
Average response rates [indicated in (*B*)] to a series of computer-generated square stimuli [as shown in (*A*)] that moved against a white background in an erratic path around the visual field center for 10 s per trial. The stimuli differed only in the number of black pixels that they contained. The fewest were in stimulus D1B1. Other stimuli were created by adding the indicated number of pixels to the border (levels B1–B3), or to the interior detail (levels D1–D3) of the stimuli. Although mantids visually tracked all stimuli, their strike rate increased as pixel number (i.e., average stimulus-to-background contrast) increased. Compared to the stimulus with the most pixels (D3B3), mantids struck at a solid black square of the same size at twice the rate. (Redrawn from Prete and McLean, 1996, with the kind permission of S. Karger AG, Basel and Johns Hopkins University Press.)

by some vertebrate predators, most notably the toad, *Bufo*. For the toad, application of the algorithm is supported in great part by the activity of class T5(2) tectal neurons, which is correlated with the animal's behavioral responses to preylike stimuli. In turn, T5(2) neurons project to contralateral hindbrain motor centers that are involved in the prey-capture sequence (see chapter 4 in this volume). Because the activity of the T5(2) neurons is strongly correlated with both the presence of preylike stimuli and the toad's prey-catching behavior, the cells are considered to be prey selective. That is, they are neurons that respond maximally to a limited combination of stimulus parameters and serve to distinguish between biologically important and unimportant objects.

Prete and McLean (1996) argued that mantid prey recognition is also underpinned by prey-selective cells, in this case, a large movement-sensitive cell in the lobula complex, which they called the mantid lobula giant movement detector or LGMD. They argued that the putative mantid LGMD is immediately presynaptic to a descending, contralateral projecting interneuron, which they called the mantid descending contralateral movement detector (DCMD). The DCMD, then, would act as the interface between the prey-selective LGMD and the motor neurons responsible for initiating the strike. This hypothesis was based on four facts. First, an LGMD–DCMD complex exists in some other orthopteroidea and it is responsive to the same fundamental stimulus parameters that define a preylike stimulus for mantids, although in the other insects the information is used quite differently (e.g., for initiating escape behavior; chapter 10 in this volume; also see O'Shea and Rowell, 1976; Rowell and O'Shea, 1976a,b; Rowell et al., 1977; Rind and Simmons, 1992a,b, 1997; Simmons and Rind, 1992; Judge and Rind, 1997). Second, predatory strikes by mantids can be elicited or suppressed by many of the same stimuli that have been shown to elicit or suppress responses of the LGMD–DCMD complex in other orthopteroidea (e.g., Prete and McLean, 1996; Prete, 1999). Third, artificial neural network (ANN) computer models of LGMD–DCMD systems "learn" to respond to the same types of stimuli that mantids recognize as prey (Prete, 1999). Finally, an apparently LGMD-like cell presynaptic to a DCMD cell has been identified (anatomically and electrophysiologically) in one species of mantid (Berger, 1985).

This hypothesis received support in a series of experiments in which Gonka et al. (1999) recorded extracellularly from the ventral nerve cords of two species of mantid while they watched precisely the same visual stimuli used to characterize the mantid prey recognition algorithm. Gonka et al. argued that because DCMD spikes follow LGMD spikes on a one-to-one basis, the activity of the latter can be determined by the former. Recordings taken from both of the cervical nerve cords of monocular mantids watching the types of computer-generated stimuli described earlier were dominated by very large spikes that traveled caudally (from the head to the thorax). This indicates the existence of a number of large descending movement-sensitive interneurons, some projecting through the ipsilateral (descending ipsilateral movement detectors, DIMDs) and some through the contralateral (DCMDs) nerve cord relative to the stimulated eye.

If an LGMD–DCMD complex does in fact exist in mantids, the activity of the DCMD component should be unequivocally identifiable in extracellular recordings taken from the cervical nerve cord (as it is in other orthopteroidea; e.g., Gabbiani et al., 1999) for two reasons. First, because of the comparatively large size of the DCMD axon, it creates unequivocally outstanding, large-amplitude spikes in extracellular recordings. Second, because it is immediately postsynaptic to the putative prey-selective LGMD, the occurrence of DCMD spikes should be strictly correlated only with the appearance of preylike stimuli and should be suppressed by the same stimulus conditions that suppress predatory striking (e.g., large-field or panoramic movement).

Large-Field versus Small-Field Movement   One of the parameters that mantids use to identify prey is the overall size of compact (e.g., square or circular) stimuli. Predatory strikes are elicited by small-field movement but are dramatically suppressed by simultaneous large-field or panoramic movement (Prete and Mahaffey, 1993; Prete and

McLean, 1996). Hence, if a mantid LGMD–DCMD complex plays a key role in prey recognition, it, too, should respond only to small-field movement. This is precisely what was found.

As predicted, Gonka et al. found that activity in the mantid's contralateral nerve cord was dominated by large DCMD spikes that appeared only in response to preylike stimuli and were suppressed by simultaneous large-field (i.e., panoramic) movement. None of the other amplitude classes of spikes identified by Gonka et al. were selectively responsive to preylike stimuli (figure 3.12).

Stimulus Location in the Visual Field   As explained earlier, mantids emit the most strikes when a small-field stimulus moves horizontally through or slightly (i.e., less than 24 deg) below their visual field center, or a vertically moving small-field stimulus moves directly through the visual field center. The strike rate falls off dramatically when a small-field stimulus is outside of this so-called "prey capture zone." Irrespective of direction, however, a small-field stimulus never elicits strikes when it is as much as 60 deg away from the visual field center (e.g., Prete, 1993). Only the mantid DCMD activity mirrors these behavioral responses. That is, in experiments done by Gonka et al. (1999) its activity was elicited only by preylike stimuli moving in the prey capture zone. The activity of other classes of movement-sensitive cells in the contra- and ipsilateral nerve cords was virtually unaffected by the elevation or lateral displacement of small-field stimuli.

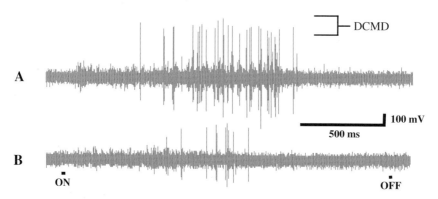

Figure 3.12
Two extracellular recordings made from the ventral nerve cord contralateral to the stimulated eye in a female *S. lineola.* The activity is in response to computer-generated square stimuli that moved horizontally through the center of the visual field at 110 deg/s. (*A*) The extremely large spikes generated by the mantid descending contralateral movement detector (DCMD) in response to a prey-sized (5 × 5 deg) square. (*B*) Activity in response to a square much larger than anything the mantid recognizes as prey (77 × 77 deg). Note the absence of DCMD activity. (Redrawn from Gonka et al., 1999, with the kind permission of S. Karger AG, Basel.)

Luminance Decreases, Target Speed, and Target Direction   As noted, mantids strike in response to decreases in moving small-field luminance (objects darker than the background) but not to increases in small-field luminance (objects brighter than the background; Prete, 1992b, 1999; Prete and McLean, 1996). Again, Gonka et al. (1999) found that only DCMD activity showed a dramatic and significant preference (i.e., a 15-fold rate difference) for luminance decreases. They also found that DCMD activity was sensitive to stimulus speed, as are intact mantids. Furthermore, DCMD activity showed the same direction preferences as mantids for downward-moving, preylike stimuli when the stimuli moved within the preferred speed range for prey-like stimuli.

Correlation of DCMD Activity with Predatory Strikes   All of the data collected by Gonka et al. (1999) indicate that only the behavior of the mantid DCMD consistently parallels the behavioral responses of mantids to preylike visual stimuli. However, in addition, they found that DCMD activity is tightly correlated with the actual occurrence of predatory strikes. In phase one of the critical experiment (the design of which was suggested by Chris Comer), a tethered mantid with an electromyogram (EMG) electrode inserted in its fast coxal promotor muscles watched a series of 10-s presentations of a computer-generated, preylike stimulus. The fast coxal promotors are the very large muscles responsible for the rapid extension of the mantid's forelegs during the strike. These muscles discharge if and only if a strike occurs. Based on the times that they fired, Gonka et al. could record the precise times that strikes occurred during the stimulus presentations and they did so over repeated trials until they had recorded 122 strikes. In phase two of the experiment, the same mantid was prepared for electrophysiological recording, after which it viewed forty-eight more trials of the same 10-s stimulus. The results were unambiguous. The peak activity of the mantid DCMD coincided precisely with the times during the stimulus presentations at which the mantid emitted predatory strikes (figure 3.13).

Is L-15 the Mantid LGMD?

As we have noted, one of the drawbacks with doing psychophysical or neurophysiological studies with highly abstracted visual stimuli (e.g., arbitrarily sized dots, gratings, and stripes) is that it can be difficult to relate the organismal or cellular responses to real-world behavior. However, this difficulty notwithstanding, one of the large lobula cells characterized by Berger (1985) in *Mantis religiosa* (his L15) is provocatively similar to the orthopteroidean LGMD in morphology, in response characteristics, and in the fact that it is presynaptic to a contralaterally projecting cell, a DCMD. Thus it could be the initial component of the mantid prey-selective LGMD–DCMD complex. Like the orthopteroidean LGMD, the mantid L15 has a primary, broad dendritic fan in the lobula and a characteristic, much smaller, anteriorly placed dendritic arborization (figure 3.14). The cell projects contralaterally within the brain where it synapses on its DCMD. The response properties and receptive field of the L15–DCMD complex in *M. religiosa* are like those of the mantid LGMD–DCMD complex described by Gonka et al. (1999) in *S. lineola* and *Hierodula membranacea*. We should also note that some

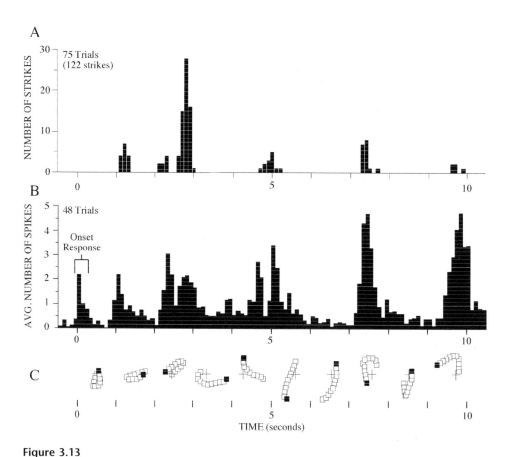

Figure 3.13
The relationship between the occurrence of predatory strikes and mantid DCMD activity in a female *S. lineola*. (*A*) The times at which a total of 122 strikes occurred during seventy-five 10-s stimulus presentations. In each trial, a computer-generated, 16 × 16-deg black square moved against a white background in an erratic path around the visual field center. (*B*) The average number of DCMD spikes (in 100-ms bins) that occurred during forty-eight subsequent, identical stimulus presentations. (*C*) The sequential positions of the computer-generated stimulus during each second of each 10-s trial in relation to the visual field center (cross; each movement sequence ends at the black square). Disregarding the stimulus onset response (discussed in the text), the peak DCMD activity was tightly correlated with the times at which the mantid emitted predatory strikes. (Redrawn from Gonka et al., 1999, with the kind permission of S. Karger AG, Basel.)

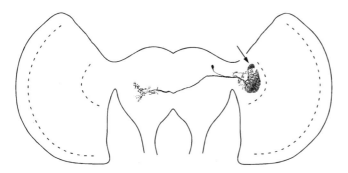

Figure 3.14
A drawing of movement-sensitive lobula cell L-15 in *Mantis religiosa* described and named by Berger (1985). This cell behaves very similarly to the putative mantid lobula giant movement detector (LGMD) described in *S. lineola* and *H. membranacea* by Gonka et al. (1999). L-15 synapses on a DCMD cell creating a movement-sensitive complex that carries visual information to the thoracic ganglia. It is particularly responsive to small dark spots and individual narrow stripes moving in and just below the visual field center (i.e., in the acute zone). This cell habituates quickly (as do the LGMD–DCMD complexes in *S. lineola* and locusts) and can be dishabituated by touching the mantis's body (as is the case in locusts). Note the small dorsal arborization (arrow), which is also characteristic of the locust LGMD. (Redrawn from Berger, 1985, with the author's kind permission.)

(as yet unpublished) data similar to Gonka's DCMD data have been collected in the Comer lab from *T. sinensis*.

Just Two LGMD–DCMD Complexes Can Underpin Prey Recognition and Localization
Prior to our work on mantid visual psychophysics, there had been a lot of speculation on just how mantids could identify and locate prey in three-dimensional space. One hypothesis that gained wide acceptance was that mantids use binocular disparity to judge the distance of an object. However, one of us (FRP) has argued that both recent experimental data and parsimony make the retinal disparity hypothesis unlikely. In brief, the main argument against the hypothesis is that it rests on a number of improbable assumptions. For instance, it assumes that the mantid actually has the neural machinery to continually compare retinal images; that the mantid's brain continually reorganizes itself to compensate for the fact that the ommatidia migrate peripherally as the mantid grows; and that the mantid can somehow compute the geometric center ("centroid") of each of two retinal images, compare the retinal locations of each "centroid," and then, based on the difference in "centroid" location, assess an object's distance. There is a good deal of experimental data indicating that these assumptions are unlikely (e.g., Gonka et al., 1999; Prete, 1999; Prete and Mahaffey, 1993; Prete and McLean, 1996). Furthermore, retinal disparity cues are ineffective at mantis-prey

distances greater than approximately 25 mm, yet mantids can locate and capture prey at distances greater than this.

One additional argument against the hypothesis is that it is unnecessary. The whole of prey recognition, localization, and correctly timed strike initiation can be explained simply by the existence of a pair of LGMD–DCMD complexes. Let us explain.

It makes sense that a pair of LGMD–DCMD complexes could underpin prey recognition and localization in mantids for a number of reasons. First, there are several key aspects of the LGMD–DCMD functional organization and response properties that are consistent with mantid prey recognition. In general, the orthopteroidean LGMD–DCMD (as described in locusts, and by Berger and Gonka et al. in mantids) is broadly tuned; it does not respond to a narrow range of stimuli. Likewise, mantids respond appetitively to a range of stimuli defined by the same parameters that define the stimuli to which the orthopteroidean LGMD–DCMD system responds. In locusts, it is believed that a feed-forward inhibitory pathway and a phasic lateral inhibitory network between incoming afferent channels presynaptic to the LGMD bias the system in favor of small moving stimuli that are in the same size range as the compact stimuli to which mantids respond. Panoramic (i.e., background) movement inhibits the locust LGMD–DCMD via the feed-forward pathway just as panoramic movement inhibits the mantid's behavioral responses to prey-sized stimuli. Similarly, large visual stimuli (e.g., greater than 40×40 deg) elicit virtually no activity from the locust or mantid LGMD–DCMD and virtually no predatory behavior from intact mantids (O'Shea and Rowell, 1976; Rowell and O'Shea, 1976a,b; Rowell et al., 1977).

Perhaps even more intriguing is the fact that the most fundamental characteristic of the orthopteroidean LGMD–DCMD complex is its keen responsivity to moving stimuli. This responsivity is a product of the spatial and temporal summation of a series of local responses in the large dendritic fan of the LGMD that are caused by a succession of changes in small-field luminance at the retina (Palka, 1967; Rowell and O'Shea, 1976a; Berger, 1985). As explained, mantid prey recognition also requires a succession of local luminance changes that meet certain spatial and temporal criteria, such as the total retinal area over which luminance decreases, the time within which the series of local decreases occur, and so on.

Finally, the orthopteroidean LGMD–DCMD complex is sufficient to explain mantid prey recognition because it is inherently sensitive to the visual field location in which a small moving object appears (and so is the mantid, behaviorally). The LGMD–DCMD complex is location sensitive by virtue of the geometry of the LGMD's dendritic fan. Because of that geometry, incoming afferent channels that are presynaptic to it have different potencies that depend upon their proximity to the LGMD's spike-initiating zone. For the locust, it has been explained like this: "The [movement detecting] system does not respond equally to identical stimuli at all points on the retina. Instead, there is a rather complex gradient of sensitivity in which responsiveness is greatest to stimuli presented to the center of the eye and declines most rapidly at the extreme edges of the visual field" (O'Shea and Rowell, 1976, pp. 305–306). In other words, the LGMD supports an acute zone. In mantids, an additional contributing factor would of course be the higher density of afferent inputs reaching the LGMD from the more tightly packed ommatidia of the (anatomical) acute zone.

Hence, if two LGMD–DCMD complexes (one in each optic lobe) are preferentially responsive to preylike stimuli moving in the acute zone, and there is a threshold number of DCMD spikes necessary to trigger a predatory strike (e.g., approximately twelve rapidly occurring spikes per strike as in figure 3.13), then a strike can only be triggered by a preylike stimulus moving in the acute zone of the visual field (figure 3.15). That is, as all of the data demonstrate, only a preylike stimulus in the prey capture zone (i.e., the area sampled by the acute zone) could maximally activate such a pair of LGMD–DCMD complexes. If their summed activity reaches a threshold level, a strike will occur. There is no need (explanatorily or physiologically) to posit an explicit comparison of retinal images or calculation of retinal disparity. The system is actually most elegant in its simplicity (figure 3.15).

This model also explains two otherwise inexplicable pieces of data. The first is the occasional predatory strike emitted by mantids when a stimulus suddenly appears far outside of the prey capture zone, sometimes as far as 120 deg from the center of their visual field (Cleal and Prete, 1996). You will notice in figure 3.13 that, as is the case for locusts, the mantid DCMD can emit a small burst of spikes when a stimulus suddenly appears in the visual field, and this characteristic "onset response" can occur even if the stimulus is far outside of the visual field area to which the DCMD is most sensitive. If, then, the onset response is sufficiently vigorous, a strike to the anomalously positioned stimulus could occur. The second piece of data is the extreme difficulty with which strikes can be elicited from monocular mantids. Put simply, in terms of our model, just one DCMD is unlikely to generate a sufficient number of spikes to trigger a predatory strike.

Visual Perception in the Natural Environment: Extracting Information from Global Image Motion and Optic Flow

Walking and Climbing
In the field, walking and climbing can be easily observed; for instance, by a male *Mantis religiosa* blown onto a shrub after a short, fluttering flight. Once landed, it will try, as inconspicuously as possible, to climb downward, to reach the shelter of the grass near the ground. The mantid will descend the branches and stems in a jerky manner, making a large movement forward, then a smaller movement backward, then another larger movement forward and a smaller one backward, and so on, moving at approximately 2 to 3 cm/s. It is clear that the wind has a significant influence on the tempo of the mantid's movements, since the frequency and amplitude of its back-and-forth rocking increases with increasing movement of the surrounding vegetation. Short gusts of wind definitely encourage activity (perhaps eliciting mimicry of the surrounding movement). This suggests that sensory information—both visual and mechanosensory—plays an important role in structuring its locomotion, which, as

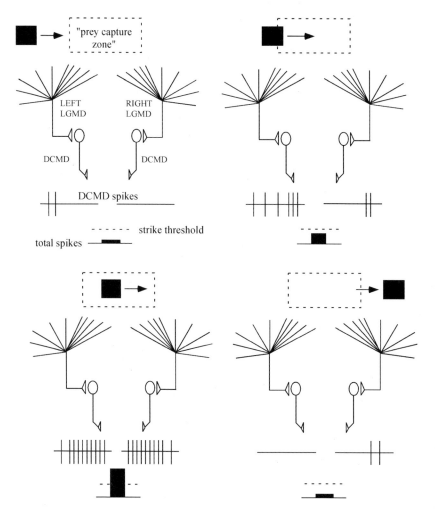

Figure 3.15

These four, sequential schematic drawings indicate how a single pair of LGMD–DCMD complexes can explain how mantids identify, locate, and strike at prey when it is centered in the visual field. Consider the following: Because the putative mantid LGMD is preferentially responsive only to preylike stimuli (represented by the square) moving (rightward, in this case) at a particular speed (i.e., at a speed indicating that the object is within catching range), and because the LGMD's broad dendritic arborization receives relatively more inputs from the densely packed ommatidia of the acute zone, which are sampling the visual field center (the so-called "prey-capture zone"), the LGMD–DCMD complex will respond most vigorously only when a preylike stimulus is moving within catching range in the prey-capture zone. Furthermore, because a threshold number of DCMD spikes is necessary to trigger a strike (strike threshold; see figure 3.13), the initiation of a predatory strike requires the summed activity of a pair of LGMD–DCMD complexes activated by the appropriate constellation of stimulus parameters (indicated by the histogram showing the number of spikes). Note that this model requires neither an explicit comparison of right and left retinal images nor a calculation of retinal disparity.

expected, cannot be explained simply as the product of a rigid central nervous system program.

In contrast to *M. religiosa*, which prefers to remain near ground level, *Empusa fasciata* often climbs from branch to branch in shrubs to reach an exposed perch in the sun. In order to move from one branch to another, it pauses before leaping or reaching and performs side-to-side peering movements with its whole body while facing its targeted branch. It may also take bearings on more than one branch at a time. This procedure is repeated several times before it grasps a branch with its forelegs or risks a leap. As a rule, the nearest and most readily accessible object is chosen. Similar behavior has been observed in other species and in some locusts (figure 3.16).

Experimentally, these types of aimed jumps are preceded by peering movements and can only be elicited when both the mantid's eyes are fully intact (see Walcher and Kral, 1994). Locusts, however, will jump with one eye blinded, although this results in overestimation of the distance (Sobel, 1990). Binocular inputs are apparently important for this type of target localization by mantids (which is analogous to the situation described for prey localization). Binocularity could also be important for linearization of the peering movement. When the insect is peering, each sideways body movement is accompanied by a compensatory counterrotation of the head about

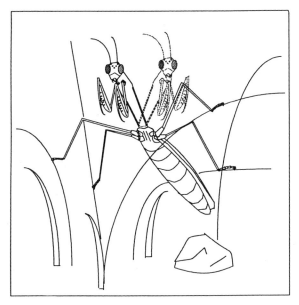
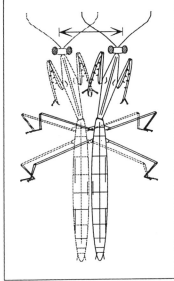

Figure 3.16
Schematic of the side-to-side peering behavior of *Mantis religiosa*. (Drawing by M. Poteser. Reprinted from Kral, 1999, with the kind permission of Johns Hopkins University Press, the author, and the artist.)

the yaw axis, so that the head is always directed straight forward and thus remains oriented toward the target's edge (Kral and Poteser, 1997). It is not yet clear what mechanisms control the linearity of the head movement, although there is some evidence of coordination between the visual system and mechanoreceptors that code head position and movement, particularly those located in the neck (the sternocervical and tergocervical hair plate sensilla; Poteser et al., 1998).

Image Motion Determines an Object's Distance   Side-to-side peering has long been assumed to be associated with estimation of distance (J. S. Kennedy, 1945). By moving a square black landing target in phase or in antiphase to a locust's peering movements, Wallace (1959) could cause it to misestimate the object's distance. The misestimation was caused by the decrease or increase, respectively, of the amplitude and speed of the image's motion. Sobel (1990) performed similar experiments with computer-controlled visual targets. Using the takeoff speed of the jump (which is proportional to an object's distance), he quantified the relationship between under- or overestimation of an object's distance and the perceived movement of a target.

Similarly, in experiments with juvenile *Tenodera sinensis* and *Polyspilota* sp., Poteser and Kral (1995) found that moving targets in antiphase to the mantid's peering caused them to jump short of the target; in-phase movements caused them to overjump. Since the velocity of the mantid's head movement is kept constant during peering, the distance to the target is inversely proportional to the velocity of the retinal image. Thus, as in estimating the distance of prey, image velocity appears to be the cue for estimating distance.

Experimental data indicate that the pendulumlike peering movements associated with walking and climbing appear to be object-related peering movements used to determine the distance of an object (Poteser and Kral, 1995; Kral and Poteser, 1997). Mantids move through their environment in a carefully controlled way, constantly using visual feedback to adjust their locomotion to the prevailing environmental conditions (Kral and Devetak, 1999).

In contrast to other mantids, the peering behavior of the empusid *E. fasciata* includes forward and backward movements containing translational components along the roll axis and rotational components about the pitch axis (Kral and Devetak, 1999). The complexity of these movements may be related to the more complex structure of the surroundings in which *E. fasciata* moves (among the branches of shrubs rather than at the base of grasses). While the translational component of sideways peering plays a role in estimating distance, the forward and backward movements may permit targets to be fixed during peering, allowing the mantid to determine their distance and direction accurately. By changing the peering axis, distance information about objects in a variety of directions could be obtained without the need for turning. Although the rotational component of the peering movements might interfere with the perception of parallax effects (Buchner, 1984), it could be beneficial in serving to intensify brightness contrast, and could permit the insect to scan a more extensive field of view.

Flying

On hot summer days, *Mantis religiosa* males fly from one grass stem to another, perhaps in search of a female. Their fluttering flights, with wingbeat frequencies of about 20 Hz, usually cover only a few meters, and their wings almost brush the heads of the grasses as they fly. The landing is always perfect, even when the target stem is swaying in the breeze. Clearly, the flight and the landing are visually controlled and probably rely to a great extent on the information provided by the optic flow created by the passing background structures.

Their landing reaction is characteristic and always predictable. It begins a few centimeters from the landing site, just at the distance at which the site comes into the binocular field of view. The mantid straightens its body for the approach, stretches its legs forward to bring them into landing position, and simultaneously slows its flight. The whole sequence of behavior lasts approximately 200 ms (figure 3.17) (Kral, 1999).

Quantitative field studies of free-flying mantids are difficult because of the overall unpredictability of their flight paths. In *M. religiosa* males, however, the initial change from a horizontal flight posture to an erect prelanding posture is related to the initial localization of the landing site. During the 120–200 ms between beginning the discrete landing reaction and the landing itself, a number of optical parameters may be

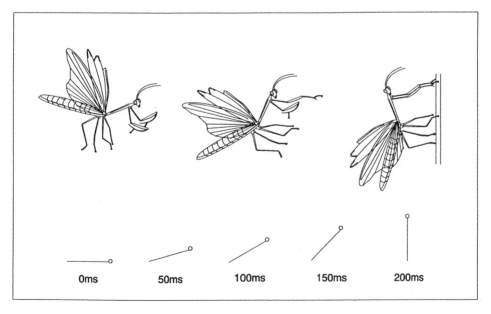

Figure 3.17
Drawings based on video recordings of the landing behavior of a male *Mantis religiosa* in the field. (Drawing by M. Poteser. Reprinted from Kral, 1999, with the kind permission of Johns Hopkins University Press, the author, and the artist.)

assessed by the mantid. These could include landing site distance (via its retinal image velocity) and/or the expansion rate of its image. Any of these cues could elicit the landing reaction.

The simultaneous change to an erect landing posture and the reduction in flight speed cause a downward movement in the retinal flow field that is counteracted to some degree by a downward movement of the head. It is conceivable that these postural changes could go so far as to eliminate the image expansion of the approaching site so as to stabilize its retinal image just prior to landing. Then, any lateral movements of the body or head during the approach would create motion parallaxes that could provide cues to localization of a perch and/or avoidance of obstacle.

Neural Mechanisms Involved in Self-Induced Image Motion

The type of neural processing involved in extracting information from motion parallax and optic flow field in mantids is still unknown. Nondirectional, nonhabituating, movement-sensitive cells that respond to relatively slow image speeds (less than 20 deg/s) may be possible candidates for motion-parallax neurons (see Kral, 1998a,b). However, neurons that are involved in movement-detecting mechanisms that measure image velocity or image displacement created by head translation, and that compare this information with head velocity or displacement, have yet to be found in mantids.

In locusts, Bult and Mastebroek (1994) identified nonhabituating nondirectional motion-detecting optic lobe cells, and Rind (1990a,b) identified a large ipsilaterally projecting movement-sensitive descending interneuron, the PDDSMD, which receives monosynaptic input from a directionally selective movement-sensitive lobular cell. The latter, in conjunction with at least two other ipsilateral, multimodal, movement-sensitive descending interneurons, allows the locust to make compensatory responses, including head movements, to movement over much of the visual field (e.g., Rind, 1987; Burrows, 1996).

Similarly, Gonka et al. (1999) recorded what appears to be several large ipsilaterally projecting movement-sensitive descending interneurons (DIMDs) in the mantid *S. lineola*. These cells responded to both small- and large-field movement over all areas of the visual field tested and in some cases became locked to the sequential 100-ms displacements of the visual stimulus as it moved across the computer screen (figure 3.18). These response characteristics suggest that these cells may play a role in coding motion velocity and/or initiating visual orientation movements. Such cells may also play a role in peering-related estimation of distance and in stabilization and navigation of flight. (See Berger, 1985, for similar cells in *M. religiosa*, and Gewecke and Hou, 1993, for locusts.)

Dynamic Integration of Visual Data Streams

At the level of the lobula complex, the dynamic features of the motion-sensitive neurons are largely determined by the inputs of the medullary elementary motion detectors. In contrast, at the behavioral level, control systems are very different in their dynamic features. For instance, consider again the landing reaction of

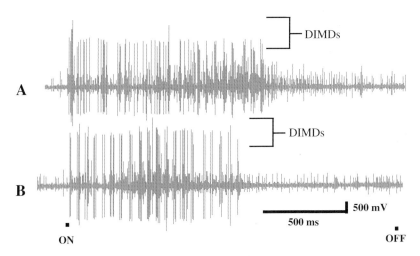

Figure 3.18
Two extracellular recordings (made simultaneously with those in figure 3.12) from the ventral nerve cord ipsilateral to the stimulated eye in a female *S. lineola*. The activity is in response to computer-generated square stimuli that moved horizontally through the center of the visual field. (*A*) The extremely large spikes generated by descending ipsilateral movement detectors (DIMDs) in response to a 5 × 5-deg square moving at 110 deg/s. (*B*) The activity elicited by a very large (77 × 77-deg square) moving at the same speed. Note that DIMD activity occurs over a broader area of the visual field than does DCMD activity (cf. figure 3.13). Furthermore, DIMD activity was tightly linked to the sequential displacements of the stimuli (i.e., the movements of the dark, vertical edges) on the computer screen. This is particularly evident in the 100-ms bursting pattern seen in (*B*). (Redrawn from Gonka et al., 1999, with the kind permission of S. Karger AG, Basel.)

M. religiosa, or the target-directed jump of *E. fasciata*. In the former case, straightening of the body for the approach to a landing site and stretching the legs into the landing position will always be initiated when some internal signal has exceeded a certain threshold. This is analogous to the point made in our discussion of how two LGMD–DCMD complexes might trigger a predatory strike.

The latency of the landing-related body and leg reflexes will vary in a gradual manner, depending on the characteristics of the eliciting stimulus. That is, reaction times will vary with, for instance, the expansion rate of the landing site's image; the faster the image is expanding, the shorter should be the latency to assume the appropriate landing posture. However, in the natural world, it is unlikely that there is a simple linear relationship between the rate of retinal image expansion and the response latencies necessary when landing after a fluttering flight or when jumping toward a nearby branch. Furthermore, we know that in some insects (*Musca*; see Egelhaaf and Borst, 1990) a subliminal stimulus can affect the landing reaction latency elicited by a subsequent stimulus. This suggests that there is a complex, dynamic integration of information in the mantid's landing system, because if only the dynamic features of the elementary motion detectors are taken into account, an initial, subliminal stimulus would have no influence over the latency of the landing reaction. A similar argument could be made regarding predatory strike latency and the associated lunge latencies.

In mantids, dynamic integration of time in landing response latencies seems to be represented in some motion-sensitive lobula output neurons; that is, neurons especially responsive to expanding stimulus patterns. The functional significance of a dynamic integrator linked to a threshold operator will be that, together, they can gradually transform a large range of stimulus values into a small range of reaction times, even if the relationship between the two is complex and/or nonlinear. Thus, a slowly expanding retinal image pattern associated with landing after a fluttering flight will lead to a relatively slow increase in the temporally integrated signals and thus to a long latency for leg stretching; while a more quickly expanding pattern, during a jump, for instance, will yield a much faster leg-stretching reaction.

Conclusion

Thanks to several decades of research in several laboratories, we now know quite a bit about mantid vision. Modern video- and computer-assisted research methods in particular have made substantial contributions in this regard. These have included studies of prey recognition using ethologically meaningful visual stimuli, of prey capture behavior using high-speed videography, and of flying and peering behavior using computer-controlled stimuli and computer-analyzed videography. These studies, in conjunction with detailed anatomical analyses, have opened our eyes to the remarkably complex and, in many ways, vertebratelike visual world of mantids.

In particular, we are struck by two capacities. The first is the mantid's ability to recognize prey based on the use of a perceptual algorithm that would be called abstract reasoning if it were described in a primate. The apparent use of what appears to be prey-selective neurons that integrate a number of key stimulus parameters suggests a new way to conceptualize prey recognition and localization in this insect. The second capacity is the mantid's ability to integrate motion parallax cues with proprioceptive information on head and body movement and position to assess the location and distance of objects in its environment. This tight linkage between visual input and body movement in the assessment of an object's distance is precisely analogous to what is seen in humans.

Of course, it goes without saying that most questions concerning mantid vision remain unanswered. We still have a long way to go before we can link the characteristics and activities of particular neurons and neural networks to specific behaviors. However, an important step forward has been made in that mantid behavior is no longer seen as simplistic, mechanistic, and stereotyped. We recognize, although we may not as yet fully appreciate, the wonderful intricacy of these insects' behavior and the complexity of the perceptual world in which they live.

Acknowledgments
Our research was supported in part by grants from the Austrian Science Foundation to Karl Kral. Frederick Prete has been supported in part by grants from Youngstown (Ohio) State University, Denison University (Granville, Ohio), DePaul University (Chicago, Illinois), The State of Ohio Board of Regents, and The Edmond and Marianne Blaauw Ophthalmology Fund (through Sigma Xi). Special thanks go to six particularly gifted students: Gerd Leitinger, Michael Poteser, Franz Walcher, Mark Gonka, Molly Bullaro, and Kristy (Cleal) Hamilton.

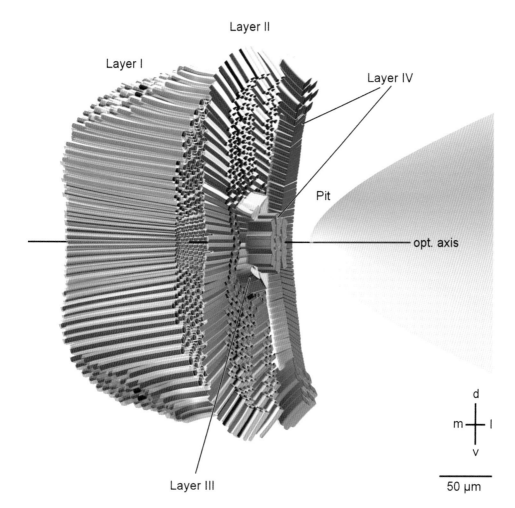

Layer II

Layer I

Layer IV

Pit

opt. axis

d
m ─┼─ l
v

50 µm

Layer III

Plate 1
Structurally complex retina of *Portia fimbriata*'s principal eye. Behind the pit (secondary lens) are four layers of receptors (I, II, III, and IV) stacked along the optical axis. Layers II, III, and IV contain more than one receptor type. Most receptors are short, with irregular transverse cross-sectional profiles. Layer I is highly ordered with well-separated receptive segments. Separation reduces interreceptor interference. Spatial acuities as low as 2.4 min arc are supported by the central fovea of layer I. The orthographic view is taken 55 deg from the inner side of the optical axis (opt. axis) of the secondary lens. d, dorsal; m, medial; l, lateral; v, ventral. Electron micrographs and structural descriptions used to construct the drawing were taken from Williams and McIntyre (1980), Blest et al. (1981), Blest and Price (1984), and Blest (1987). See chapter 1.

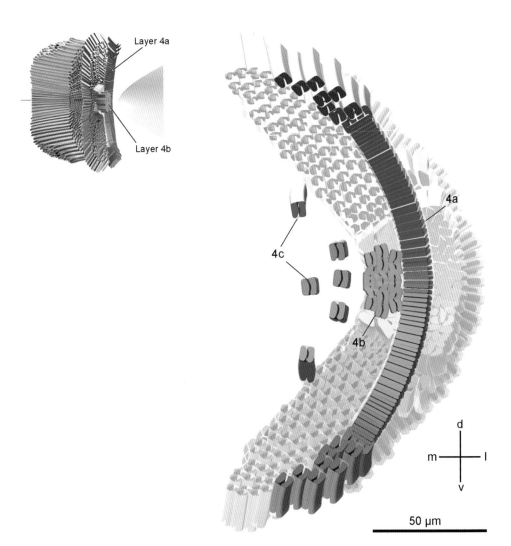

Plate 2

The retina of *Portia fimbriata*'s principal eye showing layer IV (shown in blue) in detail. The position of layer IV relative to other layers within the retina is shown at top left (view angle as in plate 1). The transverse profile of the retina is on the right. Three types of receptors make up layer IV. Type 4a receptors form a well-organized vertical strip that may act as a simple line detector and/or be used to analyze UV polarization. Type 4b receptors form a poorly organized central patch. Type 4c receptors are scattered to the side (their positions within the figure are approximate). No function has been hypothesized for type 4b and 4c receptors. m, medial; l, lateral; d, dorsal; v, ventral. See chapter 1.

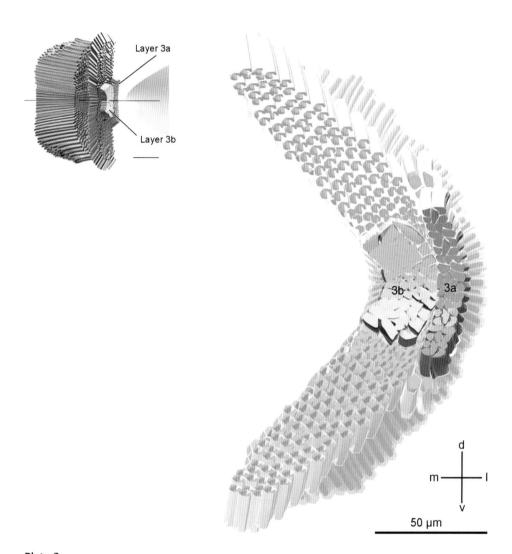

Plate 3

The retina of *Portia fimbriata*'s principal eye showing layer III (shown in yellow-orange) in detail. The position of layer III relative to other retinal layers is shown at top left (view angle as in plate 1). The transverse profile of the retina is on the right. Two types of receptors make up layer III: 3a and 3b receptors, which are large, short, irregularly disposed, and have rhabdomeres that are erratically contiguous. Layer III could receive an in-focus image in blue. The quality of any image sampled by this layer would be poor. See chapter 1.

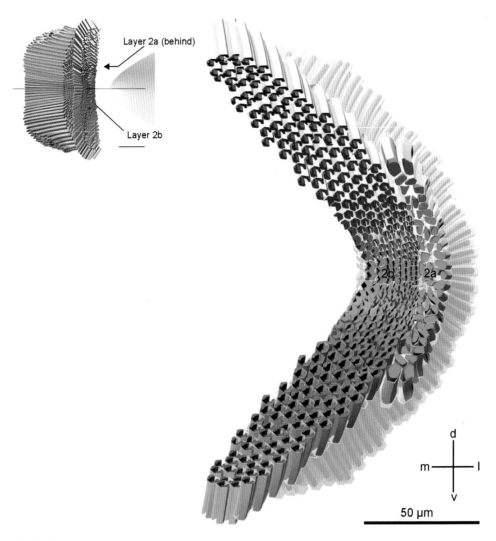

Layer 2a (behind)

Layer 2b

2b   2a

d
m ——┼—— l
v

50 μm

Plate 4

The retina of *Portia fimbriata*'s principal eye showing layer II (shown in green) in detail. The position of layer II relative to layer I is shown at top left (view angle as in plate 1). The transverse profile of the retina is on the right. Two types of receptors make up boomerang-shaped layer II. At the fovea of 2b, receptors have small interreceptor angles (although not as small as in layer I), but are arranged in a disorderly manner. The receptors increase in width toward the periphery of the boomerang arms, and the mosaic becomes more regular. Compared with layer I, receptors in layer II are short. In *P. fimbriata*, layer II does not appear to be adapted for high-acuity vision. d, dorsal; v, ventral; m, median; l, lateral. See chapter 1.

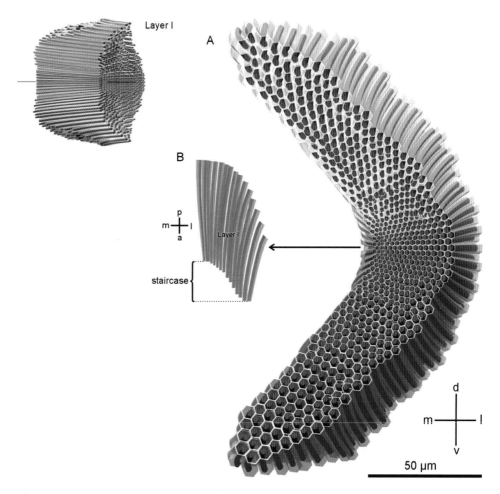

Plate 5

The retina of *Portia fimbriata*'s principal eye showing layer I (shown in red). The top left shows a view 55 deg to the medial side of the optical axis (view angle as in plate 1). (*A*) Transverse profile of the retina showing detail of layer I's boomerang-shaped mosaic. Layer I receptors are characteristically long, with hexagonal cross-sections. The mosaic is regular, formed by rows of receptors. Receptive segments (rhabdomeres) tend to be well separated (reducing interreceptor interference) with spacing as little as 1.4 μm at the fovea. There is a gradual increase in receptor size (and spacing), and gradual decrease in receptor length toward the periphery of the boomerang arms. (*B*) Longitudinal view from above of a row of foveal receptors. These receptors are longest and arranged like a staircase. Images of objects located a few body lengths distant and up to infinity come into focus on the distal (anterior) tips of one or more receptors. d, dorsal; v, ventral; m, median, l, lateral. See chapter 1.

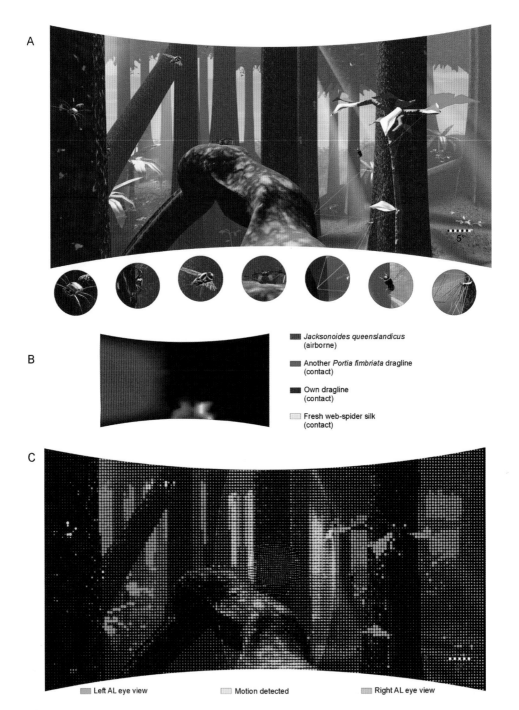

Jacksonoides queenslandicus
(airborne)

Another Portia fimbriata dragline
(contact)

Own dragline
(contact)

Fresh web-spider silk
(contact)

Left AL eye view   Motion detected   Right AL eye view

Plate 6
(Caption on overleaf)

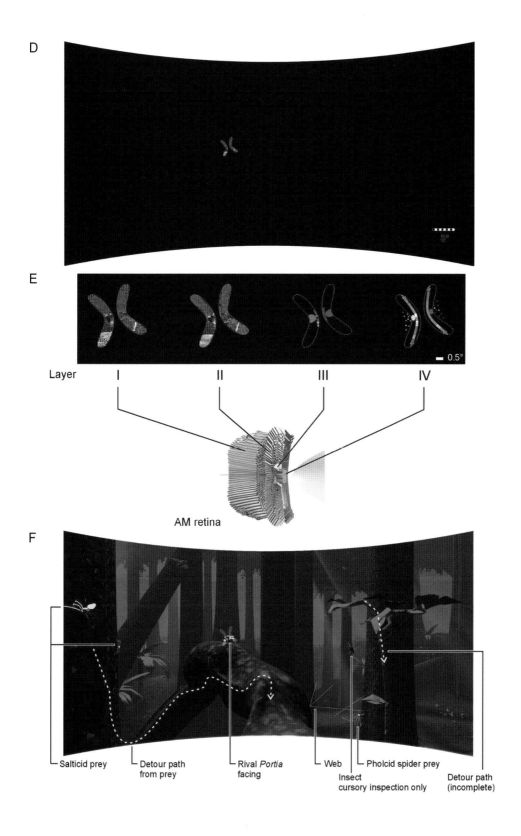

D

E

Layer   I   II   III   IV

0.5°

AM retina

F

Salticid prey   Detour path from prey   Rival *Portia* facing   Web   Pholcid spider prey   Insect cursory inspection only   Detour path (incomplete)

Plate 6
Portia fimbriata's view of the world. (*A*) *Portia*'s forest habitat (approximately 90 deg wide). The circles show some key points of interest for *Portia*. (*B*) Representation of *Portia*'s chemoreceptive environment. (*C*) Representation of the view seen by anterior lateral eyes. Note the region of binocular overlap used in range-finding and foveal regions. (*D*) Field of view provided by anterior median eyes. (*E*) View seen by the four layers of the AM eyes during inspection of other *Portia*. (*F*) View showing elements that *Portia* has abstracted from the scene using its AM eyes during several minutes of looking around. See chapter 1.

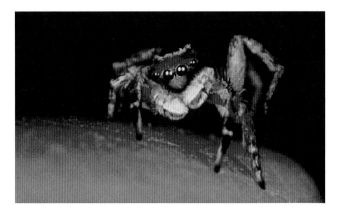

Plate 7
Undescribed adult male salticid from Sri Lanka showing colored patches associated with courtship, including red patches on the femur of each front pair of legs (Photo by D. Harland). See chapter 1.

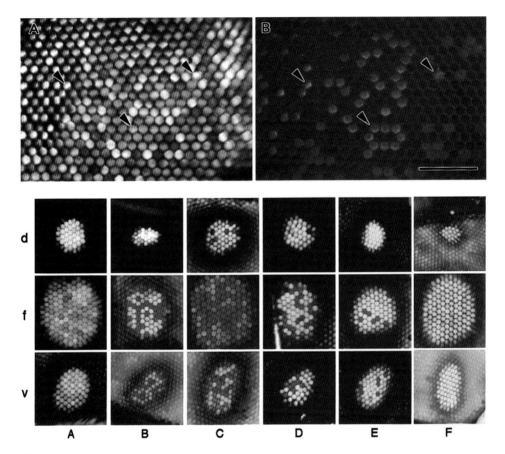

Plate 8

(*A*) Ommatidial pigmentation seen in a fresh eye slice observed in transmitted light, i.e., under antidromic illumination. (*B*) Ommatidial fluorescence observed with ultraviolet epi-illumination of the same preparation as in (*A*). Arrowheads indicate identical ommatidia. The fluorescing ommatidia are pale red or pink in transmission. Scale bar: 100 µm. See chapter 6.

Plate 9

Epi-illumination microscopy showing ommatidial heterogeneity via eye shine in the eyes of various butterfly species: (*A*) *Hypolimnas bolina*, (*B*) *Cyrestis thyodamas*, (*C*) *Argyreus hyperbius*, (*D*) *Euploea mulciber*, (*E*) *Parantica aglea*, (*F*) *Precis almana* (*A–C, F*: Nymphalidae; *D, E*: Danaidae). Dorsal (d), frontal (f), and ventral (v) eye regions were all photographed with the same microscope objective. Because eye shine is observable only in ommatidia that have their visual field coincident with the aperture of the microscope, the density of visual fields (i.e., their spatial acuity) is highest frontally. The eye shine color depends on the species, and the different colors reflect strong heterogeneity. Each figure is 400 x 400 µm². See chapter 6.

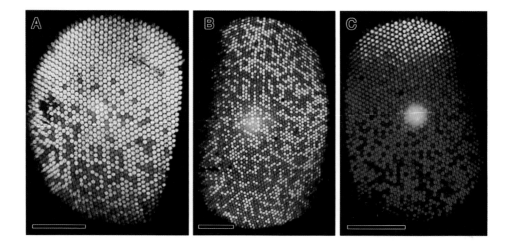

Plate 10

The eye shine pattern in the eyes of (A) the satyrine *Bicyclus anynana*, (B) the heliconian *Heliconius melpomene*, and (C) the small, white *Pieris rapae* observed with a large-aperture optical setup. The ommatidia in the three species reflect either predominantly yellow or red light. The red reflection is absent in a large dorsal area in the eye of *Bicyclus anynana* and in a small dorsal area of *Pieris rapae*. In *Heliconius melpomene*, both reflection types coexist throughout the eye. The central hot spot is due to reflection on the lens surfaces of the microscope objective. The dark areas in (A) and (B) are due to dust specks; the dark facets in (C) have a strong deep-red reflection. Scale bars: 300 μm. See chapter 6.

Plate 11

(*a*) The relative spectral transmittance of the water where the crayfish normally live. (*b*) The shape of the chelae. The female chela (*top*) leaves a space when closed. (*c*) Dorsal view of female and male crayfish. (*d*) Dorsal view of female and male crayfish through a red cut-off (<640 nm) filter. Arrows indicate the bright area in the chelae and telson. (*e*) Spectral reflection curve of the chela from the front and back sides. See chapter 7.

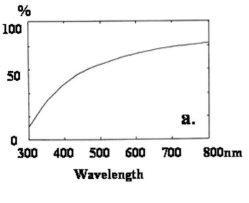

a.

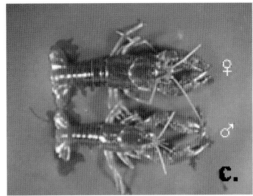

c.

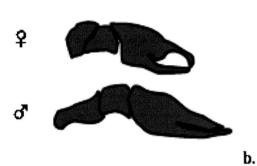

♀

♂

b.

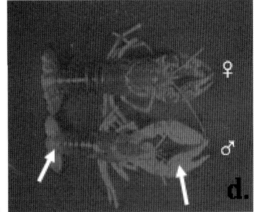

d.

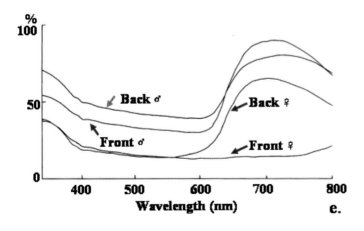

e.

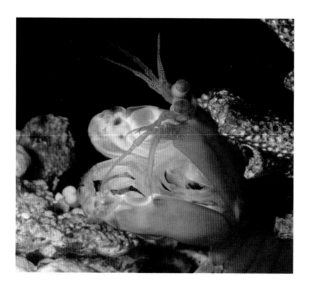

Plate 12

The stomatopod *Gonodactylaceus glabrous*, which is found in the Indo-Pacific. This species is a typical smasher, living on coral reefs. Note how colorful the animal is (particularly the yellow meral spots used in signaling), and the prominent compound eyes at the front end of the cephalothorax. (Photograph by R. L. Caldwell.) See chapter 8.

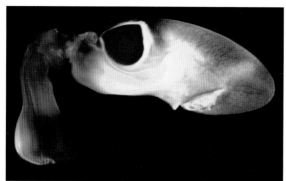

Plate 13

Medial view of the raptorial appendage of *Gonodactylus smithii*, a smasher. Note that the dactyl (the terminal segment) is folded back and that its "heel" is both expanded and armored for hitting prey. The purple meral spot, characteristic of this species, is very prominent. See chapter 8.

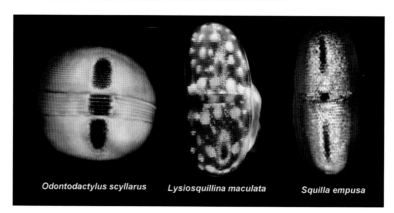

Odontodactylus scyllarus   *Lysiosquillina maculata*   *Squilla empusa*

Plate 14

Eyes of the gonodactyloid stomatopod *Odontodactylus scyllarus*, the lysiosquilloid *Lysiosquillina maculata*, and the squilloid *Squilla empusa*. Gonodactyloids and lysiosquilloids have six-row midbands, while squilloids have only two ommatidial rows here. Note also the three pseudopupils in each eye (the dark spots in particular groups of ommatidia), which indicate the eye regions looking directly at the camera. Three pseudopupils indicate that each eye has trinocular vision. See chapter 8.

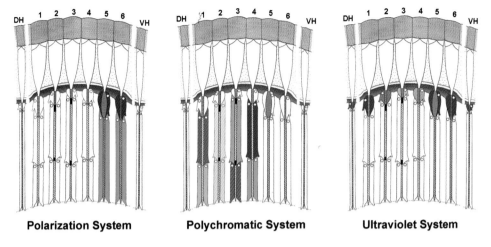

Polarization System **Polychromatic System** **Ultraviolet System**

Plate 15

Schematic views of ommatidia from typical six-row midbands, showing the polarization system (*left*), the polychromatic system (*middle*) and the ultraviolet system (*right*), using the Caribbean species *Neogonodactylus oerstedii* as a model. Midband rows are numbered 1–6 from dorsal to ventral; DH, dorsal hemisphere of the compound eye; VH, ventral hemisphere. In the polarizaion system, blue indicates the eighth (UV sensitive) retinular cells; green indicates cells of the main rhabdom. In the polychromatic system, each color suggests the wavelength range (seen by humans) to which the corresponding receptor class is most sensitive, from violet to red. The right schematic shows the ultraviolet receptors of the midband and peripheral retina, wherein different colors suggest ultraviolet-sensitive cells operating in different spectral regions (the color indicated for R8 cells of row 3 is putative, as these have not yet been characterized). See chapter 8.

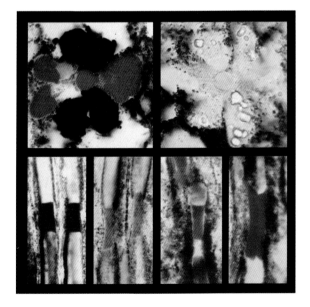

Plate 16

Filter pigments occurring in mid band photoreceptors (rows 1–4) of various stomatopods, to illustrate the spectral diversity as seen in fresh-frozen cryosections. The top two panels are cross sections, while the lower four panels are filters sectioned longitudinally. See chapter 8.

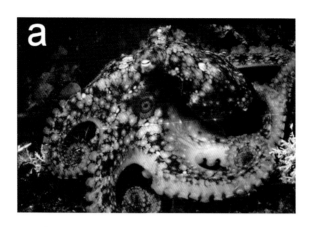

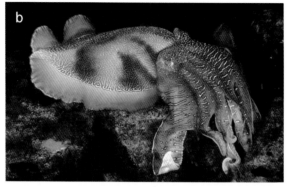

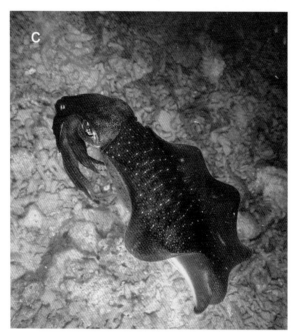

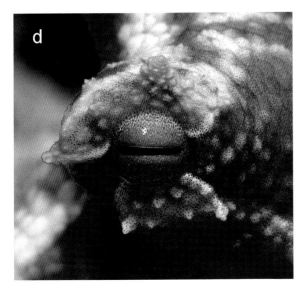

d

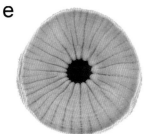

e

Plate 17

(*a–c*) Representatives of modern cephalopods to illustrate some of the main features of these animals. (*a*) *Octopus bimaculatus*, viewed from the left side, with skin color and pattern providing good camouflage against a rocky seabed. The blue and red "bulls-eye" near the center of the picture is an ocellus ("false eye-spot"); the animal's left eye is above this ocellus. Note the lightly coiled arms with many pale-colored suckers. (*b*) A giant cuttlefish (*Sepia apama*, which reaches a body length close to 1 m when fully grown) seen from the right side, hovering just above the seabed. Note the undulating fins (not present in octopuses) and the dark blotches on its back, which are waves of expanding chromatophores moving like the shadows of passing clouds over the otherwise pale body. Note also the arm extending toward the bottom of the picture. Its flattened appearance and different coloring from the other arms are part of a courtship display. (*c*) The loliginid squid *Sepioteuthis lessoniana*. Note its more slender, tubular shape compared with the cuttlefish, the relatively small and slender arms, and the metallic greens and reds of iridescent coloration, particularly on the head. (*d*) Close-up of an octopus's eye with its rectangular, slit-shaped pupil. (*e*) A sucker, 3 cm in diameter, from the arm of *Octopus conspadiceus*. (*a–d* reprinted with permission from M. Norman, *Cephalopods, A World Guide*; a courtesy of Roger Hanlon and Conchbooks, Germany; *b–d* courtesy of Mark Norman, Aquanautica.) See chapter 9.

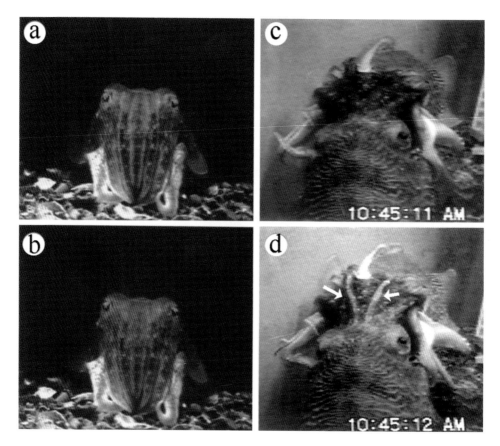

Plate 18

Examples of polarization displays in the cuttlefish, *Sepia officinalis*. (*a*) Full color image. (*b*) False color rendering of the same image. Polarization orientation is coded to hue (horizontal polarization presented as red); the percentage of polarization is coded as saturation: full saturation, fully polarized; gray shades, nonpolarized light; and lightness is proportional to the intensity of light reflected from the object. (*c, d*) Example of a male switching on the polarization pattern during mating (images photographed through a filter transmitting horizontally polarized light). (*c*) No polarization pattern visible. (*d*) Polarization pattern displayed 1 s later (indicated by arrows). (Modified after Shashar et al., 1996.) See chapter 9.

4 Motion Perception Shapes the Visual World of Amphibians
Jörg-Peter Ewert

Lack of Eye Movements: A Challenge for Movement Detection

Dining in a gourmet restaurant, we visually enjoy the arrangement of food items on our plate. A hungry toad faced with this plate would probably see nothing, because no item moves. If a fly landed on the plate, however, the toad would immediately snap at the walking fly. What made this scene different for the toad?

Sensory systems address the perception of changes in the environment. Before the fly appeared, nothing on the plate changed its position. For the toad, the only changes in sensory input would be caused by displacements of its retina relative to the items on the plate. A toad sitting quietly will see nothing because nothing seems to make its retinae move. Unlike toads, however, humans view the stationary scene with moveable eyes. We collect visual information in terms of stimulus changes in a way comparable to a blind man exploring an object with his moving fingertip, collecting information from a constantly changing stream of tactile sensations. Hence, a prerequisite of visual perception is an interaction between vision and motor systems.

Although toads and frogs have eight extraocular eye muscles, their eyes display no information-collecting movements comparable to those of mammals. However, certain kinds of saccades are responsible for optokinetic nystagmus (e.g., Grüsser and Grüsser-Cornehls, 1976). Furthermore, their eyes can be re- and protracted to prevent the cornea from drying out or to aid swallowing. The question of whether passive "respiratory" eye movements (Schipperheyn, 1963) coupled with periodic pressure changes in the buccal cavity allow frogs or toads to monitor their stationary visual world is disputed (Ewert and Borchers, 1974). Toads and frogs must move, or just have moved, their head or body to detect a stationary object.

This lack of information-collecting eye movements creates a particular salience for objects that move. Three main types of behavior correspond to this perceptual specialization: catching prey, avoiding predators, and approaching mates (for reviews see Muntz, 1977b; Ingle, 1983; Ewert, 1984, 1987, 1997; Grobstein, 1991). Hence, a number of experimental questions arise. (1) Since moving objects are typically associated with prey, predator, or mate, how are these objects categorized and discriminated? (2) Since information on a stationary obstacle can be obtained from retinal shifts caused by the toad's movement, how are retinal images of moving objects discriminated from self-induced moving images? (3) Since humans must learn to identify things, whereas toads seem to "know" many things, do toads have internal representations of prey or do they use abstract schemas and what, if anything, do toads learn? (4) Since toads have no cerebral neo(iso)cortex, where and how are visual stimuli analyzed? (5) Does vision integrate with other sensory modalities? (6) How is vision integrated into networks, the mammalian homologues of which are responsible for directional attention and learning?

Investigations of these questions are multidisciplinary, and span levels of analysis from behavior to the neuron and back. The advantage of this approach is that a number of questions are directed at the same topic, creating an integrated body of data that can be understood from many points of view.

What a Toad Sees in Terms of Visually Guided Behavior

We can hardly imagine what a toad sees, but the type and the frequency of its response to an object can tell us how the toad treats and evaluates that object in a behavioral context.

Catching Patterns Used in Prey Capture

A toad sits in the twilight in front of its shelter. A millipede crosses its visual field. The toad responds with orienting (o), approaching (a), binocular fixating (f), and snapping (s) (Schneider, 1954). The release of each response requires recognition of the millipede as prey, and the decision to snap requires the localization of the prey in three-dimensional space. If the prey appears near the toad, o, s or f, s or just s occurs. If the prey flees, then $o, o, o, a, o, a, f, a, f, o, f, s$ may be the pattern.

Questions of "what" and "where" precede the ballistic responses. Once triggered, orienting toward prey proceeds to completion based on both visual and proprioceptive input (Comer et al., 1985) without feedback from the target during the movement (Grobstein et al., 1983). Toads also preprogram a route before they start to move (Collett, 1983). Frogs may display "compound motor coordinations" (jumping and snapping; Ingle, 1970) that involve feedback-guided correctional maneuvers (Gans, 1961). Internal feedback enriches the behavioral variability and adaptability of such sensory and motor tasks (Nishikawa and Gans, 1992; Nishikawa, 1999). This feedback includes afferent information from the tongue and visual information regarding the type of prey, which can interact and create the appropriate catching pattern (e.g., jaw or tongue grasping; C. W. Anderson, 1993; C. W. Anderson and Nishikawa, 1993, 1996, 1997a,b; Weerasuriya et al., 1994; Valdez and Nishikawa, 1997; Harwood and Anderson, 2000). In addition, both frogs and toads often use their forelimbs to capture and transport prey, and some species even use limb grasping in place of tongue grasping (Gray et al., 1997).

Visual Features in Prey Recognition

Investigations of stomach contents show that most anurans feed on earthworms, slugs, wood lice, millipedes, various kinds of beetles, and other small invertebrates (Porter, 1972; also see Clarke, 1974). All these have one feature in common—they move in the direction of their longer body axis. Hence, because an object must move to be categorized as prey, the distinction between prey and nonprey is based on the object's size and shape relative to its direction of movement.

Shape and Movement   During evolution, a visual processing structure emerged that allows terrestrial amphibians to discriminate moving objects in terms of their extensions parallel to (*ep*) and across (*ea*) their direction of movement (Ewert, 1968, 1974; for a review, see Ewert, 1984; see also Wachowitz and Ewert, 1996). Relating the features *ep* and *ea* to each other provides a key for categorizing objects. Experiments using flat, two-dimensional stimuli have shown how efficiently such an *ep/ea* features-relating algorithm operates (figure 4.1, top). Extending a bar along *ep*, within limits, signals prey. Extending a bar along *ea* reduces its prey value. Hence, in discriminating between prey and nonprey, the feature *ea* is decisive. In fact, prey selection is sharpest for stimuli of maximal configurational contrast; that is, a bar moving in the direction of its long axis (prey configuration) versus the same bar oriented across its direction of movement (nonprey configuration). In this configurational paradigm, the preference prey versus nonprey increases with bar length and is invariant under changes of speed, movement dynamics, and direction of movement in the *x*, *y*, *z*-axes (Ewert, 1984). However, the configurational selectivity is significantly sharper for dark objects moving against a bright background than for the reverse. This suggests the importance of neural *off*-systems.

Luthardt and Roth (1979) repeated our studies using the urodele *Salamandra salamandra*. They assumed that at high speed a horizontal bar moving in the horizontal direction should be a weaker prey-catching releaser in salamanders than the same bar oriented across the direction of movement. Unfortunately, this phenomenon could not be reproduced in other laboratories (e.g., Himstedt, 1982; Finkenstädt and Ewert, 1983a).

If stimuli are configurationally neutral (i.e., $ep:ea = 1$), as with squares, the influences of *ep* and *ea* interact and the area $ep \times ea$ is decisive for prey selection. This requires the estimation of absolute size in conjunction with depth perception (Ingle, 1972; Ingle and Cook, 1977; Ewert, 1984; Wiggers and Roth, 1994). Testing various anuran species of different body sizes, we found that $l = 0.43j$ (cm) describes the relation between the optimal edge length *l* of a square prey dummy and the snout width *j*.

The *ep-ea* features-relating algorithm is present after metamorphosis to terrestrial predatory life and it is common among members of an anuran species. However, it displays species-specific variation, is subject to the effects of maturation during ontogeny, and can be modified by learning (Ewert, 1984, 1992; Ewert et al., 2001).

Evaluating *ep* and *ea* is clearly not the only way amphibians characterize visual objects. For instance, looming patterns release avoidance behaviors and stationary obstacles elicit detouring behavior (Ingle, 1971, 1976a, 1977, 1983). Furthermore, the pattern of stimulus movement can dramatically influence the efficacy of a prey object (Borchers et al., 1978). In addition, frogs exhibit different capture strategies for visually different types of prey, where *ep* versus *ea* provides only part of the necessary pattern recognition attributes (C. W. Anderson, 1993; C. W. Anderson and Nishikawa, 1993, 1996; Weerasuriya et al., 1994; Valdez and Nishikawa, 1997; Gray et al., 1997).

Prey catching also depends on other visual stimulus qualities (such as color) and other sensory modalities (such as touch and olfaction) that contribute to, rather than

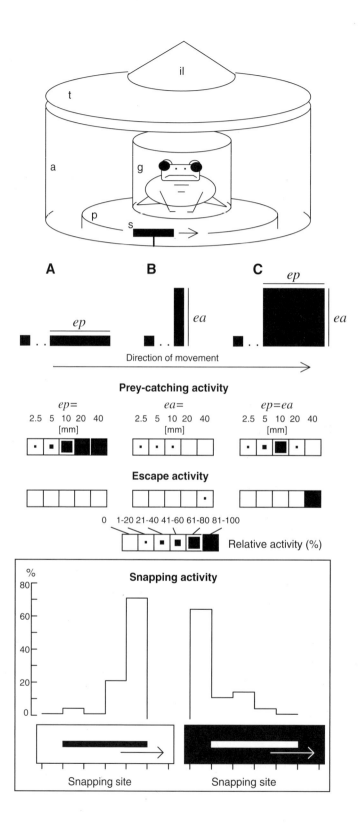

A   **B**   **C**

ep   *ea*   *ep*   *ea*

Direction of movement

Prey-catching activity

ep=   *ea=*   *ep=ea*

2.5   5   10   20   40   2.5   5   10   20   40   2.5   5   10   20   40

[mm]   [mm]   [mm]

Escape activity

0   1-20   21-40   41-60   61-80   81-100

Relative activity (%)

Snapping activity

%

80

60

40

20

0

Snapping site   Snapping site

detract from, the visual configuration preferences described here (e.g., see Dole et al., 1981; Grobstein et al., 1983; Kondrashev, 1987). For example, the effects of stimulus-specific habituation show that toads can discriminate a variety of visual cues, such as the shapes of a leading edge versus the trailing edge and isolated dots and striped patterns (figure 4.2) (Ewert, 1984; Wang and Ewert, 1992).

Concerted Action of Shape, Movement, and Contrast   Ingle and McKinley (1978) described one other kind of configurational cue. If a black prey like bar is moved against a white background, toads and frogs snap predominantly at its leading edge (figure 4.1, bottom). This "head preference" is independent of stimulus velocity (within physiological limits), the length of the stimulus, and the background texture. However, if the stimulus background contrast is reversed (white bar, black background), Burghagen and Ewert (1982) showed that common toads snap preferably toward the trailing edge. How can this phenomenon be explained? As mentioned, *off*-stimuli from contrast borders are important cues for prey selection. *Off* effects occur at the leading edge of a black bar moving against a white background and at the trailing edge of a white bar moving against a black background. Actually, in the latter case, toads snap behind the white bar.

Self-Induced Moving Images   Does a toad ignore a nonmoving prey? Toads (Ingle, 1971) and salamanders (Himstedt et al., 1978) may snap at a motionless prey-sized object after it has moved. In salamanders, snapping toward stationary prey also occurs if another nearby moving stimulus has just elicited an approach (Himstedt, 1982).

The environment of the toad is variegated. It includes leaves, branches, and stones, many of which are prey size. Why does the toad ignore these other prey-sized

◀ **Figure 4.1**
A features-relating algorithm in the visual perception of toads. (*Top*) Experimental procedure for quantitative measurements of the toad's prey-catching orienting activity toward a rectangular, black, visual stimulus (s) circling around the toad *Bufo bufo* at a constant visual angular velocity (v =) of 10 deg/s. a, opaque arena; g, cylindrical glass vessel; il, diffuse illumination; p, pedestal; s, motor-driven stimulus of black cardboard; t, transparent screen. Starting with a small square of 2.5 × 2.5 mm, various dimensions were changed in three stimulus sets at four steps in each set: (A) the length *ep* parallel to the direction of movement, (B) the length *ea* across the direction of movement, and (C) both *ep* and *ea* (*ep* = *ea*). In each set the stimuli were presented at random. The behavioral activity (prey-catching or escape responses per 30 s for *n* = 20 individuals) are expressed as a percent of the responses to the optimal stimulus of each stimulus set (A, B, or C). (Adapted from Ewert, 1997.) (*Bottom*) The contrast-dependent head or tail preference phenomenon. Distribution of *B. bufo's* snapping rates across a 2.5 × 40-mm bar moving preylike at 18 deg/s horizontally from left to right: black bar versus white background (left) or white bar versus black background (right). Averages for *n* = 20 individuals in percent of the total snapping rates. (Adapted from Burghagen and Ewert, 1982.)

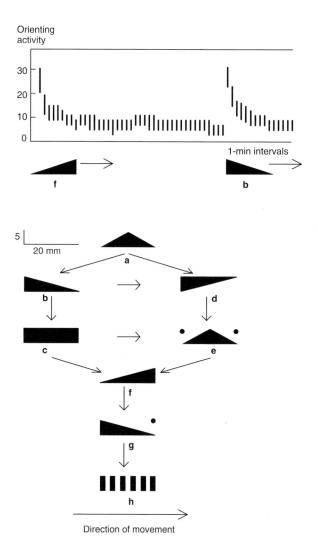

Figure 4.2
Visual cues discriminated by learning. Stimulus-specific habituation shows that *Bufo bufo* toads can discriminate various details within the preylike shape of a 5 × 20-mm stimulus moving at *v* = 20 deg/s in the direction of the arrow. (*Top*) Average prey-catching orienting activity (responses ± S.D. per 1-min interval) toward a triangle (stimulus f). After a decrease in response as a result of habituation, the triangle's mirror image (stimulus b) is presented and it immediately elicits full prey-catching activity (dishabituation). (*Bottom*) Dishabituation hierarchy. The arrows indicate that a stimulus (e.g., a) dishabituates another stimulus (e.g., b), but not vice versa. For stimuli linked by horizontal arrows, dishabituation is mutual, with a preference indicated by the arrow. (Adapted from Ewert and Kehl, 1978, cited in Ewert, 1984.)

objects when a head movement makes their retinal images move? There are two possible explanations. The first is based on the "reafference principle," which would claim that information about the toad's own body movement will cancel the effects of voluntary movements on the retinal image signal (von Holst and Mittelstaedt, 1950). The second explanation involves surround inhibition, by which the self-induced simultaneous movement of the many retinal images suppresses prey capture (e.g., see Frost, 1982).

A simple experiment invalidates the first hypothesis. If the toad moves in a homogeneous (untextured) environment, the self-induced moving retinal image of a stationary prey object readily elicits orienting and snapping responses (Burghagen and Ewert, 1983). Tests of the second hypothesis have shown that retinal images from a number of simultaneously moving preylike stimuli also inhibit prey capture (Schneider, 1954; Ewert, 1984). Furthermore, if an object and its background texture move in phase, the object is masked by the background.

Nonvisual Cues Used in Prey Recognition

Orienting and snapping responses can also be elicited by tactile stimuli to the snout, the forelimbs, or the hindlimbs (Grobstein et al., 1983). It is also the case that olfactory and gustatory cues—in combination with visual cues—play a role in the toad's learning how prey recognition should be generalized or made more discriminating (Sternthal, 1974; Shinn and Dole, 1979a,b; Dole et al., 1981; Merkel-Harff and Ewert, 1991). For instance, toads and frogs learn to avoid distasteful red earthworms (Ewert, 1984), to retreat from bombardier beetles after chemical irritation (H. Dean, 1980a,b), and to escape hive bees after even just one painful sting (Cott, 1936; S. O. G. Lindemann and Roth, 1999; see also L. P. Brower et al., 1960; H. V. Z. Brower and Brower, 1962).

Predator Avoidance

Natural predators include some snakes, predatory birds, and hedgehogs. Hedgehogs can tolerate toad venom in relatively high concentrations, and they use this venom in their own defense (Brodie, 1977). The hognose snakes, *Heterodon* spp., are primarily toad predators. Under captive conditions these snakes will not eat frogs unless they are "scented" by rubbing them with fresh toad skin.

Depending on the visual features of a predator and its location in space, toads display different types of avoidance (Eibl-Eibesfeldt, 1951; Schneider, 1954; Ingle, 1976a; Ewert, 1984). For instance, in an ambiguous but threatening situation (e.g., when viewing a nonpreylike moving bar), the toad sits motionless in a "frozen" posture, while it activates poison-secreting skin glands. If it is faced with a terrestrial predator, the toad blows up its lymphatic sacs, making its body appear bigger than normal. Flying predators elicit defensive ducking and entrenching movements with the hind legs. A predator that appears in the visual field may elicit jumping or, if it appears in a localized area of the visual field, it can elicit turning or escape movements that are directed away from the predator's location. Finally, in the case of a predatory snake, the toad assumes a stiff-legged posture, presenting its body in a shieldlike display.

The visual releasers of escape behavior are manyfold and include large moving areas, looming objects, or shadows (figure 4.1, top) (Schneider, 1954; Ingle, 1976a; Ewert, 1984). Snakes that are the toad's archenemies have certain configurational features that involve elongated shapes oriented perpendicular to their direction of movement (Ewert and Traud, 1979).

Detecting the Stationary World

The toad's or frog's stationary environment includes apertures, barriers, and textures. These may be associated with obstacles, shelters, or hiding places; or they may serve as cues for orientation.

Textures in the Use of Orientation   In the field, threatened frogs escape from a grassy bank toward a pond (Ingle, 1976b). This pond-seeking behavior is explained by positive phototaxis. For instance, *Rana pipiens* is strongly attracted by the short (blue) wavelength of the sky reflected in water (Kicliter and Goytia, 1995; see also Muntz, 1962a,b; 1977a,b; Reuter and Virtanen, 1972). Having entered the pond, frogs usually respond with a reorientation toward the bank, suggesting a perception of the bank's texture.

In fact, tadpoles of *Rana aurora* that are exposed to vertical stripes early in their lives will, after metamorphosis as frogs, prefer vertical stripes when reorienting toward a pond bank. In contrast, tadpoles of the same species exposed to black squares or those reared without any specific experience of patterns will, after metamorphosis as frogs, show no preference for the striped test stimulus (Wiens, 1970, 1972). Hence, vertically striped textures are an effective stimulus for this sort of imprinting. In *Rana cascade* it is not vertical stripes but black squares that are most effective for imprinting. This species difference can be interpreted as adaptations to the different habitats of the two frogs. *Rana cascade* lives in a mountain biotope with a patchy substrate, and *R. aurora* lives in a valley biotope among vertical plant stems.

Striped Patterns May Signal Obstacles or Shelters   Ingle (1971, 1982) showed that in *Rana pipiens* vertically oriented edges play a role in barrier detection. Frightened frogs even jump away from a vertically patchy striped texture, but approach an appropriate horizontally patchy striped texture (Ingle, 1983). In fact, frogs show a preference to orient toward and jump through horizontal apertures.

We confirmed Ingle's data in a different experimental paradigm (H.-G. Meyer and J.-P. Ewert, unpublished results). A toad sat in the center of a cylindrical homogeneous white arena, in a small starting corridor whose orientation was changed randomly (figure 4.3). The arena wall consisted of sixteen equidistant sectors. At sector 1, various 7.5×7.5-cm stationary patterns could be attached: a horizontal grid, an oblique grid, a vertical grid, a Julesz texture, and a white surface or a black surface. We measured the number of wall contacts by the toad after the animal spontaneously left the

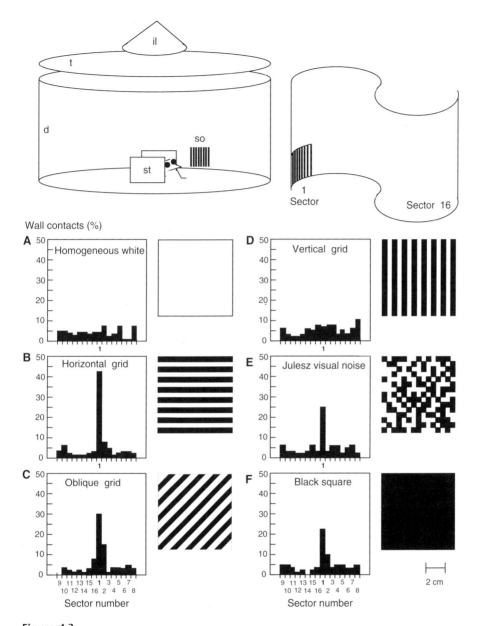

Figure 4.3
Certain stationary objects encourage toads to approach them. *Bufo bufo*, sitting in the center of a white drum, has the opportunity to walk spontaneously toward the wall, which is divided into sixteen equidistant sectors (cf. schematic view of the inner part of the drum, right). d, opaque drum of 189-mm diameter; il, diffuse illumination; t, transparent screen; st, starting corridor with toad; so, stationary object, 75 × 75 mm, attached to sector 1. Different objects can be attached to sector 1: (*A*) white sector, (*B*) horizontal grid, (*C*) oblique grid, (*D*) vertical grid, (*E*) Julesz texture, (*F*) or black square. Average number (percent) of wall contacts by different toads: (*A*) *n* = 25, 125 trials; (*B*) *n* = 20, 100 trials; (*C*) *n* = 20, 100 trials; (*D*) *n* = 25, 175 trials; (*E*) *n* = 25, 125 trials; and (*F*) *n* = 20, 100 trials.

corridor. Toads showed a strong preference for sector 1 if the horizontal grid was attached to it. Preferences were less strong to the oblique grid, the Julesz texture, or the black surface. However, they showed no preference if the vertical grid or the white surface was attached to it.

Vertical Grid in the Use of Conditioned Place Responses   Can toads be trained to approach the aversive vertical grid? After toads were fed several times with mealworms placed in front of the vertical grid, they did indeed approach it if (1) both the grid and the familiar odor of mealworms were offered, (2) only the grid was present, or (3) the location of the previously presented grid was scented with the familiar prey odor. Although the percentage of direct approaches decreased from (1) to (3), it was significantly higher than in experiments in which no associated visual or olfactory cue was offered (H.-G. Meyer and J.-P. Ewert, unpublished results).

These results are in accord with suggestions that in the wild, olfactory cues associated with landmarks may be important orientation labels, for example, during toads' migration toward ponds in the mating season (Ishii et al., 1995). Similarly, Himstedt and Plasa (1979) showed that homing salamanders use stationary visual patterns such as trees and stones as orientation markers.

What a Toad Sees in Terms of Neuronal Responses

In anuran amphibians, the visual field of the retina is retinotopically mapped mainly in the contralateral mesencephalic optic tectum (figure 4.4A) and the pretectal thalamus. These retinal projection fields are connected with each other directly or indirectly (Gaze, 1958, 1984, 1989; Trachtenberg and Ingle, 1974; Wilczynski and Northcutt, 1977; Ewert, 1984; Montgomery and Fite, 1991; Montgomery et al., 1991; Dicke and Roth, 1996). Retinotopic order means that each portion in the visual field corresponds to appropriate areas, respectively, in the retinal projection fields.

First let us describe the properties of retinal ganglion cells and neurons of the retinal projection fields in terms of their receptive fields. The (visual) receptive field of such a neuron is morphologically determined by the area of (photo-) receptors whose outputs converge via interconnected neurons toward that neuron. The physiological property of that neuron is determined by the computations of the corresponding neuronal network in which this neuron is integrated.

Retinal Ganglion Cells

Retinal ganglion cells (R) mediate the output of the retinal network. Recording studies reveal at least four different ganglion cell classes, R1 to R4 (table 4.1). Each cell expresses the computation of a functional unit of cell assemblies and sends this information primarily contralaterally along its axon via the optic nerve to the superficial tectal layers (classes R1–R4; Barlow, 1953; Lettvin et al., 1959; Grüsser et al., 1967; Ewert and Hock, 1972; Székely and Lázár, 1976; Scalia, 1976; Lázár, 1984), pretectal

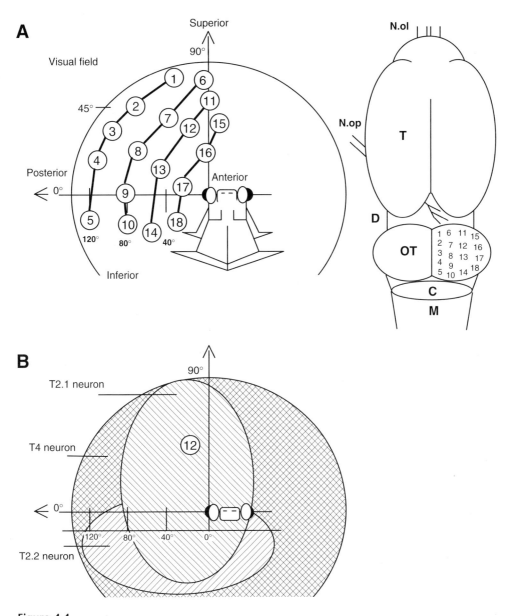

Figure 4.4
(*A*) The visual field of the common toad's eye (left) is mapped on the superficial layers of the contralateral (right) optic tectum (cf. numbers). The fiber endings of retinal ganglion cells recorded from tectal site 12, for example, respond when a visual object is moved at the visual field locus 12. (*Right*) Dorsal view of the toad's brain. T, telencephalon; D, diencephalon; OT, optic tectum; C, cerebellum; M, medulla oblongata; N.ol. olfactory nerve; N.op., optic nerve. (*B*) Receptive fields of tectal wide-field neurons encompassing the anterior visual field (T2.1 neuron), the inferior visual field (T2.2 neuron), or the entire visual field (T4 neuron). (Adapted from Ewert and Borchers, 1971, cited in Ewert, 1984.)

Table 4.1
Response properties of examples of retinal ganglion cells (R), tectal neurons (T), and pretectal thalamic neurons (TH) in anuran amphibians

Type	Response properties
R1	Monocular excitatory receptive field (ERF) of 2–3 deg diameter; optimal stimulus size 2–3 deg; very sensitive to moving contrast stimuli; minimal detectable stimulus velocity, 0.02 deg/s; after stopping the stimulus in the ERF center, the sustained responses are erasable after darkening and brightening the visual field; responsive to chromatic stimuli
R2	Monocular ERF = 4–6 deg; similar to R1 except optimal stimulus size is 4–6 deg; no erasability of sustained responses after stopping the stimulus in the ERF; strong neuronal adaptation after repetitive ERF traverses; weak responses to moving large textures
R3	Monocular ERF = 8–10 deg; optimal stimulus size is 8–10 deg; very responsive to changes in stimulus contrast; minimal detectable stimulus velocity, ~0.1 deg/s; brisk *on/off*-responses to sudden changes in general diffuse illumination; strong responses to moving large textures; responsive to chromatic stimuli
R4	Monocular ERF = 12–16 deg; responses to moving dark objects, optimal stimulus size is larger than 16 deg; lasting *off*-responses to dimming of the entire visual field
T1.3	Nasal binocular ERF = 15–30 deg; responsive to objects moving at a narrow distance; involving properties of T5.1 neurons
T3	Nasal monocular ERF = 20–30 deg; sensitive to approaching small objects; involving properties of R3
T4	ERF encompassing the visual field of the contralateral eye or of both eyes; sensitivity like that of T5.1 or T5.2; showing no (or weak) responses to moving large textures
T5.1	Monocular ERF = 20–30 deg; sensitive to moving objects of small or intermediate size; configurationally, preferring object extension parallel to the direction of movement; involving some properties of R2 and R3, but showing no (or weak) responses to moving large textures
T5.2	Monocular ERF = 20–30 deg; sensitive to small objects, with special preference to objects elongated parallel to the direction of movement; involving some properties of T5.1, showing no responses to moving large textures
T5.3	Monocular ERF = 20–30 deg; sensitive to moving large objects; configurationally, preferring object extension across the direction of movement; involving some properties of R3, R4, and TH3
T5.4	Monocular ERF ~35 deg; sensitive to moving large compact objects; involving some properties of R3 and R4
T6	Monocular dorsal wide ERF; sensitive to moving large objects; involving properties of R4
TH3	Monocular ERF = 40–50 deg; sensitive to moving large objects; configurationally, preferring object extension across the direction of movement; strong responses to moving large textures; involving properties of R3 and R4

Table 4.1 (continued)

Type	Response properties
TH4	ERF encompassing the visual field of the contralateral eye or of both eyes; sensitive to moving large objects; involving visual properties of R3, R4, and TH3; there are neurons also showing sensitivity to cutaneous stimuli
TH6	Monocular wide ERF; sensitive to approaching large objects; involving some properties of T3
TH10	Frontal ERF = 30–90 deg; sensitive or specifically responsive to large stationary objects; involving some visual properties of R1, R3, or R4; there are neurons also showing sensitivity to cutaneous stimuli
TH11	ERF encompassing the visual field of the contralateral eye; response property similar to TH3 or TH4; unlike TH3 and TH4, movement of an object only from temporal to nasal visual field positions is effective
X	Hypothetical tegmental neurons computing retinal topography and body segment orientation

Monocular ERFs refer to the eye contralateral to the neuron's recording site.

neuropil (classes R1, R3, and R4; Ingle, 1983; Ewert, 1984), or other diencephalic targets such as the anterior thalamus (e.g., class R3; Muntz, 1962a,b, 1977a,b; Lázár, 1971; Grüsser and Grüsser-Cornehls, 1976).

The R-type neurons are tuned to objects of different sizes owing to the different sizes of their roughly circular excitatory receptive fields (ERF), which are surrounded by an inhibitory receptive field (figure 4.5A). These neurons are best activated by objects that fill their ERF (figure 4.5E,F). The diameters of their ERFs are as follows: R1 neurons, 2–3 deg; and R2 neurons, 4–6 deg; R3 neurons, 8–10 deg; and R4 neurons, 12–16 deg. A walking fly, for instance, will activate R2 and R3 strongly and a hedge-hog will activate R4 and R3 strongly.

The R-type neurons prefer different ranges of stimulus velocity; R1 and R2 are very sensitive to relatively low speed, and R3 and R4 are sensitive to relatively high speed. Class R1 and R2 neurons not only discharge if an object enters their ERF, they continue to fire for several seconds after the object stops in the ERF center, probably telling the brain "a small object approached and it is still there."

The R-type neurons display different sensitivities to abrupt diffuse darkening (*off*) and brightening (*on*) of the visual field. The R1 neurons show no response; R2 may show a weak *on* response; R3 neurons show a brisk *on-off* activity; and R4 neurons respond with lasting *off* discharges. Whereas R4 neurons detect mainly shadowing, R3 neurons monitor different stimulus events, such as the flickering water turbulences of a pond, moving textures, or moving contrast borders. For example, *off* dominating R3 neurons display a similar contrast direction-dependent head versus tail (or tail versus head) preference, as observed in the toad's snapping behavior (Burghagen and Ewert,

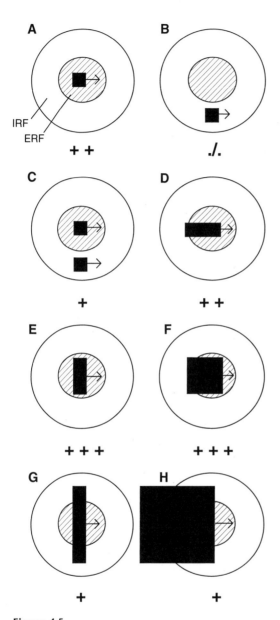

Figure 4.5
The responses of a retinal ganglion cell to moving objects depend on the traverses of portions of the neuron's excitatory receptive field (ERF) and portions of its inhibitory receptive field (IRF). The example is of a class R2 neuron. (A) Moderate response to a small black square that traverses the center of the ERF. (B) No response if the same object traverses a portion of the IRF. (C) The response to the object traversing the ERF is inhibited if at the same time a second object traverses the IRF at the same velocity. (D,E) A bar traversing the

1982; Tsai and Ewert, 1987). Among R3 cells there are also wavelength-sensitive neurons that show opponent color responses: *off* response to red, *on* responses to blue (Reuther and Virtanen, 1972). Such neurons may be involved in phototaxis through their projections to the anterior thalamus (Muntz 1962a,b, 1977a,b; Kicliter, 1973).

Toward a first synopsis, we might conclude that R-type neurons contribute to the analysis of various objects in the anuran's visual world. Visual perception, however, involves parallel distributed and convergent processing of retinal outputs in the retinal projection fields of the brain.

Tectal and Pretectal Thalamic Neurons

Morphological Survey   Morphologically distinct types of tectal neurons are suitable for collecting various retinal inputs, processing them by intrinsic and extrinsic links, and mediating the output to diencephalic, tegmental, or bulbar-spinal targets (figure 4.6) (e.g., Székely and Lázár, 1976; Weerasuriya and Ewert, 1981; Lázár et al., 1983b; Lázár, 1984; Tóth et al., 1985; Matsumoto et al., 1986). In the pretectal thalamic region, certain neurons pick up retinal input from the adjacent pretectal neuropil (Lázár, 1979, 1984, 1989; Matsumoto, 1989). The pretectal thalamic nuclei are divided into a lateral posterodorsal (Lpd), a lateral posteroventral (Lpv), and a dorsomedial posterior (P) nucleus (Neary and Northcutt, 1983). Neuroanatomical investigations of thalamic-tectal connections showed that pretectal thalamic cells project to the tectum (Wilczynski and Northcutt, 1977; Neary and Northcutt, 1983; Weerasuriya and Ewert, 1983; Kozicz and Lázár, 1994), whereas some tectal cells send axons to thalamic nuclei (Lázár et al., 1983b; Bieger and Neuman, 1984; Antal et al., 1986). With a different method, these data were confirmed and compared for frogs and salamanders by Roth et al. (1990, 1999), Dicke and Roth (1996), and Dicke (1999).

Response Properties   Extracellular microelectrode recordings in awake, immobilized toads and frogs revealed different tectal T-type neurons. The classification T1 to T9 by Grüsser and Grüsser-Cornehls (1976) considers shape, size, and location of the ERF of the neuron and the presence of monocular or binocular input (table 4.1). Binocular class T1 neurons may be involved in depth perception. Class T3 is suitable for

---

◄ ERF center in the direction of its longer axis is less responded to than the same bar whose longer axis is oriented across the direction of movement. (*E,F*) A moving large square— nearly filling the ERF—elicits the same neuronal activity as a bar of the same extension across the direction of movement. (*G,H*) A large moving square extending from the ERF into the IRF, or a bar of the same extension across the direction of movement elicits a weak response. In the ERF, *on* and *off* patches are irregularly distributed (see Grüsser and Grüsser-Cornehls, 1976). Note that the IRF is larger than shown. The arrows indicate the direction of movement; $v = 7.6 \, \text{deg/s}$. (Adapted from Grüsser and Grüsser-Cornehls, 1976 and Ewert and Hock, 1972.)

Optic tectum, surface

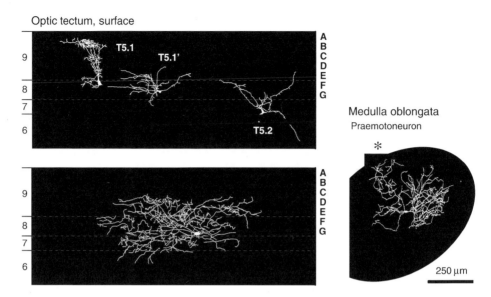

Medulla oblongata
Praemotoneuron

250 µm

Figure 4.6
Dendritic arborization patterns of frog tectal neurons and of a medullary neuron are suitable for information convergence at different processing levels. Camera-lucida reconstructions of intracellulary recorded movement-sensitive neurons labeled with cobalt-lysine. (*Top*) Fibers of retinal ganglion cells terminate in the contralateral optic tectum in laminae B and C (class R2 neurons), C through F (class R3 neurons), and F and G (class R4 neurons). A subtype of tectal T5.1 pear-shaped cell of layer 8 (top, first neuron) shows dendritic arborizations suitable for integrating retinal input from laminae B through G. Pretectotectal projections mediated by neuropeptide Y terminate mainly in laminae B and C. Another subtype of T5.1 neuron (top, second neuron) shows an arborization pattern suitable for intratectal lateral interaction. The tectal T5.2 pyramidal cell (top, third neuron), at the boundary between layers 6 and 7, may integrate input from layers 8 and 9; it projects its axon (distorted in this illustration) via layer 7 toward the medulla oblongata. (*Bottom*) The huge dendritic tree of another type of tectal cell—responsive to any moving visual stimulus—provides a substrate for general integrative processes. (*Right*) In the medulla oblongata—the motor nucleus of the trigeminal nerve—there are neurons responding best to preylike stimuli. The richly arborized dendritic tree of this cell extends into the lateral and the medial reticular formation and into the vestibular and spinocerebellar complexes, one branch extending toward the cerebellum (see the asterisk, rostral to the level of the transverse section half-segment of the medulla oblongata). Neurophysiological data suggest di(poly-)synaptic connections between efferent neurons of the tectal "snapping-evoking area" and medullary motor neurons involved in snapping. (Adapted from Ewert, 1997; cf. Matsumoto et al., 1986.)

detecting relatively small objects approaching on the z-axis. The large ERFs of tectal T2 and T4 neurons, which are responsive to moving objects, focus on different sections of the visual field (figure 4.4). The relatively small ERFs of neurons of the types T5.1 to T5.4 are retinotopically mapped. They are suitable both for analyzing and localizing moving objects (Ewert, 1974, 1984, 1987).

Among the pretectal thalamic TH-type neurons TH1 to TH11 (Ewert, 1984; Buxbaum-Conradi and Ewert, 1995), many are responsive to stimuli that release avoidance behaviors: ducking or turning away from a large moving object (e.g., classes TH3 and TH4), retreating from a looming approaching object (class TH6), or detouring around a stationary obstacle (class TH10) (For data on frogs, see W. T. Brown and Marker, 1977.) The perception of the stationary world—through which an exploratory animal like the toad must move while pursuing prey or seeking safety—requires a certain kind of motion perception during the animal's movement (e.g., that detected by R3, TH3, and TH4 neurons) or after the animal or an object stops moving (e.g., that detected by R1 and TH10 neurons). To the walking toad, an obstacle "addresses" two potential signals: a visual stimulus that it should be avoided and a tactile stimulus in case the object is not avoided. Actually, many subtypes of stationary object-detecting TH10 neurons are responsive in complex stimulus situations, so that body touch facilitates visual sensitivity. After the visual response has faded, touching the skin can even restore the neuron's visual activity toward the obstacle (Ewert, 1971).

The ERFs of other pretectal thalamic neurons include the visual field of both eyes (e.g., class TH4). They are flexible (e.g., class TH5.2), are bimodal (e.g., TH5.3), or seem to have memory (class TH9). In TH5.3 neurons, bimodal perception is divided: "looking at moving objects" with a visual ERF that initially encompasses the visual field of the ipsilateral eye and "sensing touch" with a mechanoreceptive ERF that includes the contralateral body skin. After contralateral touch, the visual ERF extends toward the side of cutaneous irritation.

Recently, Roth and Grunwald (2000) applied the TH-type classification to the salamander's thalamic neurons in *in vitro* preparations. However, these authors studied thalamic neurons in response to electrical stimulation of the optic nerve and not to visual stimuli, which are the critical criteria of the original TH-type classification (see Ewert, 1984), so that comparisons are not possible.

Subtectal Neurons
The subtectum below the optic tectum also provides a substrate for multimodal convergence (Grüsser and Grüsser-Cornehls, 1976; Ewert, 1984). Many neurons have visual receptive fields similar to T2 and T4 and therefore will be referred to as class T'. Besides vision, T'2.1 neurons are activated by vibration, for example, that caused by distant steps. Substrate-borne sound can even enhance the neuronal response to a moving visual stimulus, a property suitable for an alarm system. Besides vision, Class T'4 neurons receive cutaneous input from the contralateral body skin. They show locus-specific habituation to repeated visual or tactile stimulation. In fact, after visual habituation, a tactile stimulus dishabituates, i.e., facilitates the response to the

previously habituated visual stimulus. Class T'2.2 neurons are even trimodal, obtaining visual and vibrational input and tactile input from the contralateral body skin, especially the head region.

Computation of Moving Objects

Having discussed some qualitative aspects of neuronal receptive field properties, we now focus on neuronal correlates of the *ep-ea* features-relating algorithm.

Moving Configurational Stimuli

Since monocular input is sufficient for recognition of prey or predator, we consider the monocularly driven retinal ganglion cells (R2–R4), tectal neurons (T5.1–T5.4), and pretectal thalamic neurons (TH3) (see also table 4.1). All these have approximately circular ERFs. The *ep-ea* configurational paradigm provides a simple and efficient tool to experimentally trace and compare both behavioral and neuronal response properties. Figure 4.7 illustrates the activity patterns of R-, T-, and TH-type neurons in response to changes in *ep* and *ea*.

The R cells prefer different ranges of stimulus area (figure 4.7, R2–R3). They are most responsive to changes in *ea* or to squares of a comparable edge length (figure 4.5; see E and F or G and H) (Ewert and Hock, 1972; Grüsser and Grüsser-Cornehls, 1976). Consequently, chronic recordings in behaving toads show that an R2 or R3 retinal ganglion cell cannot be regarded as a prey detector, as suggested by Barlow (1953) and Lettvin et al. (1959). If a small black bar of *ep* ≈ ERF traverses the ERF center in a nonprey orientation, R2 or R3 neurons are optimally activated, but the probability of catching prey is zero. The same bar moving in a preylike orientation elicits only weak neuronal activity, but the toad readily responds with prey-catching behaviors (Schürg-Pfeiffer, 1989; Schürg-Pfeiffer et al., 1993) (cf. also figure 4.5D,E).

Figure 4.7 ▶

Behavioral and neurophysiological aspects of feature analysis. (*Top*) The toad's prey-catching activity in response to changes in configurational features of moving objects of different sets (*A–C*) is shown in panel P (1 mm corresponds to 0.8 deg visual angle). Escape activity is shown for comparison in panel A. Prey selection is altered after pretectal thalamic lesions (panel P_{TH}) or after visual associative learning in the course of hand-feeding conditioning (panel-L). Learning effects after hand-feeding are abolished after lesions to the posterior ventral medial pallium (panel L_{MP}). Following lesions to the caudal ventral striatum, the prey-catching response fails to occur. (*Bottom*) In response to changes in the configurational features of moving objects of the sets (*A–C*), retinal ganglion cells (R2, R3, R4), pretectal thalamic neurons (TH3), and tectal neurons (T5.1, T5.2, T5.3, T5.4) show different patterns of discharge activity. Note that the response pattern of T5 neurons is altered after pretectal thalamic lesions (panel $T5_{TH}$) in a manner similar to the alteration of prey-catching activity after pretectal thalamic lesions (panel P_{TH}). (Adapted and completed from Ewert, 1984, 1997.)

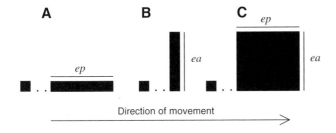

Direction of movement

Prey-catching activity

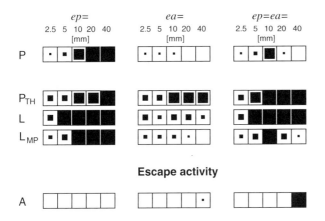

Escape activity

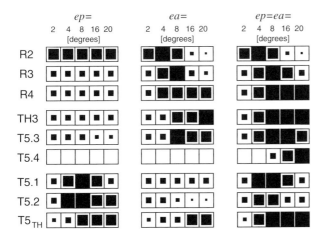

Neuronal discharge activity

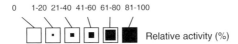

Relative activity (%)

At tectal and pretectal levels (figure 4.7, T5.1–T5.4, TH3), the feature *ea* is coded on a broad scale in T5.3 and TH3, probably owing to a pooling of information parceled in R3 and R4 cells. The T5.1 neurons code for *ep* and for squares of a comparable extension; this could be explained by a pooling of R2 and R3 outflow in connection with intratectal lateral excitation.

Tectal T5.2 neurons differentiate between *ep* and *ea*. Their responses to changes in *ep* and *ea* resemble the toad's prey-catching activity (cf. P and T5.2 in figure 4.7) (von Wietersheim and Ewert, 1978; Borchers and Ewert, 1979; Schürg-Pfeiffer et al., 1993). In this respect, T5.2 neurons are prey selective, which could be explained by excitatory input from T5.1 and inhibitory input from TH3 cells.

Tectal T5.4 neurons, on the other hand, display a sensitivity to compact (e.g., square) objects like the large ones that elicit avoidance and escape behavior (figure 4.7, panel A).

There are three additional points to consider. The first is velocity. Roth and Jordan (1982) confirmed that the various degrees of *ep-ea* discrimination in tectal neurons corresponding to T5.1, T5.2, and T5.3 were velocity invariant in the tested range of v = 2 to 20 deg/s. Only 4% of the total sample of tectal neurons switched at high speed from *ep* versus *ea* preference to *ea* versus *ep*. The second point is size constancy. In awake, pharmacologically immobilized toads, R-type and T5-type neurons are sensitive to the visual angular size of a moving object. In free-moving toads, T5.1 and T5.2 neurons—but no R types—are sensitive to an object's real size (Spreckelsen et al., 1995). Presumably these tectal cells obtain the required information on stimulus depth by motion parallax and/or the lens accommodation mechanism (Ingle, 1976a; Collett, 1977; Ingle and Cook, 1977), which is not functioning in immobilized animals. The third is tectal efferents. Antidromic stimulation and recording studies showed that many types of tectal neurons project their axons directly toward the bulbar-spinal premotor-motor systems. Among these neurons are prey-selective T5.2 and predator-sensitive T5.4 cells (Satou and Ewert, 1985; Ewert et al., 1990).

Background Texture

The R2 neurons are much less activated by a large moving texture than are other R-type neurons. Unlike most tectal wide-field and small-field neurons (T2, T4, T5.1, T5.2), thalamic pretectal TH3 and TH4 neurons readily responded to large moving textures, independent of their direction of movement (Tsai and Ewert, 1988). In addition, TH11 neurons of the large-celled pretectal nucleus display movement-direction selectivity suitable for optokinetic nystagmus (Katte and Hoffmann, 1980; Buxbaum-Conradi and Ewert, 1995).

If a prey stimulus is moved in phase with a textured background, the responses of R2 cells are moderately inhibited by the background and T5.1, T5.2, and T4 neurons are strongly inhibited (figure 4.8) (Tsai and Ewert, 1988). However, if a textured background is moved behind a stationary prey object, about half of the tectal small-field neurons investigated start to discharge after the background stops (Tsai, 1991). This suggests a postinhibitory rebound excitation.

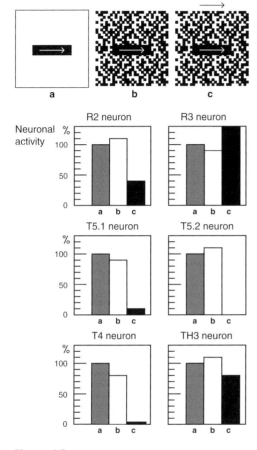

Figure 4.8
Effect of a moving background texture. The discharge activities of retinal (R2, R3), tectal (T5.1, T5.2, T4), and pretectal thalamic (TH3) neurons in response to a stimulus object are influenced differently by a background texture. (*a*) A 2.5 × 8-deg black bar moving at $v = 7.6$ deg/s against a white background. (*b*) The same bar moving against a stationary Julesz texture (minimal pixel size, 0.46 deg). (*c*) The same bar moving in phase together with the Julesz texture at the same velocity of $v = 7.6$ deg/s. Ordinate: neuronal discharge activity in percent of the activity in response to stimulus (*a*). Retinal R2 neurons: $n = 10$, ERF = 5.3 deg diameter; R3 neurons: $n = 10$, ERF = 8.5 deg diameter; tectal T5.1 neurons: $n = 5$, ERF = 26.1 deg diameter; T5.2 neurons: $n = 6$, ERF = 25.2 deg diameter; T4 neurons: $n = 6$, ERF > 180 deg diameter; pretectal thalamic TH3 neurons: $n = 5$, ERF = 47.2 deg diameter. (Adapted from Tsai and Ewert, 1988.)

Pretectal Perceptual Sharpening

At this stage in our consideration of the neuronal correlates of configurational perception, let us pose a hypothesis: The visual response properties of tectal T5.2 neurons (preference *ep* versus *ea*; inhibition by a moving textured background) are determined by inhibitory input of thalamic pretectal TH3 neurons (preference *ea* versus *ep*; excitation by a moving textured background). Could the TH3 neurons influence retinotectal transfer? We can answer this question indirectly by making four points. First, among the eleven TH-type neurons, the TH3 neurons and TH4 wide-field neurons project to the ipsilateral tectum, as shown by antidromic stimulation recording and collision techniques (Buxbaum-Conradi and Ewert, 1995). Second, a pretectotectal projection, suitable for controlling retinotectal input, is mediated by neuropeptide Y (NPY). Kozicz and Lázár (1994) and Chapman and Debski (1995) showed that NPY immunoreactive fibers in the frog superficial tectum originate from ipsilateral pretectal thalamic Lpd and Lpv nuclei. Third, both pretectal nuclei in toads contain TH3 and TH4 pretectotectal projection cells (Buxbaum-Conradi and Ewert, 1995). Finally, administration of NPY to the tectal surface attenuates the tectal surface field potential evoked by electrostimulation of the contralateral optic nerve or by visual *on-off* stimulation (Schwippert and Ewert, 1995; Schwippert et al., 1995, 1998). Testing NPY fragments, Schwippert et al. (1998) showed that NPY_{13-36} (a Y_2 receptor agonist) but not NPY_{18-36} (a Y_2 receptor antagonist) attenuated the *on-off* responses of tectal field potentials (figure 4.9). An attenuation of the visual tectal field potential was also evoked by electrostimulation of the pretectum (Schwippert et al., 1995).

The question of whether ipsilateral pretectotectal projections inhibit tectal neurons was tested by cutting these connections or by lesioning the pretectal Lpd-P region with the axon-sparing excitotoxins kainic acid or ibotenic acid. The result was that tectal neurons showed a strong increase in their discharge rates to moving visual stimuli and there was an impairment of the *ep* versus *ea* preference (figure 4.7, $T5_{TH}$), and strong responses to moving textures (Ingle, 1973; Ewert, 1974, 1984; Ewert et al., 1996).

The ultimate evidence that pretectotectal projections make T5.2 neurons selective for prey was provided by recording T5.2 neurons in behaving toads (Schürg-Pfeiffer et al., 1993; Ewert et al., 1996). In response to a bar moving in a preylike

---

Figure 4.9 ▶

One pretecto-tectal channel is mediated by neuropeptide Y, NPY. (*A*) Administration of porcine NPY to the tectal surface in cane toads (*Bufo marinus*) attenuates the initial excitatory wave of the tectal surface field potential evoked by abrupt changes in diffuse illumination at *off*-set. (*B*) Administration of the fragment NPY13-36. (*C*) Administration of NPY18-36. The initial *on* and off response showed comparable effects. Abscissa: administration time, start at 0 min. Ordinate: tectal field potential (mV); average values ±S.E.M. of *n* = 14 toads (*A*,*B*) or *n* = 12 toads (*C*). (From Schwippert et al., 1998.)

A 1st *off* response of tectal field potential after administration of porcine NPY

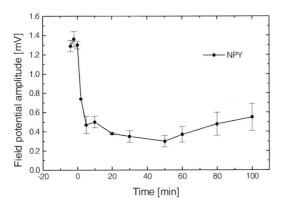

B 1st *off* response of tectal field potential after administration of the fragment NPY13-36, a Y2 receptor agonist

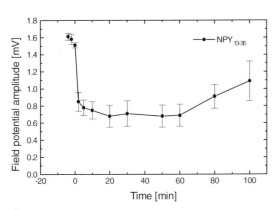

C 1st *off* response of tectal field potential after administration of the fragment NPY18-36, a Y2 receptor antagonist

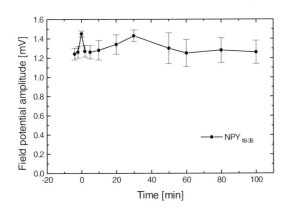

configuration, there was a strong burst of spikes that preceded the toad's prey-catching orienting movement (figure 4.10A). The same bar moving in a nonpreylike configuration was neglected both neuronally and behaviorally. However, shortly after an electrolytic lesion was made in the ipsilateral pretectal Lpd-P region (via a second implanted electrode), strong firing rates of the same T5.2 neuron introduced prey-catching behavior directed to both the prey or nonpreylike stimulus (cf. also T5.2 and T5$_{TH}$ in figure 4.7). The pretectal lesion thus impaired the ability to distinguish between prey and nonprey, both neuronally and behaviorally (cf. also panel P and P$_{TH}$ in figure 4.7).

In salamanders, too, the visual response properties of certain tectal neurons depend on an intact pretectal thalamus (Finkenstädt and Ewert, 1983b). Luksch and Roth (1996) showed that pharmacological (glutamate) stimulation of the pretectum attenuates the amplitudes of tectal field potentials in response to optic nerve stimulation. Luksch et al. (1998) described in terminal branching axon collaterals in pretectotectal projection neurons. In toads such divergence was postulated by Ewert (1987) to explain functional recovery of prey-selection behavior after small pretectal lesions.

Stimulus-Response–Mediating Pathways and Their Modulatory Loops

Stimulus-response mediation in toads and frogs is managed by sequentially connected processing. For example, visuomotor behavior related to prey catching is mediated by retino-tecto-bulbar–spinal processing streams. Besides the direct tectobulbar–spinal tracts, there are indirect tecto-tegmento-bulbar–spinal pathways that contribute to locating prey or predators in space (Grobstein et al., 1983; Masino and Grobstein, 1989a,b, 1990; Grobstein, 1991; Roche King and Comer, 1996).

The pathways for prey orienting and snapping responses, respectively, are to some extent segregated. Ingle (1983) showed that cutting the crossed tectobulbar–spinal projections at the level of the ansulate commissure of the tegmentum abolishes orienting toward but not snapping at prey if the prey moves in a horizontal plane. The frog will then snap straight forward, no matter what the direction of the prey. Cutting the ipsilateral tectobulbar–spinal projections, on the other hand, abolishes snapping toward prey, but not orienting.

The processing stream that mediates barrier avoidance involves a retino-pretecto (P)-bulbar–spinal pathway. This is segregated from the pathways that mediate prey catching. Whereas tectal ablation does not impair barrier avoidance behavior (Ingle, 1977), lesions to the pretectal P nucleus abolish barrier detection (Ingle, 1979, 1983). The lesion site in P is congruent with the recording sites of barrier-detecting TH10 neurons (Buxbaum-Conradi and Ewert, 1995).

All these stimulus-response-mediating circuits basically function after telencephalic lesions. Such lesions, however, may produce impairments in visual perceptual tasks, response gating, learning, and motor skills (for a review, see Ewert et al., 2001). This suggests that the processing streams mediating stimulus and response can

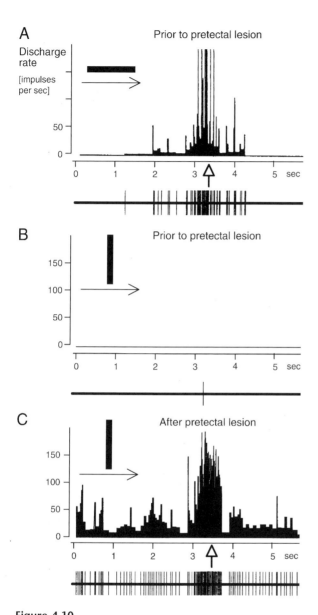

Figure 4.10
Correlation between prey stimulus, neuronal activity, and prey-catching response. (*A*) With chronic recording techniques in behaving toads it can be shown that the animal's orienting response (see vertical arrow) toward a bar moving in prey configuration (2.5 × 20 mm in size) is preceded by an increase in the discharge rate of a T5.2 neuron. (*B*) Toward the same bar moving in nonprey configuration, the T5.2 neuron is almost silent and a prey-catching response fails to occur. (*C*) After a pretectal thalamic lesion is delivered with a second electrode ipsilaterally to the tectal recording site, the same T5.2 neuron discharges strongly toward the nonprey stimulus and a very strong burst of spikes precedes the onset of prey-catching response toward that stimulus. Note that the neuron displays background activity postlesion. (From Ewert et al., 1996.)

be modulated, modified, and specified by neural loops that involve various structures of the forebrain (see Doty, 1987). The pretectal Lpd-P nuclei, for example, are important in processing and relaying forebrain influences to the optic tectum.

Gating an Orienting Response toward Prey
Since it is known that the pretectum controls certain retinotectal computations and, thus tectomotor output, the question arises of what controls the pretectum. Various evidence suggests that such a function of response gating depends on a loop involving the telencephalic caudal ventral striatum (vSTR) (Ewert, 1992; Ewert et al., 2001).

Visual Responses of Striatal Efferents   The toad's caudal vSTR contains different types of visual neurons. Among these there are neurons whose steady streams of discharges are modulated up or down, depending on the moving visual stimulus (Gruberg and Ambros, 1974; Buxbaum-Conradi and Ewert, 1999). Their visual receptive fields encompass either the whole visual field of the contralateral eye or the entire field of vision. Antidromic stimulation and recording studies show that striatal visual output running in the lateral forebrain bundle (LFB) is mediated mainly by such "visual motion-detecting neurons" (for neuroanatomical data, see Wilczynski and Northcutt, 1983b; see also Lázár and Kozicz, 1990; Marín et al., 1997a,b).

Properties of a Tectal Loop Involving the Ventral Striatum   Among the different connections from the striatum to the optic tectum (OT) (Marín et al., 1997a,b), the striato-pretecto-tectal pathway offers interesting neuroethological perspectives. Studies applying the ^{14}C-2-deoxyglucose (^{14}C-2DG) technique in prey-catching toads showed that glucose utilization was strongest in the vSTR and OT, whereas the pretectal Lpd nucleus displayed a utilization decrease (Finkenstädt et al., 1985, 1986; Finkenstädt and Ewert, 1985). One explanation is that striatal activity reduced pretectotectal inhibition, thus gating the tectomotor output involved in prey catching.

Is there evidence of striatopretectal inhibitory influences? Intracellular recording and labeling experiments showed that electrical stimulation of the vSTR or LFB evoked mainly inhibitory postsynaptic potentials in pretectal neurons (Matsumoto et al., 1991). Distinct sets of striatal cells as well as LFB fibers terminating in the ipsilateral pretectum contain the inhibitory neurotransmitter and neuromodulator, methioninenkephalin (Merchenthaler et al., 1989; Lázár and Kozicz, 1990; Schwerdtfeger and Germroth, 1990; Lázár et al., 1993; for chemoarchitecture in basal ganglia organization, see Marín et al., 1997b, 1998a, 1999).

The available evidence suggests (figure 4.11B) that the vSTR obtains retinotectal visual excitation ($\rightarrow$) via the lateral anterior (La) thalamic nucleus. In turn, the vSTR facilitates OT via a striato-pretecto-tectal disinhibitory pathway. This disinhibitory connection involves both an inhibitory (-|) striato-pretectal route and an inhibitory (-|) pretecto-tectal route:

R $\rightarrow$ OT $\rightarrow$ La $\rightarrow$ **vSTR** -| Lpd -| OT

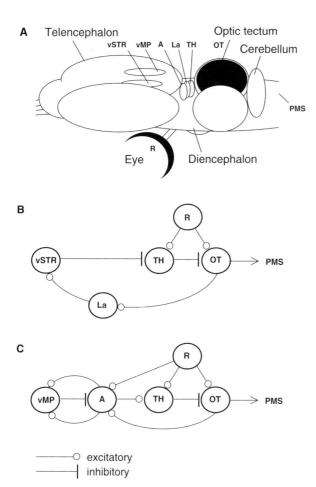

Figure 4.11
Stimulus-response mediating circuits and examples of their modulating loops. (*A*) Structures of the anuran brain involved in the mediation and modulation of visually guided behaviors. A, anterior thalamus; La, lateral anterior thalamic nucleus; OT, optic tectum; PMS, premotor-motor systems; R, retina; TH, pretectal thalamus; vMP, posterior ventral medial pallium; vSTR, caudal ventral striatum. TH includes the lateral posterior dorsal and the posterior thalamic nuclei. The PMS includes the medial reticular premotor structures and cranial nerve motor nuclei. (*B*) Modulatory loop suggested to be involved in gating an orienting response toward prey; R feeds in parallel to TH and OT; vSTR obtains input of OT via La and in turn activates OT by the disinhibitory pathway vSTR–TH–OT. (*C*) Modulatory loop suggested to be involved in modifying prey selectivity after hand-feeding conditioning; R feeds in parallel to A, TH, and OT; vMP obtains concurrent input of A related to the prey stimulus and the hand stimulus, respectively. As a result, certain vMP neurons are sensitized and stimulate OT by the disinhibitory pathway vMP–A–TH–OT. (Adapted from Ewert, 1997.)

The appropriate anatomical data are provided by Wilczynski and Northcutt (1983a,b) and Marín et al. (1997b).

Let us now discuss the striato-pretecto-tectal disinhibitory pathway in connection with results from brain lesion studies (Finkenstädt, 1989; Patton and Grobstein, 1998a,b). After striatal lesions, prey-capture behavior fails to occur, probably because the striato-pretectal inhibition is absent, so that pretectotectal inhibition overrides the release of the tectal prey-catching system. After pretectal lesions, the tectal prey-catching release system is disinhibited, probably because pretectotectal inhibition fails to occur.

In the intact toad, striatal activity may control the toad's readiness to orient toward prey. If striatal activity is weak, pretectotectal inhibition is strong and the toad hesitates; if striatal activity is strong, pretectotectal inhibition is reduced and the orienting release system is gated. For example, the striatal "visual motion detector" channel may sensitize the tectal neurons responsible for orienting. If an object traverses the visual field, the striatopretectal connection attenuates pretectotectal inhibition, thus raising directed attention and, in the case of a prey stimulus, gating the translation of perception into action.

Associative Conditioning of Threat with Prey

The Hand-Feeding Paradigm   If an experimenter offers a mealworm to a toad by hand, the hand, which is initially threatening, comes to be associated with the prey and will alone come to elicit prey-capture behavior (Brzoska and Schneider, 1978; Ewert et al., 1983; Finkenstädt and Ewert, 1992; Ewert et al., 1994a). This conditioning is generalized, so that other nonprey stimuli such as a large, black, moving square or a bar in nonprey configuration will also elicit a prey-catching response (cf. figure 4.7, panels P, L). In this case, ^{14}C-2DG uptake is increased both in the telencephalic posterior ventromedial pallium (vMP) and in OT, but reduced in Lpd.

How can the training-induced impairment of prey selectivity be explained? We know that configurational prey-selection behavior is based on the evaluation of the stimulus features ep and ea, and the area $ep*ea$. If these features are within a certain range, the object is seen as prey. We suggest that during evolution, objects extended along ea or with large $ep*ea$ areas, analyzed in the pretectal thalamus, became linked with threat. If this link, ultimately stored in pretectotectal connections, is broken, prey versus threat discrimination is impaired. Experimentally, this link can be broken if a large moving area is associated with prey, as in the case of hand-fed toads. A hand-conditioned toad with reduced Lpd activity behaves in a way similar to that of a pretectally lesioned toad with no Lpd activity (cf. panels L and P_{TH} in figure 4.7).

Properties of a Tectal Loop Involving the Ventromedial Pallium   Our working hypothesis suggests that during hand-feeding, information on both the unconditioned stimulus (prey) and the conditioned stimulus (hand) coincide in the vMP (figure 4.11C):

visual prey $\rightarrow$ R $\rightarrow$ OT $\rightarrow$ A $\rightarrow$ **vMP** $\leftarrow$ A $\leftarrow$ OT $\leftarrow$ R $\leftarrow$ visual threat

As a result, certain vMP neurons may be sensitized and, becoming responsive to hand/threat stimuli, alter tectal prey-selective properties via the anterior thalamic (A) and pretectal Lpd nuclei by a disinhibitory pathway:

$$vMP + A \rightarrow Lpd + OT.$$

After vMP lesions are made prior to learning, the toad will not learn. If this lesion is made after hand-feeding, the learning effect is abolished and species-common prey-selective properties reemerge (cf. panel L_{MP} and P) (Finkenstädt, 1989; Ewert et al., 1994a). The vMP is probably not the only telencephalic structure involved in associative learning, however. The lateral nucleus amygdalae may participate, particularly in paradigms associated with fear (e.g., S.O.G. Lindemann and Roth, 1999).

Conditioning Visual and Olfactory Cues

Prey-Associated Odor   Toads in the wild are not familiar with mealworms. However, after being fed on mealworms in the laboratory, they associate the mealworm odor with that of prey (Dole et al., 1981; Ewert, 1984; Merkel-Harff and Ewert, 1991; Ewert et al., 2001). In the presence of the familiar mealworm odor, prey-catching motivation increases greatly. Concomitantly, prey selectivity decreases to include nonprey items also. In the absence of prey-associated odor, prey-selection behavior is normal.

Associative Convergence of Visual and Olfactory Information   Neuroanatomical studies show that various brain structures and their connections are involved in visual-olfactory learning (figure 4.12) (Ebbesson, 1980a; Vanegas, 1984). In addition, studies using ^{14}C-2DG (Finkenstädt, 1989; Ewert et al., 2001) suggest that in the presence of prey and familiar prey odor, visual information (mediated by the anterior thalamus and olfactory information mediated by the main olfactory bulb (MOB) coincide in the vMP:

olfactory stimulus $\rightarrow$ MOB $\rightarrow$ **vMP** $\leftarrow$ A $\leftarrow$ OT $\leftarrow$ retina $\leftarrow$ visual stimulus

As a result, certain vMP neurons may be sensitized and in turn inhibit neurons of the ventral hypothalamus (vHYP) that normally attenuate the tectal (OT) prey-catching release system (Ewert et al., 2001). Hence, prey-catching responsiveness will be increased. In conditioned toads, vMP lesions abolish visual-olfactory conditioning (Finkenstädt, 1989).

How a Toad Sees: Models Simulating Aspects of the Amphibian Visual World

Conceptualizing Action-Related Visual Perception

Sensorimotor Codes: Translating Perception into Action   If a certain tectal area is stimulated electrically, snapping is triggered, or commanded, as if this area were

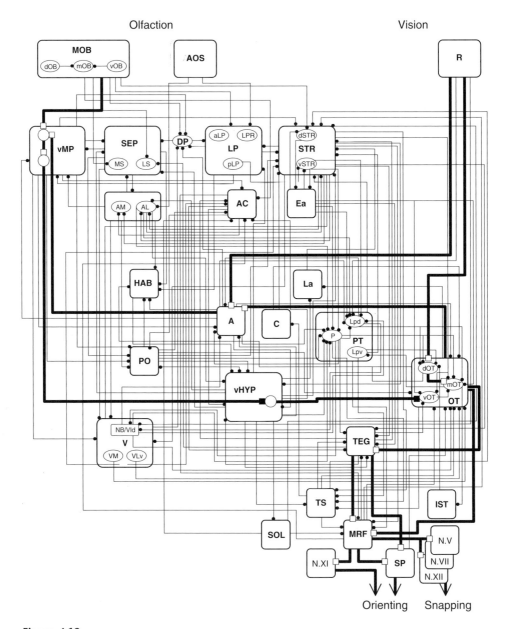

Olfaction   Vision

Figure 4.12
Associating visual and olfactory cues. The neural structures and connections shown
in heavier type, integrated into a macronetwork, are suggested to be involved in visual-
olfactory conditioning. In studies of visual-olfactory conditioning of prey and prey odor,
these structures showed significant changes in local cerebral glucose utilization monitored
with the [14]C-2DG method. It is suggested that vMP obtains concurrent visual input from
the retina and optic tectum (via A) and olfactory input (via MOB). As a result, certain vMP
neurons are sensitized and inhibit certain neurons of vHYP that normally attenuate certain
neurons of OT. A, anterior thalamus; AOS, accessory olfactory system; HAB, habenula

excited by an appropriate visual input (Ewert, 1974). By "commanded," we refer to the triggering of a rapid, ballistic response. Command functions provide a sensori-motor interface that translates a specific pattern of sensory input into an appropriate spatiotemporal pattern of activity in premotor and motor neurons and involves a motor pattern generator (MPG). Depending on the sensorimotor function, DiDomenico and Eaton (1987) envision a spectrum of possibilities by which com-mands can be executed. It is commonly accepted that ballistic behavior organized in distributed networks is triggered by populations of commandlike interneurons (command elements, CEs) that form a command system (CS) (Kupfermann and Weiss, 1978; Eaton, 2001; Ewert, 2002).

The concept of a command-releasing system (CRS) considers the combinatorial aspects of stimulus perception (Ewert, 1987, 1997; Comer, 1987). Different types of CEs, each type monitoring a certain stimulus aspect, cooperatively trigger an MPG (figure 4.13; table 4.1) (Satou and Ewert, 1985; Ewert et al., 1990). A certain combi-nation of CEs provides a sensorimotor code, whereby input from motivational systems is also required for MPG activation. The notion of coded commands suggests a number of ideas. For instance, the code {T4, X, T5.2} may tell the toad, "An object is moving in the visual field (T4); it is located at position x-y (X); and it has prey features (T5.2) →orient!" Alternatively, the code {T4, T1.3, T3, T5.2} may say, "An object is moving in the visual field (T4), specifically in the frontal binocular field at a short distance (T1.3); it is approaching (T3) and it has prey features (T5.2) →snap!" Or the code {T6, TH6} may indicate that "A large object is moving in the dorsal visual field (T6), and it is approaching (TH6) →duck!"

In this multifunctional network, the same MPG can be activated by differently combined CRSs whose CEs may be distributed in different brain structures; on the other hand, CEs may be shared by different CRSs.

Behavioral choice may depend on mutual excitatory or inhibitory actions of the respective CEs and/or MPGs (Ewert, 2002). A "behavioral hierarchy" can be determined by hormonal modulation: during summer, predator-avoiding behavior in toads dominates prey-catching behavior, whereas mate-approaching behavior fails to occur (see also Guha et al., 1980; Laming and Cairns, 1998). During spring, mate-approaching behavior dominates avoidance of predators whereas prey-catching behavior fails to occur.

◄ nucleus; LP, lateral pallium; MOB, main olfactory bulb; MRF, medullary medial reticular formation; N.V.-N.XII, cranial motor nerve nuclei; OT, optic tectum; R, retina; SP, spinal motor nuclei; TEG, tegmentum; vHYP, ventral hypothalamus; vMP, ventral medial pallium. Putative excitatory influences are labeled by open squares and putative inhibitory influ-ences by solid squares. For explanations, see the text and Ewert et al. (2001).

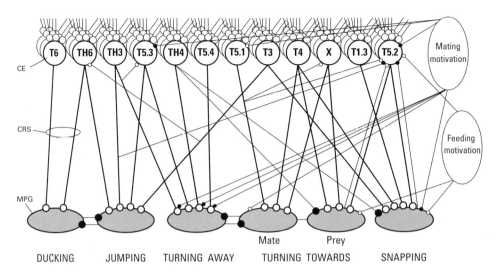

Figure 4.13

The hypothesis of sensorimotor codes suggests that certain combinations of (distributed) sensory processing streams collectively activate a motor pattern generator (MPG) involving principles of convergence and divergence at different levels. Owing to the convergence of inputs, different response properties emerge in tectal (T) and pretectal thalamic (TH) neurons (cf. table 4.1). The release of a behavioral motor pattern may depend on the adequate activation of different types of T and/or TH neurons (command elements, CE) that converge on an MPG. In such a system, one CE may contribute to the activation of different MPGs (divergence). Motivational systems may influence CEs and/or MPGs. The descending character of most CE neurons was determined by antidromic stimulation and recording techniques (collision test). The open circles denote putative excitatory connections; the solid circles indicate putative inhibitory connections. (Adapted from Ewert, 1997.)

Schema Theory

A CRS can be regarded as the neurobiological correlate of Nikolaas Tinbergen's (1951) concept of "releasing mechanism," originally called "releasing schema" by Konrad Lorenz (cf. Schleidt, 1962; Baerends, 1987; Ewert, 1997). Schema theory (Arbib, 1989; Cervantes-Pérez, 1989) offers an interdisciplinary science that allows one to treat principles of neuroethology and neural engineering in the same language. In this language, the sensorimotor code of a CRS (Ewert, 2002) embodies a perceptual schema that exists for only one purpose: to determine the conditions for the activation of a specific MPG embodying a motor schema. The CRS must also ensure that the resultant movement is directed in relation to the target. A schema and its instantiation usually are coextensive; that is, instantiation of a schema appears to be identifiable with appropriate activity in certain populations of neurons of the brain; each schema may involve several brain regions and cell types, while a given cell type may be involved in several schemas.

The motor schemas of directed appetitive behaviors (orienting, approaching, fixating) and consummatory behavior (snapping) need not occur in a fixed order. Rather, each may proceed to completion, followed by perceptual schemas that will determine which motor schema is to be executed next. Schemas may be linked by so-called "coordinated control programs." Motor schemas, for example, can take the form of compound motor coordinations (e.g., a frog's programmed jump-snap-gulp sequence), which make up a set that will proceed to completion without intervening perceptual inputs (e.g., in such a way that schema A proceeds to completion, and completion of schema A triggers the initiation of schema B, or that schema A passes a parameter x to schema B). It is also possible that two or more motor schemas may become coactivated simultaneously and interact through competition and cooperation to yield a more complicated motor pattern.

Functional Models of Prey Selection

Various models are suitable for explaining how neuronal networks solve the problem of configurational prey recognition.

Interacting Neural Filters   Based on quantitative behavioral data (Ewert, 1968, 1974) a systems-theoretical model consisting of interacting homogeneous neuronal nets was proposed by Ewert and von Seelen (1974) (figure 4.14A). In this model retinal output is passed in parallel to a type-I tectal filter sensitive to the stimulus area and configurationally to its extension *ep*, and to a pretectal thalamic filter sensitive to the stimulus area and configurationally to its extension *ea*. The output of the pretectal filter inhibits the response of a type-II, tectal filter which receives the excitatory input of type I. The type-II tectal filter thus relates *ep* and *ea* to each other (*ep-ea* is the feature-relating algorithm).

In this model, a preylike moving bar would optimally excite tectal type I, whose influence on tectal type II is weakly attenuated by the pretectal response, thus yielding a strong type-II output. A bar moving in a nonprey configuration would yield little

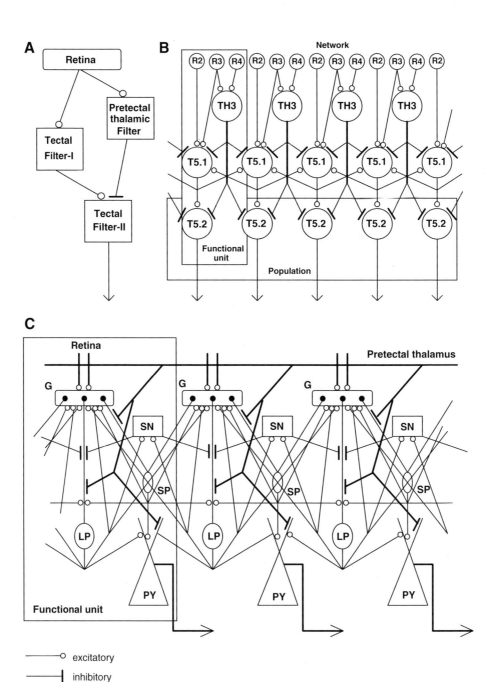

Figure 4.14
Models suitable for explaining neural correlates of the *ep/ea* feature-relating algorithm. (*A*) Concept of interacting pretectal and tectal filters (see Ewert and von Seelen, 1974). (*B*) Neurophysiological correlates of the filter hypothesis (see Ewert, 1987). (*C*) Computer simulation of neuroanatomical functional units of cell assemblies (see Arbib, 1989, and Cervantes-Pérez, 1989). G, glomerulus; LP, large pear-shaped cell; PY, pyramidal cell; SN, stellate neuron; SP, small pear-shaped cell. For explanations, see the text.

type-I activity, strong pretectal activity, and a resultant weak type-II output. A square stimulus would yield an intermediate response.

The tectal type II can be regarded as a "prey filter." It compares, or cross-correlates, information related to visual configural features with stored information provided by the neural circuitry in which T5.1 neurons (tectal type-I filter), TH3 neurons (pretectal filter), and T5.2 neurons (tectal type-II filter) participate. When the parameters in this model are adjusted, it fits the behavioral data over a linear subrange.

Up to this point the model would predict that after pretectal lesions, T5.2 neurons respond like T5.1 neurons. However, this was not the case (cf. T5.1 and T5$_{TH}$ in figure 4.7), which suggests an advanced model in which both T5.1 and T5.2 neurons receive inhibitory influences from TH3 (figure 4.14B). Thus far the network involves a purely feed-forward computation. Mutual facilitation across neighboring T5.1 neurons and mutual inhibition of TH3 neurons on adjacent T5.1 and T5.2 would allow *ep-ea* discrimination across space and time as the target traverses the visual field (Ewert, 1987).

Functional Anatomical Units of Cell Assemblies

One drawback of the previous models (figure 4.14A,B) is that they neither explain the spatial locus nor the time at which the toad snaps. This was overcome in a computer simulation by Arbib and co-workers (Arbib, 1989; Cervantes-Pérez, 1989). Their model is derived from the tectal anatomy of Székely and Lázár (1976) and Lázár (1984) that suggests continuous functional units of cell assemblies (figure 4.14C). In the present context, the output of such a unit is expressed by one pyramidal cell (PY) (corresponding to T5.2), which receives excitatory input both from large pear-shaped (LP) and small pear-shaped (SP) cells (corresponding to subtypes of T5.1). Retinal input (mainly from R2 and R3) activates the unit through a glomerulus via the dendrites of LP and SP cells. The axons of LP and SP return to the glomerulus, providing a positive feedback. A collateral of LP axons also contacts stellate neurons (SN) that are inhibitory to LP. There is thus competition between recurrent excitation and recurrent stellate inhibition. The SP cells also excite the LP cells to recruit the activity of the unit. Adjacent units (an 8 × 8 array in the model) are linked by SP, LP, and SN through lateral excitatory and inhibitory connections, respectively. The retina projects R3 and R4 axons to pretectal thalamic TH neurons in parallel R2 and R3 axons to tectal neurons. Pretecto-tectal inhibitory input arrives at SP and LP, and mainly at PY cells.

With the parameters appropriately set, the model precisely describes the experimentally measured neuronal and behavioral stimulus-response relationships. It was extended to include modulatory properties with respect to learning.

Backpropagation-Instructed Artificial Neural Networks

Werbos (1995) points out that artificial neural networks (ANNs) trained by the backpropagation algorithm may help us to understand the functions of neurons in biological neural networks, such as feature detection (see Prete, 1999 for an analogous application to mantid prey recognition).

Consider a simple two-layered ANN consisting of an input matrix (of 10×10 elements), a hidden layer (of five neurons), and an output layer (of two neurons) (figure 4.15). In this topology, each element of the input matrix is connected to each hidden-layer neuron, and each output neuron obtains input from all hidden-layer neurons. By means of a special program involving backpropagation (Disse et al., 1992), the net can be trained to evaluate bars moving in prey configuration (P) as "prey" (feature ep) and bars moving in nonprey configuration (N) as "nonprey" (feature ea). This is expressed by two output neurons, whose evaluation indices, i_P and i_N, range between 0.0 and 1.0.

To transform the dynamic process of moving bars into a static pattern, a difference picture measures the difference between two consecutive pictures of a moving object (figure 4.15, top). In the training phase, the program allows one to feed difference pictures of P and N bars of different lengths randomly to different sites of the input matrix for horizontal and vertical directions of movement, and to minimize the errors of their evaluation at the output side until a 5% error is reached. Figure 4.16a shows the evaluation indices of the trained net in detecting horizontally moved bars of different lengths: P bars with $i_P = 0.95$ and $i_N = 0.08$, and N bars with $i_N = 0.99$ and $i_P = 0.01$.

To check the function of hidden-layer neurons, the program allows the elimination of single neurons of the trained net (figure 4.16b–d). Elimination of neuron 3 actually improved prey detection and left nonprey detection unchanged (figure 4.16b). Hence, this neuron probably contributed to training, but is dispensable in the trained net. Elimination of neuron 4 abolished prey detection and left nonprey detection unchanged (figure 4.16c). Elimination of neuron 5 left prey detection unchanged but affected nonprey detection, depending on the length of the bar: an N bar two pixels long was classified as prey; nonprey detection improved with increasing bar length (figure 4.16d). Lesions applied to neurons 1 or 2 showed similar results. The lesion-induced effects were independent of the input site on the matrix. Studies of ANNs with larger matrices and hidden layers yielded comparable data.

These studies suggest some neurobiological parallels. The artificial neuron 4 is associated with the analysis of feature ep (cf. tectal T5.1, T5.2 neurons), whereas neurons 1, 2, and 5 are involved in the analysis of ea (cf. tectal T5.3 and pretectal thalamic TH3 neurons). The analysis of feature ea involves more hidden-layer neurons than the analysis of ep. During the evolution of biological networks, such "need" may have led to an amplification in the evaluation of ea by involving both tectal (T5.3) and pretectal (TH3) neurons in the stimulus analysis.

Evolutionary Aspects of Visual Perception in Amphibians

Transition from Aquatic to Terrestrial Life
With the transition of vertebrates from aquatic to terrestrial life, the biotope changes. For predatory amphibians living at the boundary, so to speak, visual perception acquires a new quality. Developmental studies in *Salamandra salamandra* suggest that

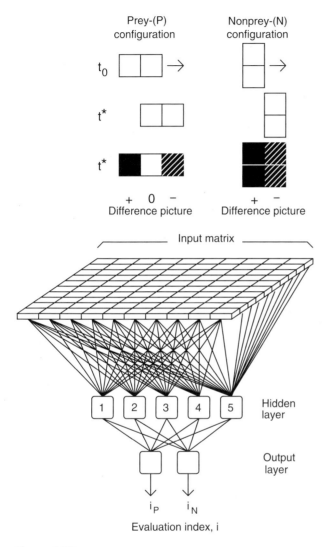

Figure 4.15

A two-layered artificial neural net (ANN)—instructed by a backpropagation algorithm—can be trained to classify and evaluate bars of different lengths moving in prey (P) or in nonprey (N) configuration. (*Top*) Principle of transforming a moving bar (of one-pixel width and two-pixel length) into a static "difference picture" shown for the P and N configuration. The bar is displaced in the horizontal direction by one pixel; the bar starts to move at time t_0 and stops at t^*; the third group shows the difference between the pictures of the bar at t_0 and t^*. (*Bottom*) An ANN consisting of an input matrix, hidden layer, and output layer. Not all connections from the input layer to the hidden layer are shown in this illustration. For further explanations, see the text. (Adapted from Disse et al., 1992.)

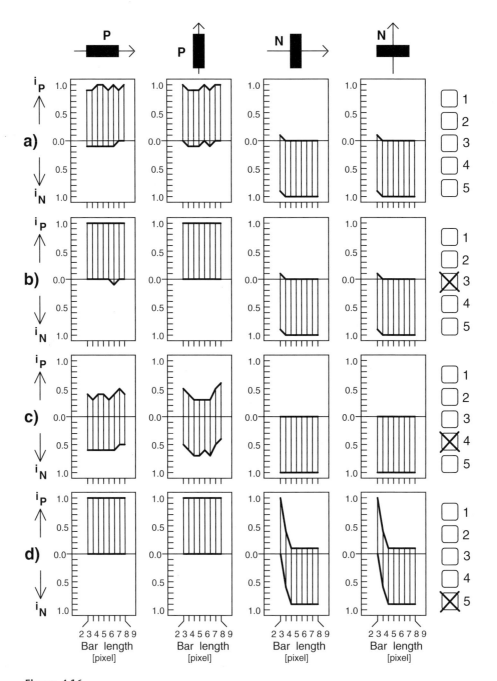

Figure 4.16
Lesion studies with a trained artificial neuronal net (cf. figure 4.15). Elimination of different neurons of the hidden layer allows us to determine the function of these neurons for the detection of bars moving in prey (P) or nonprey (N) configuration. The arrows denote horizontal or vertical directions of movement. Abscissa: length of the bar. Ordinate: evaluation index (i) of the bar as prey (i_P) or as nonprey (i_N). (*a*) Evaluation indices for an intact hidden layer. (*b*)–(*d*) Evaluation indices when either neuron 3 (*b*), or neuron 4 (*c*), or neuron 5 (*d*) is eliminated. For explanations, see the text.

food filters prior to and after metamorphosis are adapted to the different stimulus situations in water and on land (Himstedt et al., 1976). Aquatic salamander larvae capture small invertebrates that, in conjunction with water turbulences, do not display special visual configurational cues. When tested experimentally, bars moving in prey or nonprey configurations are chosen equally often. After metamorphosis, configurational prey selection matures in salamanders, as is also known in toads (Ewert, 1968). Experimentally it was shown that prey selection in common toads improves during the first ten postmetamorphic days, independent of experience with prey (Ewert et al., 1983). Perceptual sharpening and estimation of absolute size are fully established 6 to 8 months after metamorphosis.

Thalamic filtering systems appear to display a parallel development (Clairambault, 1976). The differentiation of the dorsal thalamus starts before metamorphosis and is completed 6 months to 1 year thereafter. In anurans, a cellular migration beginning from the area of the dorsomedialis gives rise to the new area of the dorsolateralis. This proceeds only in the presence of the anterior tectum (Straznicki and Gaze, 1972). In accordance with Ebbesson's (1980b, 1984, 1987) parcelation theory, the ontogenetic parcelation of the caudal dorsal thalamus in pretectal Lpd and P nuclei probably results in a finer tuning of circuits involved in visual computation.

The NPY immunoreactivity of frog pretectal cells occurs in tadpoles in stages 24–25, becomes very conspicuous in advanced larval stages 28–30, and shows maximal values during and after metamorphosis (D'Aniello et al., 1996).

Implicit versus Explicit Computation

In amphibians, the three fundamental behaviors—feeding, escape, and courtship—are directed to stimuli that are living objects, and "living" is associated with movement. An object that does not move will be attributed to the "stationary" world. Moving objects, monitored by movement-detecting neurons, can be abstracted into their shape in relation to the direction of movement. These parameters are analyzed in terms of their different spatiotemporal features. A neural network consisting at least of TH3, T5.1, T5.2, T5.3, and T5.4 neurons is suitable for computing a quantity of spatiotemporal features within one bounded continuum (figure 4.17). This suggests that prey, predators, and mates are not represented explicitly, but rather are implicit in structures of shared spatiotemporal features, at least as far as species-common pattern recognition is concerned. Figure 4.17 depicts an organization of feature relationships that can be modulated by many factors, including motivation. In coming to understand the networks that underpin such structures of relationships (and these are certainly far from template comparisons), Arbib (1987) pointed out that we may do well to consider (whether on the time scale of evolution, development, or learning) the Markov chain training models for nonseparable classes of patterns given in Sklansky and Wassel (1981).

The principle of implicit computation emerges in the selectivity for moving elongated shapes travelling in the orientation in which they are elongated versus same shapes oriented across the direction of movement. This selectivity is independent of

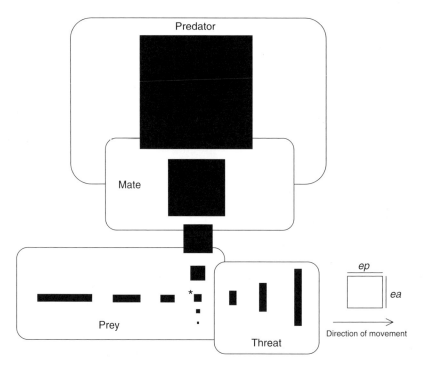

Figure 4.17
Complex visual world of a toad abstracted by the toad's brain in terms of simple features and feature combinations. Stimulus continuum of moving configurational features: starting with a small 5 × 5-mm square object (marked by an asterisk), its extension *ep* or *ea* or both (*ea* = *ep*) is varied. Different ranges of sets of features determine the categories of prey, threat, mate, or predator. An overlap between mate and prey categories and mate and predator categories is avoided in the mating season by hormonal influences that raise the thresholds for prey-catching and predator-avoiding responses (cf. figure 4.13).

the direction of movement. Explicit computation of the many possible bar orientations would require a highly redundant brain structure with different asymmetric
processors like the ones organized in orientation columns in the visual cortex of
mammals (Hubel and Wiesel, 1962).

The "trick" by which evolution in amphibians seems to circumvent this need
(Stevens, 1987) is to compute bar orientation implicitly with symmetric processors
that take advantage of the asymmetry in the time domain of the stimulus. The bar
moving in a nonprey configuration displays spatial effects across the direction of
movement, averaged by TH3. The bar moving in a preylike configuration displays
both spatial and temporal effects along its elongation in the direction of movement,
averaged by T5.1 and T5.2 (sharpened by TH3).

The solution of implicit computation is both efficient and economical. It shows
how a relatively small brain may solve a large problem. The "cleverness" obviously
lies in the abstract algorithm (software) and not in the cytological network structure
(hardware), since it was shown that such an algorithm can be implemented in the
very different brains of quite different predatory animals such as the amphibious fish
Periophthalmus koehlreuteri (Ewert et al., 1983) or the praying mantids, *Sphodromantis
lineola* and *Tenodera aridifolia sinensis* (Prete, 1992a, 1999; chapter 3 in this volume).

Processing Streams
Visual perception in amphibians involves neural structures that are homologous to
the ones of phylogenetically advanced tetrapods. The functions of these structures are
adapted to the needs of the species. The optic tectum–superior colliculus is one of the
most ancient structures of the vertebrate visual system and is concerned with visual
processing, multisensory integration, the influence of forebrain systems on sensory
processing, and generation of motor commands for approach and avoidance (for data
in mammals, e.g., see Mize, 1983; Vanegas, 1984; Meredith and Stein, 1986; Foreman
and Stevens, 1987; Sparks and Nelson, 1987; P. Dean et al., 1988a,b; Westby et al.,
1990; P. Dean and Redgrave, 1991; Binns, 1999; Sparks, 1999; Brandao et al., 1999;
Krout et al., 2001).

Segregation and Interaction   In amphibians, the integrated view derived from behavioral, electrophysiological, neuroanatomical, and neuropharmacological studies has
led to a number of conclusions. Retinal output is processed by corresponding brain
structures in a parallel distributed fashion. The neuronal mechanisms responsible for
formation of a stimulus category, localization, and release of behavior take advantage
both of distributed processing and convergence at various brain levels. Such processes
range from the very basic in the retina to the complex at the tectal, pretectal, and
premotor or motoneuronal levels.

Whereas retinal ganglion cells scan the visual world and carry prefiltered information on elementary features (blinking, darkening, moving, contrasting, etc.), tectal
and pretectal thalamic neurons abstract feature combinations, such as shape in relation to the direction of movement. There are various retinofugal pathways in which

retinal output may be pooled. First, retinotectal processing is involved in approaching and acquiring prey or a mate and in avoiding predators (e.g., Ewert, 1974, 1984; Ingle, 1983). Second, retinopretectal (Lpd) processing is involved in avoiding predators (Ewert, 1971, 1984). Third, retinopretectal (P) processing is involved in avoiding stationary obstacles (Ingle, 1983). Fourth, retinoanterior thalamic processing is involved in phototaxis (Muntz, 1962a,b). Finally, the retinopretectal nucleus lentiformis mesencephali and retinobasal optic route nucleus are involved in optokinetic nystagmus (Lázár, 1973; Montgomery et al., 1982; Montgomery and Fite, 1991; Z. Li et al., 1996).

Certain processing streams need to interact at sensory and/or motor levels. Visual perceptual tasks thus may result from different kinds of interaction within the same macronetwork. This implies that a neural structure is not necessarily made for (dedicated to) a single perceptual task; it may contribute to other perceptual tasks as well. For example, whereas the different retinopretectal processing streams for obstacle avoidance and optokinetic nystagmus, respectively, function independently of tectal input, various kinds of pretecto-tectal interactions are responsible for prey recognition, predator recognition, and discrimination between an object's motion and self-induced motion (for a discussion, see Ewert, 1997).

The differentiated processes in the pretectum and tectum are transmitted via different pretecto- and tectomotor channels (Ingle, 1983; Tóth et al., 1985; Satou and Ewert, 1985; Ewert et al., 1990) that may interact in medial reticular (premotor) and bulbar-spinal (motor) nuclei to select a motor program in conjunction with modulatory input (Satou et al., 1985; Matsushima et al., 1989; Weerasuriya, 1989; Nishikawa et al., 1991, 1992; Ewert et al., 1994b; Dicke et al., 1998; Nishikawa, 1999).

Modulation and Modification   The differentiated processes in the tectum can be modulated and modified by telencephalic nuclei either directly or indirectly via thalamic nuclei. For one, there are tectal loops involving the posterior ventral medial pallium. This structure is homologous to portions of the mammalian hippocampus (Herrick, 1933; Neary, 1990; Northcutt and Ronan, 1992; Bruce and Neary, 1995; Roth and Westhoff, 1999). It participates in stimulus-specific habituation, classic conditioning, and instrumental conditioning (Finkenstädt, 1989; Finkenstädt and Ewert, 1992; Papini et al., 1995).

Stimulus specificity in habituation is a property not observed among invertebrates. In mammals, habituation is stimulus-specific, so that dishabituation is mutual. If a stimulus B can dishabituate stimulus A, the stimulus A can dishabituate stimulus B as well. Since a toad's dishabituation is not necessarily mutual, this characteristic might represent an intermediate evolutionary step (Wang et al., 1991).

After vMP lesions, modifications of visual perception by learning disappear while the species-common capabilities reappear (Finkenstädt and Ewert, 1988; Finkenstädt 1989; Ewert et al., 1994a). This shows that the vMP is not part of, but is associated with, the stimulus-response mediating system. Another telencephalic structure involved in learning in amphibians concerns the amygdalar complex. S.O.G.

Lindemann and Roth (1999) suggest that fear conditioning in *Bombina orientalis* after a single bee sting is linked with the expression of the immediate early gene *erg-1* in certain components of this complex.

Gating the Translation of Perception into Action   Gating an action via directed attention seems to require a tectal loop involving the caudal ventral striatum that is homologous to a portion of the amniote basal ganglia (Marín et al., 1997a–d; González et al., 1999; Smeets et al., 2000).

Marín et al. (1998b) and Medina et al. (1999) put forward the notion that elementary structures of the basal ganglia were present in the brain of ancestral tetrapods and that they were organized according to a general plan shared by all extant tetrapods. Anurans, reptiles, and birds possess various pathways by which basal ganglionic influences can be exerted on the tectum (for anurans, see Marín et al., 1997a–d). One connection is mediated by pretectal structures (Reiner et al., 1980, 1982a,b, 1984, 1998; Reiner, 1987; Medina and Reiner, 1995; Medina et al., 1999). More specifically, a bird's nucleus pretectalis and a reptile's dorsal pretectal nucleus (equivalent to an anuran's pretectal thalamic Lpd nucleus) give rise to terminals in superficial retinorecipient tectal layers. In pigeons it was shown that such pretectotectal projection involves neuropeptide Y (Gamlin et al., 1996), comparable to a frog's pretecto(Lpd)tectal projection (Kozicz and Lázár, 1994; for recent reviews on neuropeptides in frog brain areas processing visual information, see Lázár, 2001 and Kozicz and Lázár, 2001).

In anurans, a disinhibitory striato-*pretecto*-tectal pathway is suggested to be involved in an attentional gating function, as described earlier. In mammals, a comparable gating function is described for a disinhibitory striato-*nigro*-tectal(superior collicular) pathway (Chevalier and Deniau, 1990). Wilczynski and Northcutt (1983b) and Reiner et al. (1984) suggest that in the line of evolution of amniotes, the "pretectal leg" was greatly deemphasized, so that in mammals it may have been lost. Or perhaps may it not as yet have been found (Mengual et al., 1999)?

Concluding Remarks

Visual perception in amphibians has been well investigated from various points of view, so that an integrated multidisciplinary presentation of behavioral, neurophysiological, neuropharmacological, and neuroanatomical data with evolutionary perspectives, including computer modeling of the processing structures, is now possible.

Amphibians are phylogenetically basal tetrapods at the border of aquatic and terrestrial life. The peculiarities of the amphibian's visual system specialize it for motion perception and, consequently, determine the general characteristics of the amphibian's visual world.

Motion perception presumes a discrimination between motion and self-induced motion. "Surround-inhibition" is (part of) the mechanism that allows this distinction.

The three fundamental behaviors—feeding, escaping, and breeding—are addressed to living objects, and "living" is associated with movement. The corresponding behaviorally relevant objects, preys, predators, and mates are not represented explicitly in the brain; rather, they can be abstracted into their shapes in relation to the direction of their movement. Such objects are thus not detected explicitly; rather, they are implicit in structures of different, partly shared spatiotemporal features within one bounded continuum of feature relationships. The classification of objects (categorization) can be implemented by feature-relating algorithms.

Implicit computation is regarded as an evolutionary "trick" by which a relatively "small" brain can solve a large problem; namely, by circumventing the need for explicit computation, which would require an enormous processing structure.

The principle of the prey feature-relating algorithm probably results from an adaptation of an organism to terrestrial predatory life. This algorithm is generalized since it is implemented by the different brains of different animal groups like anuran amphibians such as *Bufo bufo*, the amphibious fish *Periophthalmus koelreutheri*, and mantid insects such as *Sphodromantis lineola*.

Visual categorial perception involves neural processing streams. Depending on the function (prey orienting, mate orienting, prey snapping, predator avoiding, obstacle avoiding, etc.), the corresponding processing streams may be (partly) segregated and may interact at certain levels of integration beyond the retina, e.g., in tectal, pretectal, tegmental, and/or premotor structures.

Categorial perception, based on certain combinations and/or relations of features, can be modulated and modified by many factors, including attention, motivation, and learning. This presumes that there are basic stimulus-response-mediating circuits (processing streams) whose mediation can be modified by modulating neural loops that involve various forebrain structures, such as the ventral medial pallium, a structure that is homologous to portions of the mammalian hippocampus.

Gating perception into action obviously takes advantage of a modulating forebrain loop that involves the caudal ventral striatum, a structure that is homologous to portions of the amniote basal ganglia.

Translating perception into action involves a command-releasing system that consists of different command elements in a combination suitable for selecting the appropriate type of motor pattern, the behavior. The CEs analyze a stimulus and/or localize it in space. Depending on stimulus situations, the same behavior may be activated by different CRSs. Different CRSs may share the same CE. A CRS can be regarded as the neurophysiological equivalent of a "releasing mechanism" according to the classic terminology of Nikolaas Tinbergen.

II ENHANCING THE VISUAL BASICS: USING COLOR AND POLARIZATION

INTRODUCTION
Thomas W. Cronin

For us humans, vision is the sense that seems most directly connected to "reality." Human vision is unquestionably complex, with two receptor sets (rods and cones) operating in parallel, a rich sense of color based on three primary receptor classes, and an occasionally overwhelming experience of shape, space, and motion. Understanding the neural basis of human vision is clearly a daunting challenge for the neuroscientist. Hence the hope that by studying vision in animals with "simpler" nervous systems we will gain insights into potential bioengineering solutions that have applicability beyond the animal being studied.

In this part of the volume, several scientists review their work on animal visual systems that serve as models for the complex processing of information on color and distribution of light. Surprisingly, the chapters leave the impression that human vision is actually simple compared with the visual systems of the small invertebrates discussed here. Human color vision does in fact lose some of its impressiveness when compared with smaller, even tiny, systems that are based on three (honeybees), five (butterflies), or as many as sixteen (mantis shrimps) receptor spectral classes. Even more impressive, however, is the fact that these small invertebrates have access to sensory experiences that are unavailable to humans, including the perception of ultraviolet light and the perception created by the complex processing of polarized light. This overall complexity is amplified by the fact that in some invertebrate species, receptor types vary with the season (crayfish) or habitat (mantis shrimps), and that, in the case of mantis shrimps, eye movements are so complex that they appear horrendously confusing to the human observer.

Ironically, studying these supposedly simpler visual systems poses many unique challenges. Because invertebrate nervous systems are small and contain many fewer neurons than ours, it is often difficult to conceptualize their functional organization. In addition, the constituent neurons are small and, consequently, difficult to acquire and hold with standard electrophysiological techniques. Finally, of course, it is difficult to imagine what the world looks like to an animal that sees ultraviolet and polarized light. Nevertheless, despite the conceptual and technical challenges, the study of invertebrate color and polarization vision continues to provide richly rewarding perspectives on the design and function of visual systems.

The chapters that follow introduce themes that reappear in many different invertebrate visual systems. The eyes are often regionalized, permitting different receptor classes or functional groups to specialize for different tasks. Invertebrate vision is often surprisingly flexible, varying significantly among even closely related species, or over time within single individuals. Finally, the anatomy of the invertebrate visual system is often very approachable, and can reveal much about its functional organization to the careful observer. In particular, the anatomical organization can reveal how incoming visual stimuli are initially, sometimes immediately, processed, or how different types of information are separated and isolated into distinct information streams that flow into the central nervous system.

Invertebrates provide particularly clear examples of visual evolution designed to solve unique environmental challenges, and many species are surprisingly easy to train for studies of visual function in action. And, of course, invertebrates are fully worthy research subjects in their own right, giving us the satisfaction of seeing beautiful and successful creatures making the best of the sensory challenges that they face.

5 Color Vision in Bees: Mechanisms, Ecology, and Evolution
Lars Chittka and Harrington Wells

The fact that many animals see the world in colors and in ways that are very different from those of human vision has long fascinated scientists. These differences underscore the fact that the world we see is not the "real," or physical world. The world that any organism experiences is a product of the specific sensory filters that the animal has acquired during its evolution.

It was a hymenopteran species that first provided this insight. More than 100 years ago, Lubbock (1889) discovered that ants had ultraviolet sensitivity, demonstrating for the first time a sensory capacity not held by humans. Then, just a few decades later, UV vision in bees was discovered (Kühn, 1924). Subsequently, several generations of bee vision *aficionados* have produced a wealth of information on neural color processing in the tiny brains of these insects. In fact, our knowledge of color vision in bees is more extensive than that of any other animal besides primates. However, there are still many intriguing questions to be asked, some very fundamental. These questions are not limited to the mechanisms of color coding by bees, they also have to do with why bees see colors the way that they do.

Much of early sensory ecology was shaped by a naive panadaptionism, a version of the early twentieth-century naturalists' belief that there is a creator who wields unlimited power and creativity. However, in this case the creator was natural selection. This belief slowed progress in the field substantially. That is, to demonstrate evolutionary adaptation, adaptation itself cannot be the null hypothesis. One needs to consider alternative hypotheses such as an organism's evolutionary history, molecular and phylogenetic constraints, and chance evolutionary events.

In this chapter, we discuss what has been discovered in recent decades about bee color vision and suggest some promising avenues for future research. After our discussion of several key issues in understanding color vision in bees, we will turn to the question of how bees use color signals during foraging. Essentially, we will use bees as a case study of how color vision is used in the economy of nature.

The Spectral Sensitivity and Phylogeny of Bee Photoreceptors

The complex eyes of bees contain between 1000 and 16,000 ommatidia, depending on the species. Honeybees have some 5000 ommatidia (U. Jander and Jander, 2002). Each ommatidium contains nine photoreceptor cells. Eight of these elongated cells are arranged side by side so that they form a quasi-circle. Their rhabdomeres, brush-shaped microvillous extensions that contain the photopigments, protrude into the center of the circle. In bees, these extensions form a fused rhabdom, which means that the rhabdomeres from all eight photoreceptor cells are functionally fused to form a single light-guiding structure (A. W. Snyder, 1979). In honeybees, it was traditionally thought that four of these receptors are green receptors with maximum sensitivity (λ_{max}) at about 540 nm, two are blue receptors ($\lambda_{max} \approx$ 440 nm), and two are UV receptors ($\lambda_{max} \approx$ 340 nm). The ninth photoreceptor cell is small and is located near the base of the ommatidium. It is presumably a UV receptor (Menzel and Backhaus, 1991). Recent molecular biological work, however, appears to indicate that there are three types of ommatidia, each with a different set of spectral receptors (Kurasawa et al., 2002).

In bees, each class of spectral receptor contains a distinct visual pigment, which consists of two components. One is the chromophore, retinal (or one of its congeners), which changes its configuration when it absorbs a single quantum of light (Seki and Vogt, 1998). The other component is a protein, the opsin, consisting of about 370 amino acids. Opsins are integrated into the membrane of rhabdomeric microvilli (Deeb and Motulsky, 1996). They consist of seven transmembrane helices in a circular arrangement so that they form a pocket, which contains the chromophore. Specific amino acids in the transmembrane helices oriented toward the center of the pocket (and thus interacting electrostatically with the chromophore) are responsible for spectral tuning (Hope et al., 1997). Spectral sensitivity curves have a roughly Gaussian shape, with a halfbandwidth of approximately 100 nm. The absorption spectra of short-wavelength pigments are generally narrower than those of long-wavelength pigments. This is an intrinsic photopigment characteristic in plots using a linear wavelength scale (figure 5.1).

Long-wavelength pigment absorption spectra have two peaks in the range from 300 to 700 nm, a large α peak and a smaller β peak in the UV. The β peak is caused by the *cis* band of the chromophore. As the visual pigment peak wavelength (λ_{max}) value is shifted toward shorter wavelengths, the β peak gradually is consumed by the larger α peak.

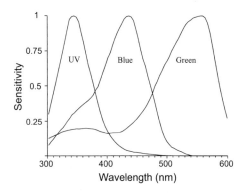

Figure 5.1
Spectral sensitivity of photoreceptor cells in the honeybee *Apis mellifera* (Peitsch et al., 1992). The UV-, blue-, and green-sensitive photoreceptors of the genus *Apis* have spectral sensitivity curves typical of many insects.

In order to understand how visual pigments in bees have changed over evolutionary time, it is important to understand the phylogeny of arthropod opsins. To this end, Briscoe and Chittka (2001) compared the amino acid sequences of the opsins of fifty-four species of arthropods available in the literature, including the different opsins found within each of these species.

Invertebrate opsins fall into distinct functional clades according to their spectral sensitivity (figure 5.2). There is one cluster of UV pigments, a distinct group of blue pigments, and a third group of long-wave pigments, which includes pigments with peak sensitivity from green to red. (For a discussion of the blue-green cluster, see Chittka and Briscoe, 2001) Of particular interest is the fact that chelicerate and crustacean green-sensitive pigments are more similar to insect green pigments than they are to either UV or blue pigments. This suggests that the opsin clades diverged from one another before the major groups of arthropods had diverged, and it is therefore likely that ancient arthropods already possessed (at least) UV and green visual pigments.

The Hymenoptera are especially interesting in terms of visual ecology because the species studied come from a wide variety of habitats, with very different lifestyles and feeding habits (figure 5.3). Nevertheless, there is surprisingly little variation in photoreceptor spectral sensitivity. All species, with the exception of ants, possess UV, blue, and green receptors. The few species for which data on UV and blue receptors are absent (e.g., Symphyta and Ichneumonidae), as well as, for example, *Colletes* and *Lasioglossum*, presumably represent cases where such cells exist but have not as yet been recorded (Peitsch et al., 1992). Some species possess additional red receptors, for example, three species of Symphyta (hence red receptors were probably present in their ancestor species) and one andrenid bee. There are pronounced differences in lifestyle among these species with red receptors; while *Tenthredo* oviposits on leaves, *Xyphidria* is a wood-boring wasp (figure 5.3). *Callonychium* is a solitary bee that appears to visit purple *Petunia* flowers exclusively (Wittmann et al., 1990). Therefore, different selective pressures presumably drove the evolution of red receptors in these species.

The remaining species, those with only UV, blue, and green receptors, also inhabit diverse habitats and have varied life histories. They include not only several generalist nectarivores (such as honeybees, stingless bees, and bumblebees), but also a few species that specialize on a narrow range of flowers (*Andrena, Lasioglossum, Colletes*). In addition, this group contains generalist (*Vespa*) and specialist (*Philanthus*) predators. Some of these species are ground nesting (e.g., most bumblebees) others nest in trees (*Apis*), and still others utilize termite nests (*Partamona*). All species featured here are primarily diurnal, but some are known to forage at night (Warrant et al., 1996). Some members are obligatorily Alpine species (e.g., *Bombus monticola*), and so forage in a very UV-rich environment, whereas others (e.g., some stingless bees) may do much of their foraging in dense tropical forests, which have relatively little UV light (Endler, 1993).

Peitsch et al. (1992) suggested that the only case of adaptive tuning evident in the Hymenoptera is a long-wavelength shift in the UV receptor of forest-dwelling

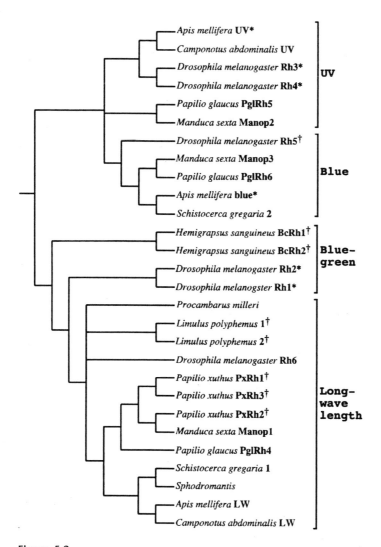

Figure 5.2
Phylogeny of insect, chelicerate, and crustacean opsins, based upon a maximum parsimony analysis of opsin amino acid sequences. The tree shown is simplified from the analysis of a larger data set of fifty-four opsin sequences. Only representative species from available orders or suborders are shown. The brackets indicate measured (asterisk) or inferred (dagger) spectral properties of the visual pigments in each clade. Inferred spectral properties are based upon in situ hybridization or immunohistochemistry in combination with electro-physiological studies. For references for the measured spectra, see Chittka and Briscoe (2001). (From Chittka and Briscoe, 2001, with permission from Springer-Verlag.)

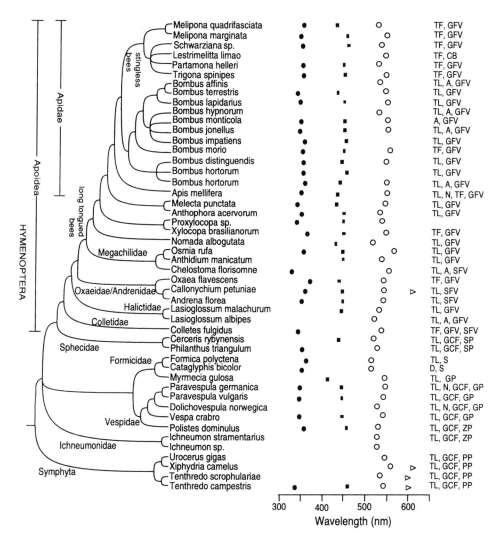

Figure 5.3
Spectral sensitivity of Hymenoptera, superimposed on their phylogeny, and ecological specializations for which vision is important. The values of maximum sensitivity are shown for each known receptor type in each species. For references, see Briscoe and Chittka (2001). Light habitat or type of activity: A, alpine; D, desert; N, nocturnal activity (in addition to diurnal, which is primary in all these species); TF, tropical forest; TL, temperate lowland. Feeding specialization: GFV, generalist flower visitor; SFV, specialist flower visitor; GCF, generalist carbohydrate forager (flowers, fruits, tree sap, and honeydews); GP, generalist predator; SP, specialist predator; CB, cleptobiotic (*Lestrimelitta limao* obtains its food exclusively by robbing the nests of other bees); S, scavenger; PP, phytoparasitism; ZP, zooparasitism (in the latter species, the larvae are parasitic, and the imaginae need to identify appropriate hosts). Circles, squares, and arrows indicate wavelengths of peak sensitivity for UV, blue, green, and red receptors.

stingless bees. An inspection of the λ_{max} values superimposed on the Hymenopteran phylogeny does not reveal strong support for this hypothesis, however. The UV receptors of all stingless bee species fall well within the scatter of other apid bees. In conclusion, despite a wide variety of visual-ecological conditions under which the Hymenoptera live, we find few differences in color receptors among most species, and in the few cases where we do find differences, a convincing adaptive explanation has yet to be found.

Optimal Sets of Photoreceptors for Natural Color Coding

A dozen years ago, one of us (LC), in collaboration with R. Menzel, set out to identify the adaptive significance of bee color vision. The idea was to generate a set of theoretically optimal color receptors for the task of color coding flowers, and to compare this with the system really implemented in bees. We hypothesized that because bees obtain most of their food from flowers, their color vision should be adapted for optimal detection and identification of flower colors. Our evolutionary model calculations consisted of moving three color receptor sensitivity curves along the wavelength scale. For each theoretical combination of receptors so generated, the quality of the color vision system for color coding flowers was determined. The result was striking; the optimal color receptors generated by the evolutionary model invariably occurred near λ_{max} = 330, 430, and 550 nm, values very close to the most common λ_{max} found in flower-visiting bees (figure 5.4) (Chittka and Menzel, 1992). This result was independent of whether we varied one, two, or all three photoreceptors. It was also independent of the particular set of flowers used (Chittka, 1996). Since the optimal set of color receptors might also depend on the particular kind of opponent coding in the brain, the mode of this processing, too, was varied, and the result remained unchanged (Chittka, 1996).

An engineer could hardly design a better receiver for flower colors than the color receptor set of bees. But does this mean that flower colors drove the evolution of bee color receptors? Our findings led some to think that bee color vision was an adaptation to flower colors, although we explicitly stated that this is not necessarily the case (Chittka and Menzel, 1992).

Indeed, there are several complications. Although models are useful in generating hypotheses of optimality, a correlation between a model and certain biological traits does not resolve the question of how the traits evolved. Using models to reject a hypothesis of evolutionary causality is much more straightforward. Had the optimal color receptors derived from our model calculations been different from the ones found in extant animals, then this would have indicated that evolution has not optimized the photoreceptors according to the model's criteria. At the very least, it would mean that there are other, more important criteria, or that evolutionary constraints might have hindered the animal from evolving along the same lines as the model predicts. In fact, sets of color receptors similar to those of bees occur in animals that occupy entirely different ecological niches.

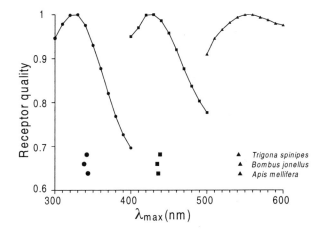

Figure 5.4
Determination of an optimal photoreceptor set for discriminating flower colors. In each of three variations, two receptors were fixed at the wavelength positions where they most frequently occur in Hymenoptera, and the third was shifted in 10-nm steps from 300 to 400 nm, from 400 to 500 nm, or from 500 to 600 nm. The spread of floral color loci in the bee's color space was determined by which set of spectral photoreceptors was used. All of these distances were summed, and the sum serves as a measure for the quality of each receptor set. The single points show the λ_{max} actually found in three species of bees (Peitsch et al., 1992).

Postreceptor Neural Processing

Basic Neuroanatomy of the Optic Lobes

To understand the specifics of color processing in bees, we should first take a general look at arthropods. The basic architecture of the optic lobes in malacostracan crustaceans and insects is extremely similar and was most likely present in a common ancestor (Osorio et al., 1995). The visual information is passed from the receptor level to three successive ganglia, called the lamina, medulla, and lobula (figure 5.5). Of the eight or nine photoreceptors present in each ommatidium, six to seven terminate in the lamina (short visual fibers), while one to three project to the lobula (long visual fibers) (Osorio et al., 1995). Based on comparisons among fruit flies, honeybees, locusts, and crayfish, Osorio et al. (1995) concluded that the ancestral *bauplan* (body plan) of these animals involved long-wavelength sensitivity (blue-green) in the short visual fibers, and at least one long visual fiber with UV sensitivity.

The internal wiring of the lamina, as well as the lamina-medulla connections, are highly conserved across insects from different orders, and even many crustaceans (Osorio et al., 1995). One widespread type of neuron that appears to be central in color vision consists of the large monopolar cells, which relay the information from the

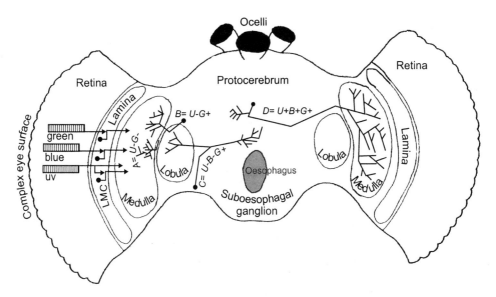

Figure 5.5
Frontal section through the brain of a honeybee showing the neuronal pathways that are most likely involved in color coding. Each ommatidium contains four green and two blue receptors, which project into the lamina (short visual fibers), and three UV receptors, which project into the medulla (long visual fibers). All receptors make contact with lamina monopolar cells (LMCs) in the lamina. These cells convey the receptor signals to the medulla (de Souza et al., 1992). LMCs exist in both depolarizing and hyperpolarizing forms. The distal medulla and lobula contain several types of color-coded neurons, very few of which have been stained. The soma of neuron A (Hertel, 1980, his figure 6) was not dyed. The neuron produced a tonic inhibition (but phasic excitation) to both UV and green light at daylight intensity. Blue light was not tested. Neuron B was inhibited by UV light and excited by green light; blue light produced no response (Menzel and Backhaus, 1991). Neuron C (Hertel and Maronde, 1987, their figure 6) was strictly phasic. This neuron received the opposite input (i.e., long wavelength inhibition and UV phasic excitation from the contralateral eye). Neuron D (Hertel and Maronde, 1987, their figure 2) has arborizations almost throughout the entire medulla and is excited by light of all wavelengths from the ipsilateral eyes, but is inhibited by UV and green light from the contralateral eye. All visual neuronal pathways appear to converge on the protocerebrum, which seems to be an area of higher-level color processing. (Adapted from Menzel and Backhaus, 1991.)

photoreceptor cells to the medulla. Some of these cells appear to amplify the unprocessed signals from particular photoreceptors (de Souza et al., 1992), while others sum inputs from two or three spectral receptor types, possibly to form the initial stage of a brightness coding system used in phototaxis (Menzel and Backhaus, 1991).

The medulla and lobula of the honeybee, *Apis mellifera*, contain a bewildering variety of neurons that might be related to color coding. Such neurons can have phasic properties, which means that they respond only to the onset (and/or offset) of a light stimulus (of a particular wavelength) with a burst of action potentials. Other neurons have tonic responses; i.e., they produce a sustained series of action potentials, or are continuously inhibited, in response to light of a particular spectral domain. For color identification, it is presumably necessary that a tonic component be present. Otherwise the signal would vanish as the bee approaches the target (a flower, for example). While there are some neurons in the optic lobes of the bee that are purely phasic, all tonic neurons so far found in the bee optic lobes also have a phasic component, so that signals are amplified when a target occupies only a small portion of the receptive field.

Wavelength-Selective Behavior

The processing of spectral stimuli has been divided into two types, wavelength-selective behavior and color vision (Menzel, 1979). Wavelength-selective behavior occurs when specific behavioral responses are triggered by specific configurations of signals from the photoreceptors (Goldsmith, 1990). For example, sea anemones retract their tentacles when they are exposed to UV light, but bend them toward visible light (Menzel, 1979). This behavior has no plasticity; it cannot be altered by learning. In such cases, it is reasonable to assume that the motor circuits are connected to rather unprocessed output from the visual periphery in a hard-wired fashion.

Phototaxis in bees is an example of wavelength-selective behavior. When honeybees leave the hive or a flower, or when they are trying to escape from a precarious situation, they seek out bright daylight. This response is color-blind: when given the choice between two routes, bees will invariably pick the brighter one, irrespective of spectral content. Brightness, in this context, is the weighted sum of all three spectral receptors' responses, where the strongest input appears to come from the UV receptors (Kaiser and Seidl, 1977; Menzel and Greggers, 1985). Neurons whose activity might underlie this behavior have been found in all optic ganglia of the honeybee. These cells, phasic or tonic, sum up the signals from the UV, blue, and green receptors (Kien and Menzel, 1977a; Hertel and Maronde, 1987b; de Souza et al., 1992).

Another example of wavelength-selective behavior is related to navigation using a sun compass. If the sun itself is obscured by clouds, bees will use the polarization pattern of sky light to reconstruct the position of the sun (K. von Frisch, 1967). This is accomplished using specialized, polarization-sensitive UV receptors in the dorsal margin of the compound eyes (Wehner, 1989a). In the laboratory, bees will interpret small, nonpolarized, and long wavelength-dominated light sources as the sun, whereas extended light sources with a strong UV component (polarized or unpolarized) will be interpreted as open sky (Edrich et al., 1979; Rossel and Wehner, 1984). Neurons that are UV–bluegreen antagonistic, which might be used in this behavior, have been recorded frequently in the medulla of bees (Kien and Menzel, 1977b).

Several types of motion-related behaviors are also color blind. All appear to be driven entirely by a single class of receptor, the bees' long-wave, or green receptor.

One classic experimental paradigm used to study, for example, the temporal resolution of vision in different animals, is the optomotor response. Animals placed in a rotating drum with vertical stripes will typically turn in the direction of the drum's rotation, which stabilizes their position within the visual environment. Under natural conditions, this is equivalent to compensating for involuntary displacements from the intended position or direction of movement. However, honeybees will only follow the direction of movement if the stripes present contrast in the green domain of the spectrum (Kaiser, 1974). Other types of behavior controlled by the input from the green receptor are movement avoidance, motion parallax, and edge detection (Lehrer, 1998).

The green receptors are also important in floral detection by bees. Before honeybees are able to analyze the color of a flower, they detect the flowers by means of green contrast. This means that the bees compare the signals from the green receptors stimulated by the flower with the signals from the green receptors stimulated by the background (Giurfa and Lehrer, 2001). One might expect a phasic neuronal channel to drive these motion-related behaviors (Horridge, 2000), and indeed, phasic green-sensitive neurons have been found in each of the bee's optic ganglia (de Souza et al., 1992; Kien and Menzel, 1977b).

It is intriguing that Kien and Menzel (1977a) found a cell that responds to green light with a phasic response, but responds tonically to a mixture of UV and green light. This cell might be used both for green receptor-driven detection and for subsequent color identification of a target.

In bumblebees, the green channel appears to be used only for detection of very small flowers. For larger flowers, in a tradeoff between detection and correct identification, bumblebees seem to use the more reliable color channel for detecting flowers (Spaethe et al., 2001). In fact, bees of several genera use color vision for identification of flowers (Chittka et al., 2001) and their nest entrance (Chittka et al., 1992). They also respond to colored landmarks seen en route between the nest and a food source (Cheng et al., 1987; Chittka et al., 1995; Zhang et al., 1996), but it remains to be shown whether color (rather than, for example, the signal generated by the green receptors) is a cue used in identifying these landmarks.

Color Vision

An essential prerequisite for color vision is the presence of color opponent coding by neurons that compare inputs from different color receptor types. Menzel and Backhaus (1989) and Backhaus (1991) postulated that in honeybees the photoreceptor signals are evaluated by means of two types of color opponent processes, one of which is UV–bluegreen antagonistic, and another that is blue–UV-green antagonistic (figures 5.6 and 5.7). This model has been widely referenced and appears to be useful in predicting how honeybees discriminate colors.

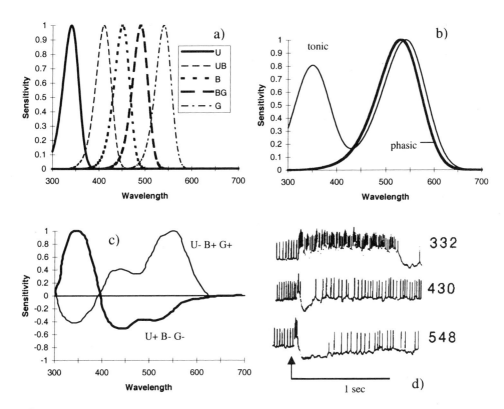

Figure 5.6
Spectral sensitivity of neurons related to color coding in the bee optic lobes (Kien and Menzel, 1977b; Hertel, 1980; Hertel and Maronde, 1987b). Sensitivity functions are smoothed and stylized to emphasize the important features. (*Upper left*) Narrow-band neurons from the lamina and medulla, most sensitive in the UV, violet, blue, blue-green, and green. These cells can be phasic-tonic or strictly phasic. (*Upper right*) A cell with different responses in different temporal phases of the stimulus; the phasic response is predominantly to green light, while in the sustained phase, UV and green wavebands excite the cell. (*Lower left*) Color opponent neurons of two types. (*Lower right*) Spike trains of a UV+ B- G- cell in response to UV (332 nm), blue (430 nm), and green light (548 nm). (From Menzel and Backhaus, 1989, with permission from Springer-Verlag.)

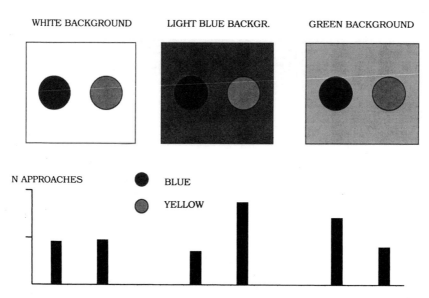

Figure 5.7
The attractiveness of yellow (bee green) and blue (bee blue) dummy flowers for bumble-bees (*Bombus terrestris*) depends on the background color. On a white background, both flower types are approached equally frequently. On a light-blue background, yellow flowers are more attractive. On a green background, blue flowers are more attractive. (From Lunau et al. 1996, with permission from Springer-Verlag.)

The neurophysiological evidence underlying Backhaus' proposed opponencies is not strong, however. Kien and Menzel (1977b) frequently found only one type of tonic color opponent neuron. These cells were excited by UV light and inhibited by blue and green light (UV+B-G-). However, the cells differed widely in the strengths of inputs from the blue and green receptors, and so the assumption of a single set of weighting factors is a simplification. A single UV-B+G+ cell was also found. However, the existence of the other type of neuron postulated by the model, a tonic neuron with excitatory input from blue receptors and inhibitory input from UV and green receptors (UV-B+G-), or its mirror image, UV+B-G+, is uncertain.

To make matters even more complicated, a number of color-coded neurons not included in the model have also been described. A strictly phasic neuron that reacted antagonistically to blue and UV-green was found by Hertel (1980). It produced a brief burst of action potentials at the onset of blue light and also a brief burst when the UV or green light was switched off. There was no inhibitory response to UV and green while the stimulus was ongoing. Hertel and Maronde (1987b) also found a phasic neuron that was green versus UV-blue antagonistic. The functions of these cells are unclear, but they might be used in coding successive color contrast (Neumeyer, 1981) or turning the bee's attention to a target seen in flight.

Single-waveband neurons, tuned to only a narrow section of the wavelength scale, were found in both the medulla and the lobula of bees (figure 5.6). Neurons with maximum signal response to UV (antagonistically $\lambda_{max} = 340$ nm), violet ($\lambda_{max} = 410$ nm), blue ($\lambda_{max} = 440$ nm), blue-green ($\lambda_{max} = 490$ nm), and green ($\lambda_{max} = 540$ nm) were found (Kien and Menzel, 1977b). All of them had very narrow spectral sensitivity functions compared with those of photoreceptor cells. For example, the green-sensitive neurons had no beta peak in the UV. This suggests that not even those cells with a λ_{max} similar to that of the photoreceptors simply relay unprocessed receptor signals to the protocerebrum. Rather, there must have been inhibition from other wavebands. A cell that responded with a tonic excitation from both UV and green light was also found (Kien and Menzel, 1977a).

The function of these neurons might be in unique hue coding or in the formation of color categories. The neurons themselves, of course, cannot code for hue any more than single receptors can (because wavelength is always confounded with intensity); but hue coding through such wavelength-tuned cells might be possible in conjunction with a color opponent system. We certainly need more neurophysiological data before we can be sure how color coding functions in the honeybee brain. And we also have to lament the complete absence of neurophysiological data for any hymenopterous species other than *Apis mellifera*.

Higher-Order Color Processing

How do bees really perceive colors? Do they actually see a colored image, or are different components of the visual scene processed in parallel, never to be reassembled into a picture, as some researchers suggest (Horridge, 2000)? Can bees process hue, brightness, and saturation independently, as do humans? Do they categorize colors, so that the hundreds of colors they might be able to distinguish (Chittka et al., 1993) are grouped into sets of similar ones? How does the bee achieve color constancy, the ability to identify colors despite changes in the spectral content of the illumination?

Spectral Purity and Saturation

Spectral purity, or the corresponding perceptual term, *saturation*, is the degree to which colors differ from being uncolored. For humans, black, white, and gray have zero saturation; pastel colors have low saturation; and monochromatic lights (which contain only a single wavelength) have the highest possible saturation (at least at optimum intensity). In color space, spectral purity can be measured as the distance from the uncolored point. Lunau (1990) assumed that bumblebees (*Bombus terrestris*) analyze stimulus saturation because he found that they preferred more spectrally pure colors over those that had a strong uncolored component. However, the most spectrally pure colors were also those that produced the strongest color contrast to the background, which makes pure colors also easily detectable (Spaethe et al., 2001). Therefore these early experiments could not unambiguously demonstrate an independent mechanism that codes for saturation.

Lunau et al. (1996) performed experiments with backgrounds of different colors and confirmed that color contrast to the background was important in determining floral attractiveness for naive bees (figure 5.7). However, in a series of tests with bicolored flower dummies (corollas with nectar guides), the authors clearly showed that color contrast alone was not sufficient to explain the data. Two types of reactions of naive bees to flower dummies were analyzed: the frequency of approach flights and the percentage of approach flights that ended in antennal contact with the nectar guide. The latter could not be explained by color contrast. Whether the approach flights were interrupted or whether they ended in an antennal contact with the nectar guide was strongly dependent on the direction (sign) of color contrast, not only its magnitude. Bees strongly preferred saturated nectar guides on unsaturated corollas, but not the reverse condition in which color contrast between nectar guide and corolla was equal. It seems, therefore, that bumblebees possess the perceptual dimension of saturation.

Dominant Wavelength and Hue
In color space, the dominant wavelength of a color locus can be measured by drawing a straight line from the center of color space through that locus and extrapolating to the spectrum locus (the line that connects the loci of monochromatic lights). The point of intersection at the spectrum locus marks the dominant wavelength. Hue is the corresponding perceptual term; it is the attribute of color perception denoted by yellow, red, purple, etc. (Wyszecki and Stiles, 1982). Clearly, bees can distinguish stimuli that differ in dominant wavelength (von Helversen, 1972), but this does not necessarily mean that hue is a meaningful concept in color perception by bees. We need to compare pairs of stimuli that have equal color contrast with one pair that has the same dominant wavelength and the another that does not. If it can be demonstrated that bees somehow group stimuli of the same dominant wavelength, we can conclude that they have the perceptual dimension of hue.

An interesting observation is that floral colors are strongly clumped in the color space of bees, so that there are some dominant wavelengths where many flower colors occur and others where there are hardly any. The reason is not that bees have a mechanism that facilitates such clustering (e.g., color categorization); rather, there is a limited number of distinct types of spectral reflectance functions (Chittka et al., 1994). It is intriguing that the dominant wavelengths at which floral colors are most common are also those at which interneurons in the bee optic lobes are most sensitive (figure 5.8). However, it is not known whether these neurons are in fact involved in coding specific, biologically relevant hues.

Backhaus (1992b) and Chittka (1992) predicted that the Bezold-Brücke phenomenon, known in human color vision, should exist in bees also. The Bezold-Brücke effect occurs mainly at high intensities: subjectively, hue changes even though the spectral distribution of the stimulus remains the same. So far, behavioral tests have only shown that the discriminability of monochromatic lights from uncolored stimuli changes with stimulus intensity, an effect that is based on the nonlinear transduction

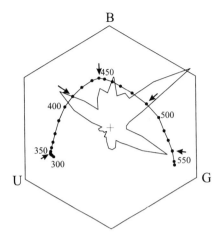

Figure 5.8
Clustering of floral hues in the bee's color space and maximum sensitivity of interneurons in the honeybee optic lobes. The relative number of flowers occurring in each 10-deg hue category is plotted as a circular histogram. A total of 1965 flower colors were evaluated. Clusters appear roughly every 60 deg. The spectrum locus is given from 300 to 560 nm, with solid circles in 10-nm steps. The cross specifies the neutral locus. Arrows mark the wavelength values at which bee interneurons are most sensitive. Note the correspondence of the angular position and peaks in the floral hue distribution.

process in the photoreceptors (Backhaus, 1992b; Chittka, 1992). The same phenomenon would also be expected for broadband reflection functions such as those of flowers (figure 5.9). Whether the predicted hue shifts are actually measurable in bee behavior remains to be determined.

Intensity and Brightness
In human color perception, stimulus brightness (the sensations by which a stimulus appears more or less intense; Wyszecki and Stiles, 1982) is an important dimension of color perception. In bees, this seems not to be the case. Numerous studies have found that it is much more difficult to train bees to attend to differences in stimulus intensity than to differences in spectral quality (von Helversen, 1972; Backhaus and Menzel, 1987; Chittka, 1999). All models of color vision in bees agree in terms of one aspect: all are two-dimensional and do not include a brightness dimension (Vorobyev and Brandt, 1997). It is important here to distinguish between a brightness dimension in color vision in the context of feeding, and intensity-dependent responses generated outside the realm of color vision. For example, honeybees will respond to stimulus intensity in their phototactic escape response (Menzel and Greggers, 1985), but this has no relationship to color vision. If they are extensively trained, however, bees can

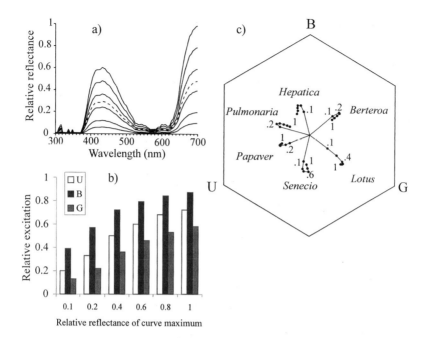

Figure 5.9

Intensity-dependent changes in flower color. (*a*) The intensity of *Hepatica nobilis* is adjusted to six values of maximum reflectance. The maximum of the original measurement is 0.53 (dashed line). (*b*) A set of three color receptor voltage signals is calculated for each curve intensity (ultraviolet, Blue, and green). (*c*) Intensity-dependent color shifts are shown for six typical flower colors. For full species names and reflectance functions, see Chittka et al. (1994). For each color, the curve starts at intensity zero in the uncolored point; it ends at intensity one. The intermediate points correspond to the intensity values 0.1, 0.2, 0.4, 0.6, and 0.8. At very high and very low intensities, the receptor signals are closer to equal than at intermediate intensities; the color locus lies closer to the uncolored point in the hexagon. At some intermediate intensity value, the receptor signals become maximally different from each other; a color with maximal spectral purity will be generated. The type of shift is different for different colors. For all colors, there is a certain intensity between zero and one that generates a maximal spectral purity. Flowers may evolutionarily optimize their detectability by adjusting their intensity. The optimal intensity is low for the UV-blue *Pulmonaria* (optimal intensity, 0.2) and the blue *Hepatica* (optimum at 0.4), whereas it is higher for all other colors.

discriminate stimuli that differ only in intensity (Menzel and Backhaus, 1991), so that bees can apparently learn to attend to cues that they do not naturally use. It is also important to bear in mind that another type of intensity-dependent signal, that produced by the green receptor, is very important in driving several kinds of motion-related behavior (Giurfa and Lehrer, 2001).

Color Categories

Humans form color categories, and cross-cultural studies find consistencies in terms of the boundaries between categorical color names (Ratliff, 1976; Kay and McDaniel, 1978; Zollinger, 1988), which suggests a physiological basis (but see Saunders and van Brakel, 1997). Clearly, the question of whether a similar categorization occurs in animals is interesting but we do not have the answer for a single nonhuman animal. One reason is that in humans, the scientist's access to perception is through language. Another reason is that standard tests to understand color perception in animals do not work for color categories. Color discrimination, for example, is independent of whether two stimuli lie within a category or on the two sides of a boundary between two categories (Heider and Olivier, 1972). Some workers have mistaken sharp discontinuities in color discrimination along the wavelength scale as boundaries of color categories (Goldman et al., 1991). But such discontinuities occur naturally because animals are particularly good at distinguishing wavelengths in spectral ranges where the slopes of two spectral sensitivity functions overlap in opposite directions (Chittka and Waser, 1997), and so they may have no relationship to color categorization. Thus, wavelength discrimination probably is an inappropriate paradigm for studying color categories. Generalization or transfer tests (in which bees are trained to one color, then confronted with two alternative colors) may reveal boundaries of categories (Neumeyer and Kitschmann, 1998), or one might use nonverbal tests that have been developed for infants (Teller and Bornstein, 1987).

Color Constancy

Color constancy is the ability of a visual system to identify a stimulus by its spectral properties, independent of the spectral distribution of the illuminant. This is an important capacity because the spectral radiant power of light varies substantially between sunlight and forest shade, and between noon and sunset (Dyer, 1998; Endler, 1993). Thus the physical quality of light reflected from an object changes, and so without a mechanism to compensate for this change, identification of an object may be compromised. Behavioral experiments, however, show that bees can compensate for the change, and so experience color constancy (Mazokhin-Porshnyakov, 1966; Neumeyer, 1981; Werner et al., 1988). Early workers generally assumed that color constancy is, and has to be, essentially perfect. This is not the case, however. Tests in humans (Maloney, 1986) as well as bees (Neumeyer, 1981) have shown that there are conditions in which color constancy is not flawless. Dyer (1998) has recently started to explore the mechanisms that might underpin color constancy in bees. While some authors have assumed that complex central nervous system operations are necessary for color constancy in bees (Werner et al., 1988), Dyer points out that a more parsimonious approach is in order.

Using an approach developed earlier for human vision (von Kries, 1905), Dyer asked whether color constancy might not simply be explained by von Kries's receptor adaptation. This simply assumes that receptors increase their overall sensitivity when the average illumination that reaches them is low in intensity and decrease their sensitivity when they are strongly stimulated. Clearly, this assumption is fulfilled in insect photoreceptors (Laughlin, 1981). Dyer (1999) showed that such a simple mechanism would yield a rather efficient color constancy mechanism. On the other hand, he predicted specific deviations from perfect color constancy under some conditions, especially in the UV region of color space. Dyer proposed that these deviations occur because of the asymmetric overlap of the spectral sensitivity curves of the spectral receptor types. There is little overlap at longer wavelengths, but the bees' long wavelength receptors, because of their β peak (figure 5.10) overlap strongly with that of their UV receptors (Dyer, 1999). Empirical evidence for these predictions has recently been found (Dyer and Chittka, 2004).

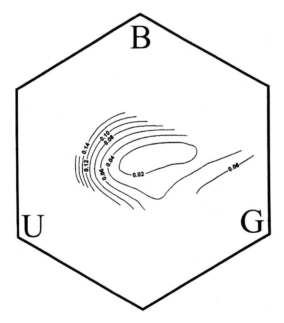

Figure 5.10
Predicted color shift in different parts of bees' color space, assuming von Kries's color constancy. The numbers on the contours indicate the distance that a color in that region of color space would shift for a change in correlated color temperature from 4800 to 10,000 K. For comparison, the distance from the center of the hexagon to any of the corners is unity. The color shift is greatest in the UV and UV-blue areas of color space. (Figure redrawn from P. G. Kevan et al., 2001.)

It should be emphasized that such failures of color constancy are as important for understanding mechanism and ecology as are the instances when color constancy works. Do flower colors "avoid" areas of color space where failures of color constancy would make them hard to identify (Dyer, 1999)? What strategies do bees use to cope with imperfections of color constancy? Do they place stronger emphasis on other floral cues, such as odor, shape, or position in space, when color constancy fails? These will be rewarding topics to explore experimentally in the future.

The Use of Color in Natural Foraging

Much of the diet that most animals consume is cryptic. Bees are fortunate because their food "wants" to be seen. Most species of bees obtain pollen and nectar from plants, which advertise these rewards with conspicuous and colorful signals, the flowers. Flower colors can contain information about the kind of reward that they offer (e.g., pollen or nectar), its quantity, its quality (e.g., nectar volume and sugar concentration), and its variability, as well as information about the handling procedures needed to exploit the flowers (H. Wells and Wells, 1986; Chittka et al., 1999).

In turn, the behavioral response to the flower's color information tells us something about the bee's information processing and, perhaps, the cognitive capacities. Foraging behavior, the repetitive decision-making process of choosing which flowers to visit, has provided a wealth of knowledge about how bees process and perceive color information.

Innate Flower Color Preferences

Many newly emerged insects that have never seen flowers prefer certain colors over others. Such innate color preferences help naive insects find food, and, possibly, select profitable flowers among those that are available.

Floral preferences can be overwritten by learning to some degree, but there is evidence that in some situations (for example, when rewards are similar across flower species), bees will revert to their initial preferences (Heinrich et al., 1977; Banschbach, 1994; Gumbert, 2000). We believe that these innate preferences reflect the traits of those local flowers which are most profitable for the bees. We also think that evolutionary changes in such preferences require changes only in the synaptic efficiency between neurons coding information from color receptors. Therefore, color preferences might adapt more readily to environmental pressures than the wavelength sensitivities of color receptors. Bee color preferences are a promising model system for appreciating, not only the use of color by animals in their natural setting, but also for understanding patterns of heredity of a basic color-related behavior.

For instance Giurfa et al. (1995) found a correlation between the color preferences of naive honeybees and the nectar offerings of different flowers in a nature reserve near Berlin. Honeybees preferred the colors violet (bee UV-blue) and blue (bee blue), which were also the colors most associated with high nectar rewards. Of course, correlation does not indicate causality. To show that color preferences evolved to match floral offerings, we need to compare a set of closely related bee species (or populations of the same species) that live in habitats in which the relationship between floral colors and rewards varies.

We did this by testing eight species of bumblebees from three subgenera: four from central Europe (*B. terrestris terrestris, B. lucorum, B. pratorum,* and *B. lapidarius*); three from temperate East Asia (*B. diversus, B. ignitus,* and *B. hypocrita*); and one from North America (*B. occidentalis*). We found that all species preferred the violet-blue range, presumably a phylogenetically ancient preference (figure 5.11). In addition, however, *B. occidentalis* had the strongest preference for red of all the mainland bumblebee populations examined. This is intriguing because this species frequently robs nectar and forages heavily from red flowers whose morphology seems well adapted for pollination by birds (Chittka and Waser, 1997; Irwin and Brody, 1999). Obviously, this red preference is derived and therefore might be an adaptation unique to *B. occidentalis.*

We also tested *Bombus terrestris terrestris* from Holland, *B. terrestris terrestris* from Germany, *B. terrestris dalmatinus* from Israel, *B. terrestris dalmatinus* from Rhodes, *B. terrestris sassaricus* from Sardinia, *B. terrestris xanthopus* from Corsica, and *B. terrestris canariensis* from the Canary Islands. The rationale for testing island populations was that islands are hot spots of evolutionary change. The effects of chance will be more manifest on islands than in large mainland populations. In addition, small populations might adapt more readily to local conditions, whereas in large populations, gene flow across long distances may prevent local adaptation. The island populations of *B. terrestris* are particularly interesting because they are genetically differentiated from each other and from the mainland population, whereas the entire mainland population, which stretches through central, southern, and eastern Europe, appears to be genetically more homogeneous (Widmer et al., 1998).

No strong differences in color preferences were found among the mainland *B. terrestris* populations; all showed the same strong preference for violet-blue shades as the other species. But some island populations showed an additional red preference (Chittka et al., 2001). In *B. t. sassaricus,* this preference is stronger than that for blue colors in some colonies and is highly significant in all colonies. In *B. t. canariensis,* four of five colonies showed a significant preference for red over yellow and orange.

Figure 5.11 ▶
The color preferences of eight species of bumblebees, with their phylogeny (P. H. Williams, 1994). Each bee was experimentally naïve at the start of the experiment, and only the first foraging bout was evaluated. Three colonies were tested per species, except for *B. terrestris,* where we tested twenty-one, and *B. occidentalis,* where four colonies were tested. The bees were individually tested in a flight arena. They were offered the colors violet (bee UV-blue), blue (bee blue), white (bee blue-green), yellow, orange; and red (the latter three are all bee green). The height that bars indicates the average of choice percentages. The whiskers indicate standard errors.

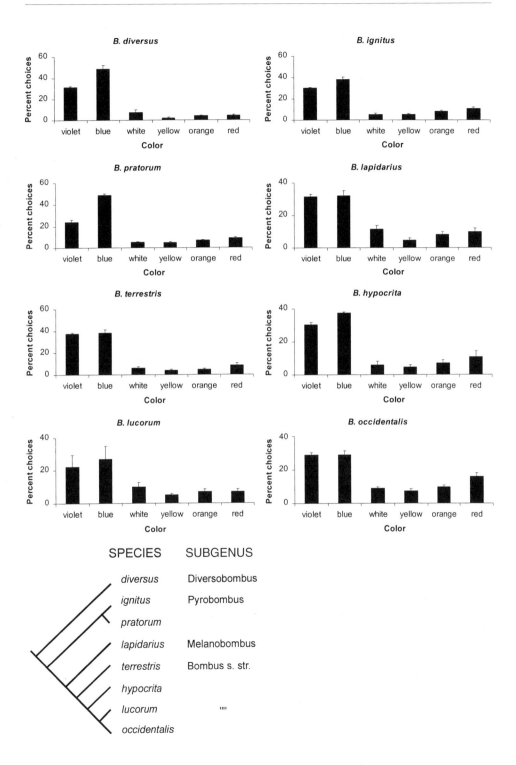

The adaptive significance of such red preference is not easy to understand. Some red, UV-absorbing, and pollen-rich flowers exist in the Mediterranean basin, particularly the eastern part, with the highest concentration in Israel (Dafni et al., 1990). In Israel, however, bumblebees do not show red preference, and the red flowers there appear to be predominantly visited by beetles (Dafni et al., 1990).

In Sardinia, red, UV-absorbing flowers are neither more common nor more rewarding than flowers with other colors (Schikora et al., 2002). The Canary Islands harbor several orange-red flower species. These are probably relics of a Tertiary flora, and some seem strongly adapted to bird pollination (Vogel et al., 1984). Bird visitation has been observed in at least some of these species, but it is not known whether bees utilize them (Vogel et al., 1984). Thus we are left with an interesting observation: Flower color preferences are clearly variable within *B. terrestris*, but we cannot easily correlate the color preferences in different habitats with differences in local flower colors. The possibility that genetic drift has produced the color preferences in some island populations certainly deserves consideration.

To test experimentally whether a trait is adaptive, we should exploit heritable variation to see if animals that have the trait in question are in fact more efficient foragers, and, ultimately, more efficient than those that do not. To this end, we need to show that the variance we find among colonies is heritable. To examine this question, we inbred queens from colonies of different populations with their brothers. The resulting F_1 colonies were practically mirror images of their parental colonies (figure 5.12). For instance, if we cross *Bombus terrestris terrestris* from Germany with *Bombus terrestris sassaricus* from Sardinia, we obtain an F_1 with intermediate red preference. This means there is a strong possibility of doing selection experiments in which we can test the influences of directional selection (Endler et al., 2001) and then perform fitness tests.

Finally, could the peculiar long-wavelength preferences of some island bees be underlain by specialized red receptors? Schikora et al. (2002) made extracellular recordings from bumblebees from Sardinia, and found that indeed their sensitivity to long-wavelength light is significantly higher than in mainland bumblebees. This could mean that some island bees could see colors differently than their mainland relatives, as a consequence of evolutionary chance processes.

Color Learning and Foraging Decisions

In simple laboratory setups where one flower type contains a large reward and alternative flower types typically contain none, bees very rapidly learn to associate floral colors with rewards. A single rewarded visit to a color target is sufficient to induce a measurable change in behavior in honeybees and bumblebees (Schulze Schencking, 1969), and three such visits are sufficient to establish a life-long memory (Menzel, 1985). Colors are first stored in a transient short-term memory, where they are sensitive to interference, and, on repeated exposure, are stored in more stable long-term memory (Menzel, 2001). Mirroring their innate preferences (Giurfa et al., 1995), honeybees learn violet and blue colors even more rapidly than others (Menzel, 1985).

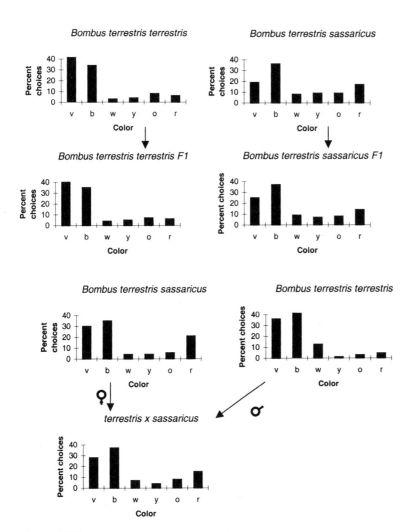

Figure 5.12
Heritability of innate color preference in *Bombus terrestris*. Individual worker bees were tested as explained in figure 5.7. (*Upper four graphs*) Queens from *B.t. terrestris* (Germany) and *B.t. sassaricus* (Sardinia) were inbred (mated with their brothers). Preferences are shown for the parental colonies and the colonies founded by the mated queens. (*Lower three graphs*) Intermediate red preference for a colony founded by a Sardinian queen mated with a German male. The preferences of the workers from the parental colonies are also shown.

Learned preferences can be rapidly reversed if the reward situation changes (Chittka, 1998).

However, when exposed to realistic situations where flowers of two or more types of different colors are intermingled and differ only gradually in rewards, bees will often choose the more rewarding flowers (Heinrich, 1979; Menzel, 2001), but there are cases in which innate preferences (Banschbach, 1994) or cognitive limitations (Chittka et al., 1999; P. S. M. Hill et al., 2001) will make bees deviate substantially from the optimal choice.

The time needed to detect flowers is strongly influenced by floral color (Spaethe et al., 2001). Thus the optimal choice of flowers is not only dependent on the reward and the handling time, but also on the search costs, which are affected by flower color. It is not known if bees take these costs into account when choosing flowers.

Bees also learn to use color to predict the variance of rewards. Tests to deduce such "risk-sensitive" foraging must involve equal average rewards, but differences in reward consistency among flower types of two colors, for example, yellow and blue. In some cases, bees have avoided the flowers with a higher variance in reward; i.e., they were "risk averse" (e.g., Cakmak et al., 1999; Waddington, 2001). The reasons for this behavior are controversial. Both mechanistic (Waddington, 2001; Chittka, 2002) and ultimate explanations (H. Wells and Wells, 1986) have been proposed. In some conditions, bees did not respond at all to reward variance (Fülöp and Menzel, 2000; Waddington, 2001). These differences in reported behavior may be due to alternative experimental designs. However, the possibility of genuine differences among populations has been left largely unconsidered. For example, when different taxa were compared under controlled conditions, differences were found not only among various *Apis* species (N. Muzaffar and H. Wells, unpublished results), but also among *A. mellifera* subspecies (Cakmak et al., 1998, 1999). Possibly the endemic taxa's environment might determine where variance-sensitive foraging occurs.

Flower Constancy

Flower constancy occurs when bees temporarily specialize on one species or morph of flower and bypass other rewarding flowers (H. Wells and Wells, 1986; Waser, 1986). Flower constancy favors an efficient and directed pollen transfer between conspecific plants (Chittka et al., 1999). Color is one important clue by which bees recognize flowers (P. S. M. Hill et al., 1997). To understand the kind of color diversity in flowers that can be expected to evolve as a strategy to promote constancy, it is critical to know the range over which a pollinator-subjective color difference is correlated with flower constancy. For example, if a barely distinguishable contrast between two flower colors can produce 100% constancy, then flower constancy may drive only small-scale color differences, such as that between two similar, but just distinguishable, shades of blue. However, character displacement across color categories, such as blue to yellow, would be harder to explain by pollinator constancy if this were the case.

Previous work allows us to predict how color discrimination improves with color distance (Chittka et al., 1992), but flower constancy and discrimination are unlikely to increase with color difference in the same way. In measuring flower constancy as a function of floral color difference, we do not ask: "How well can bees distinguish colors?" Instead, the appropriate question is: "How readily do bees retrieve memories for different flower types, depending on how similar they are to the one currently visited?" The ability to discriminate flowers sets the upper limit for constancy, but there is no a priori reason to assume that constancy is directly determined by this factor.

In order to measure flower constancy as a function of color distance between flower types, we tested six species of apid bees on fifteen pairs of plant species or color morphs of the same species, using a paired-flower, bee-interview protocol (Thomson, 1981). Even though our analysis ignores differences other than color, there is a clear relationship between bee-subjective color difference and flower constancy (figure 5.13). Constancy does not deviate from chance at color hexagon distances up to 0.1 (where bees already discriminate well between colors; A. Dyer and L. Chittka, 2004). At distances of about 0.2, constancy levels rise sharply in all pollinator species and above 0.4, constancy is generally above 80%. Thus, flower constancy is negligible at small color differences, even for some differences easily discriminated by bees; it is at its maximum only in cases of pronounced differences. In the case of such pronounced differences, such as those between yellow and blue flowers, individual honeybees will sometimes stay constant to the less rewarding flower morph without even sampling the alternative (H. Wells and Wells, 1986; P. S. M. Hill et al., 1997, 2001). But even

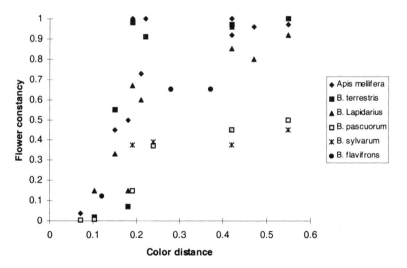

Figure 5.13
Flower constancy in several species of bees as a function of color distance between pairs of flower types. For each pair of flower types, we recorded at least eighty choices. Flower constancy data are calculated as explained in Chittka et al. (2001). (Figure reproduced from Chittka et al., 2001, with permission from Cambridge University Press.)

when rare sampling does occur, or is forced to occur, constancy results in a manner that ignores harvest rate (Hill et al., 1997).

The Relation of Flower Color with Other Cues

Floral color not only serves as a predictor of rewards but also of the particular motor pattern required to exploit flowers of complex morphology (Chittka and Thomson, 1997). In addition to this, the interactions between color and other floral cues, such as scent or pattern, are complex and often poorly understood.

In honeybees, minor changes in flower morphology or arrangement may have major effects on flower constancy, without changes in the colors of the flowers (H. Wells and Wells, 1986). Deviations in flower structure (e.g., adding pedicels; Waddington and Holden, 1979; H. Wells et al., 1986), adding a color pattern without a difference in flower structure (cf. Banschbach, 1994; P. S. M. Hill et al., 1997), and spatial arrangement (e.g., P. S. M. Hill et al., 2001) each affect behavior substantially.

Scent is clearly important in identifying flowers (Raguso, 2001), but the relative importance of scent and color depends on the particular scents and colors involved and on the individual bee (P. H. Wells and Wells, 1985). For example, in a patch of color-dimorphic flowers, some honeybees were constant to yellow and some to blue flowers when all flowers provided a clove-scented reward. The flower constancy of individual bees was not altered when the scent of all the rewards was changed to peppermint. However, when the scent of only one color morph was changed, some bees remained constant to color, whereas others switched color attachment and remained constant to odor (H. Wells and Wells, 1985). The presence of scent can also improve discrimination between rewarding and unrewarding flowers of two colors, even when both types have the same scent (J. Kunze and Gumbert, 2001).

The interaction of floral color with pattern is especially controversial (Giurfa and Lehrer, 2001). Menzel and Lieke (1983) trained bees to bicolored patterns of different orientation and found results that defied any simple explanation. Recently, Hempel de Ibarra et al. (2001) presented a center-surround model to explain how green receptor input from the retina is used in the detection of bicolored patterns. In an interesting analogy to human visual search (Desimone, 1998; Chittka et al., 1999), bees are less efficient at foraging when multiple flower types differ only along a single stimulus dimension (e.g., color), rather than along several dimensions (e.g., color, size, and pattern; Gegear and Laverty, 2001).

Conclusion

Bees, especially honeybees, have long been model organisms for highlighting how complex visual perception is achieved with miniature nervous systems. Their visual spectrum differs fundamentally from our own, as do other aspects of their vision, for example, the apparent lack of a brightness coding dimension in the bee's color space. On the other hand, bee color vision shares surprisingly many general principles with that of humans. Most bee species, just as humans, are trichromatic on the receptor level. Both humans and bees appear to use two spectrally antagonistic mechanisms for color coding. Color and motion are largely processed in parallel in humans as in well as in bees.

Because of such similarities, it was once thought that some invertebrate models might eventually help us understand neural information processing in higher vertebrates, including humans (e.g., Huber, 1983). This hope has remained largely unfulfilled, especially because research on primate color processing has progressed at such a rate that neurobiological work on insect color vision seemed comparatively frustrating. The result is that development of the field has slowed in the past decade.

We think this is unfortunate because the study of color vision in bees has tremendous potential in its own right. In no other organisms do we have as profound an understanding of color used in natural foraging as we do in bees. If we wish to understand how color vision evolves, both as a result of adaptation and chance, bees are a magnificent model system, as we hope to have shown in this review. Primates, conversely, are simply not as amenable to selection experiments and fitness tests as are bees. Other organisms, such as *Drosophila*, offer a wider variety of mutants of the visual system, but testing their fitness under biologically relevant conditions (i.e., natural densities of food, predators, and mates) is virtually impossible, whereas it is straightforward in bees. It is for these reasons that we must continue to study the mechanisms of postreceptor color processing in bees as well. For if we have no information on differences in such processing among species, populations, and individuals, we have nothing to study if we are asking questions about adaptation to the environment. We think that recognizing these shortfalls in our knowledge, rather then resting on what has already been achieved, will bring us much closer to a comprehensive understanding about color vision in the animal kingdom.

Acknowledgments
The authors wish to thank Adrian Dyer, Almut Kelber, and Mickey Rowe for suggestions and criticism.

6 Color Vision and Retinal Organization in Butterflies
Kentaro Arikawa, Michiyo Kinoshita, and Doekele G. Stavenga

Color vision is the ability to discriminate visual stimuli based on their chromatic characteristics regardless of their brightness. Because of their close relationship with flowers, many insects are believed to see colors. Whether color vision is indeed present in any insect, of course, must be demonstrated by behavioral experiments. Yet, behavioral proof of color vision in insects is surprisingly rare. Honeybees (e.g., Menzel and Backhaus, 1989), blowflies (Fukushi, 1990; Troje, 1993), and butterflies (Kelber and Pfaff, 1999; Kinoshita et al., 1999) are the only examples in this respect so far.

The current views on insect color vision are founded on the early work performed on the honeybee, *Apis mellifera*, the first insect whose color vision was convincingly demonstrated. Almost a century ago, Karl von Frisch (1914) showed that foraging honeybees rely on color vision by training them to feed on nectar put on a colored piece of cardboard. The honeybees readily learned the task and, after a learning phase, visited the colored cardboard even though nectar was no longer provided. Von Frisch (1914) then presented the bees with several differently colored pieces of cardboard and demonstrated that the trained honeybees chose the colored cardboard that had been associated with the nectar reward. Using cardboard pieces colored with different shades of gray, he also demonstrated that the honeybees discriminated the stimuli based on their chromatic characteristics rather than their brightness.

When von Frisch trained bees with red cardboard, they could not discriminate red from gray very well, indicating that they are blind to red. However, surprisingly at that time, they appeared to be sensitive to ultraviolet light.

These behavioral experiments suggested that the visible spectrum of honeybees extends from the ultraviolet to the green wavelength region. Subsequent physiological studies revealed that the spectral range of bees is covered by three classes of photoreceptors, with maximum sensitivity in the UV (335 nm), blue (435 nm), and green (540 nm) wavelength region, respectively (Autrum and von Zwehl, 1964; Menzel and Blakers, 1976). Hence these spectral receptors serve as the physiological basis of the trichromatic color vision system of honeybees (Menzel and Backhaus, 1989).

The molecular basis of the different photoreceptor sensitivity spectra is well established. Visual pigment molecules, the rhodopsins, consist of a protein (opsin) and a chromophore (retinaldehyde). The chromophore of insect visual pigments is either retinal or 3-hydroxyretinal (Vogt, 1989). Together, opsin and chromophore determine the absorption spectrum of the rhodopsin. Generally, a single photoreceptor contains only one type of opsin. Since the first cloning of complementary DNA (cDNA) of a *Drosophila melanogaster* opsin (O'Tousa et al., 1985; Zuker et al., 1985), many insect opsins are now fully known. For instance, all three honeybee opsins have been cloned (Townson et al., 1998). The opsins' primary structure has allowed the construction of evolutionary trees for the various classes of visual pigments in different insect species (Kitamoto et al., 1998, 2000; Briscoe and Chittka, 2001; Vanhoutte et al., 2002). Since the peak wavelength of the absorption spectrum of known visual pigments appears to closely correlate with the primary structure, newly cloned visual pigments can be spectrally categorized (Briscoe and Chittka, 2001).

Electrophysiological studies on various insects in recent decades have demonstrated multiple classes of spectral receptors in many species (Arikawa, 1999). Contrary to expectations from the bee work, the number of spectral receptor classes turned out not to be limited to three. Butterflies were first reported to have at least five classes of spectral receptors (i.e., *Papilio xuthus*, Arikawa et al., 1987; *Pieris rapae*, Shimohigashi and Tominaga, 1991). Dragonflies also have five classes of receptors (Yang and Osorio, 1991). Because all insects tested so far have UV receptors, sensitivity in the UV wavelength region appears to be a general feature of insect vision. Blue and green receptors are also universally found. Red receptors are rather rare, however (Briscoe and Chittka, 2001).

Rather little is known about the neuronal mechanisms underlying color vision, either for bees or for other insects (Menzel and Backhaus, 1989). Except for some anatomy (Strausfeld and Blest, 1970), and a limited number of electrophysiological recordings from a few higher-order neurons in a few scattered butterfly species (S. L. Swihart, 1970; Schumperli, 1975; Schumperli and Swihart, 1978; Maddess et al., 1991), knowledge of how color information is processed in the central nervous system is virtually nonexistent. This review on butterfly color vision therefore will be restricted to the two more extensively studied areas: first, the behavioral analyses of learning, discrimination, and color recognition and second, the structure and function of the participating retinal components.

Color Vision in *Papilio*

Color Discrimination and Learning

Butterflies are highly visual as well as highly visible animals. Their putative ability to see colors has been investigated by several workers in the past several decades. However, attempts to prove true color vision have all been unsuccessful, probably because of the difficulties in handling butterflies experimentally (Kolb and Scherer, 1982; Kandori and Ohsaki, 1996). Then, in 1999, two studies on foraging swallowtail butterflies of the genus *Papilio* were published virtually simultaneously (Kelber and Pfaff, 1999; Kinoshita et al., 1999).

Kinoshita et al. (1999) investigated newly emerged Japanese yellow swallowtails, *Papilio xuthus*. The butterflies were housed in a cage with a black cardboard floor, illuminated by halogen lamps. The butterflies were fed a 5% sucrose solution daily, which was placed on a colored paper patch (red, yellow, green, or blue) on the cage floor.

At the beginning of the training, we had to manually extend each butterfly's proboscis. However, the butterflies rapidly acquired the ability to find the patch, land on it, and feed successfully by themselves. After training, we tested the butterflies' ability to discriminate one color from another by presenting individual insects with the four colored patches used in training (red, yellow, green, or blue) but without any sucrose solution (figure 6.1A). After the test, the butterfly was given the previously rewarded patch for a few minutes with the sucrose reward, and then returned to its home cage. This testing regime lasted about 1 week. The rate at which the butterflies chose the target color increased with the number of training days (figure 6.2), and the rate of correct choices reached nearly 100% after 10 days of training.

To demonstrate that the discrimination was not based on brightness differences, we presented the insects with a disk of the target color along with seven other disks of different shades of gray (figure 6.1B). Even then, the butterflies selected the colored disk without exception, providing convincing evidence that foraging *Papilio xuthus* have true color vision (Kinoshita et al., 1999).

Kelber and Pfaff (1999) tested the Australian orchard butterfly, *Papilio aegeus*, and reached the same conclusion by using light-emitting diodes (LEDs) as the colored targets. They trained the butterflies to feed on sucrose solution at a feeder attached to a blue, green, or red LED. Together, both studies have firmly established the presence of color vision in *Papilio*.

Once a butterfly has learned to associate one color with food, can it learn (i.e., "relearn") to associate a different color with a food source? Our experiments indicate that they can, indeed, do so (Arikawa and Kinoshita, 2000). Butterflies trained to associate food with a yellow patch seldom visit a red patch. When a butterfly trained to a yellow patch for a week is fed on a red patch just once, it will not show a preference for either color in a choice test. However, additional rewards presented on the red patch strengthen the new association within minutes (figure 6.3).

Field observations suggest that relearning happens regularly in the life of flower-visiting insects (see Wehner, 1981; Weiss, 2001). This is probably an essential capacity, since flowers bloom and provide nectar for only a short time, and different colored flowers follow each other in blooming period. Newly emerged butterflies, which may have learned that yellow flowers are a good source of food in their first experiences, would rapidly starve if they continued to search for yellow flowers after they have wilted.

In all of the behavioral experiments carried out so far, the ultraviolet wavelength range has remained underilluminated: the experiments were performed in a room equipped with regular halogen lamps, whose irradiation spectrum is virtually zero in the UV range (Kinoshita et al., 1999), or with LEDs emitting light only in the human visible range (Kelber and Pfaff, 1999). So the extent to which UV light plays a role in butterfly color vision is still unknown.

Color Constancy

Color vision in humans is reinforced by color constancy. This is the ability to recognize the color of an object as constant regardless of the chromatic content of the illumination. For instance, an apple appears red under both direct sunlight and regular

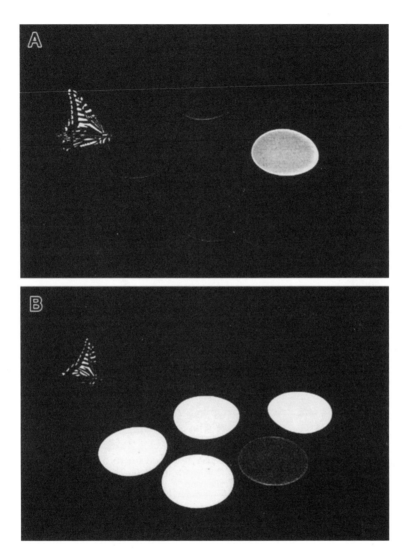

Figure 6.1
Experimental arrangement for testing butterfly color vision. A Japanese yellow swallowtail, *Papilio xuthus*, is first trained to a colored patch by drops of sucrose solution on the patch, which is on the black cage floor. Illumination is from a halogen light. When trained on a blue patch, the butterfly invariably lands on (*A*) a blue patch positioned either among patches of other colors or (*B*) on gray patches of different brightness. Hence the butterfly has true color vision.

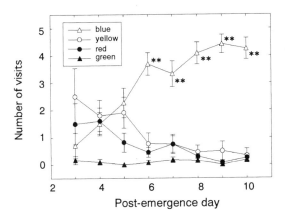

Figure 6.2
Newly emerged butterflies (postemergence day 1) were used in these color vision tests. Butterflies were food deprived until they were offered a colored patch with sucrose on postemergence day 2. On day 3, the choice frequency for visiting four colored patches (blue, green, yellow, and red; none with food) was calculated. Subsequently, the butterflies were offered the training patch. Although the initial color preference is rather random (although it is higher for longer wavelengths), the frequency of choice for the trained color rose dramatically after a few days of experience. The figure shows the results of training with a blue patch, but essentially similar results were obtained with other colors. The asterisks indicate the data where the visit frequency was significantly higher for the trained color than for any other color.

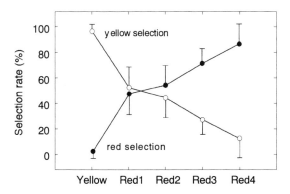

Figure 6.3
Change in color preference that is due to relearning. The choice frequency of butterflies trained to yellow was investigated with two colored patches, yellow and red. The yellow patch was highly preferred, and the red patch was neglected. Repeated offerings of a red patch containing sucrose drops rapidly changed the choice behavior, showing that learning crucially affects color preference.

room light, despite the fact that the spectral contents of sunlight and room light are very different.

Generally, color constancy is very important for animals that rely on the ability to discriminate colors. This should also be true for bees and butterflies because they forage for flowers in sunny open areas, in shaded woods, and at different times of day.

Neumeyer (1981) and Werner et al. (1988) investigated color constancy in honeybees and demonstrated the general independence of pattern discrimination from the illuminant. *Papilio xuthus* also appears to display color constancy (Kinoshita and Arikawa, 2000). We tested the color discrimination ability of foraging *Papilio xuthus* under red, green, or blue illumination. In addition to using stimuli consisting of an assembly of four colored patches (red, green, yellow, and blue), we tested the butterflies with a color collage containing red, green, yellow, blue, white, light gray, and dark gray, called a "Mondrian," a method for testing color constancy introduced by E. H. Land (1977).

We first trained the butterfly to visit a colored patch as described earlier. After confirming that it could distinguish the target color in the four-color pattern or in the Mondrian collage under white illumination, we tested its ability to discriminate colors under different spectral illuminations with different degrees of color saturation. The butterflies were generally able to discriminate well under all types of illumination tested, although some strongly saturated illuminants impaired their abilities somewhat.

One might argue that the four principal colors used (red, yellow, green, and blue) are very different from each other, and that the butterflies could have simply selected the color that looked most similar to the trained color instead of using color constancy. To examine this possibility, we tested whether butterflies could discriminate between two patches of similar colors. We used two alternative pairs of similar colors: blue-green and emerald-green and orange and red. The definition of similarity here is that the reflection spectrum of one of the patches under white illumination is nearly identical to that of the other patch under a suitably chosen colored illumination. For example, the reflection spectrum of the emerald-green patch under white illumination closely matches that of the blue-green paper under green illumination of a suitable saturation.

A butterfly trained to emerald-green discriminates the emerald-green patch from the blue-green patch under white illumination. If the butterfly selects emerald-green solely on the basis of the spectral content of the reflection spectrum, (i.e., without using color constancy), it should select the blue-green patch under the green illumination, because the reflection spectrum will be virtually the same as the training spectrum. This did not happen, however. The emerald-green-trained butterflies selected the emerald-green target under green illumination. Similarly, butterflies trained to a red patch under white illumination always selected that patch under the spectrally very different red illumination (Kinoshita and Arikawa, 2000). Hence, foraging *Papilio xuthus* butterflies do display color constancy.

The recent behavioral experiments on butterfly color vision have shone new light on the importance of color for their successful survival. Their colorful world offers essential clues to the presence of food sources as well as potential partners and plants for laying eggs (Kelber, 1999a). Of course, many experiments are waiting to be done to unravel the neural mechanisms underlying color discrimination, color constancy, and color learning. These will involve experiments done on many levels of complexity, from the retinal input level to the processing of transduced visual signals by higher-order neurons. In this chapter we discuss what is currently known about the beginning of the color vision pathway in butterflies.

The Butterfly's Eye

Spectral Characterization of Photoreceptors

One of the basic physiological requirements for color vision is to have several types of spectral receptors in the retina. The human visual system employs blue-, green-, and red-sensitive photoreceptors as the basis of its trichromatic vision. Honeybee color vision is also trichromatic, but is based on ultraviolet, blue, and green photoreceptors. The behavioral experiments described earlier reveal that *Papilio* can discriminate red. In the field, *Papilio* and a number of other butterflies (Ilse and Vaidya, 1955; C. A. Swihart and Swihart, 1970) frequently visit red flowers, whereas honeybees rarely do (H. Tanaka, personal communication see also chapter 5 in this volume). Whereas bees lack photoreceptors with peak sensitivities in the red wavelength region, which makes them insensitive to red, the butterfly's preference for red suggests that these insects have photoreceptors that are specifically tuned to red. In fact, butterflies were the first insects shown to have red receptors (Bernard, 1979; Matic, 1983).

We have investigated the spectral photoreceptor types present in the eye of *Papilio xuthus* by intracellular recording and found that there are several different types of spectral photoreceptors, including red receptors. In fact, we have identified six types of receptors in the *Papilio* retina. Five of them peak in the UV (at 360 nm), violet (400 nm), blue (460 nm), green (520 nm), and red (600 nm) wavelength region, respectively (figure 6.4). The bandwidth of the sensitivity spectra varies between 50 and 100 nm (Arikawa et al., 1987). Recently, a sixth type of photoreceptor was characterized, which has a very large bandwidth of about 270 nm, without a clear peak wavelength preference.

Anatomical Characterization of Spectral Photoreceptors

The retina of *Papilio xuthus* appears to contain at least six classes of spectral photoreceptors. On the other hand, a butterfly ommatidium, the building block of the compound eye, contains nine photoreceptors (figure 6.5). Since a *Papilio* compound eye consists of about 12,000 ommatidia, each retina contains more than 100,000 photoreceptor cells. Each of these photoreceptor cells should fall into one of the six spectral classes. This immediately raises a number of questions regarding where these spectral receptors are located in the ommatidia, whether one ommatidium contains all of the

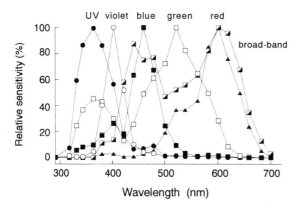

Figure 6.4
Photoreceptor sensitivity spectra of the yellow swallowtail, *Papilio xuthus*. At least six spectral types of photoreceptors can be distinguished. Five types have clear peaks in the ultraviolet, violet, blue, green, and red, respectively. The sixth type has a broadband shape with two peaks in the blue and red, respectively. The spectra result from a total of five visual pigments and three photostable screening pigments acting as selective spectral filters that are put together in three types of ommatidia.

different classes of spectral receptors, and whether there are regional differences in the eye.

Each photoreceptor cell has a crucial photoreceptive organelle, the rhabdomere, which is a stack of microvilli formed by evaginations of the photoreceptor cell's membrane. The rhabdomeric microvilli contain both the visual pigment molecules and the molecules of the phototransduction machinery. The rhabdomeres of the nine photoreceptors of *Papilio* jointly form what is called a fused rhabdom. This is a long, slender cylinder situated in the center of the ommatidium along its longitudinal axis. The rhabdomeres of the different photoreceptors are organized in a precise, regular pattern. Photoreceptor cells R1 to R4 have microvilli located exclusively in the distal two thirds of the rhabdom. Accordingly, R1–R4 are called the distal photoreceptors. The orientation of the microvilli of two of the four distal photoreceptors, R1 and R2, are along the dorsoventral (vertical) axis of the insect. The orientation of the microvilli of the other two, R3 and R4, is along the insect's anteroposterior (horizontal) axis.

The rhabdomeres of photoreceptor cells R5–R8 form the rhabdom in the proximal third of the retina and are called the proximal photoreceptors. These photoreceptors contribute diagonally oriented microvilli to the rhabdom. Photoreceptor R9, the basal photoreceptor, adds vertically oriented microvilli to the rhabdom, immediately distal to the basement membrane (figure 6.5).

An important characteristic of the rhabdom is that it acts as an optical waveguide. This is due to the high concentration of proteins and phospholipids that it contains,

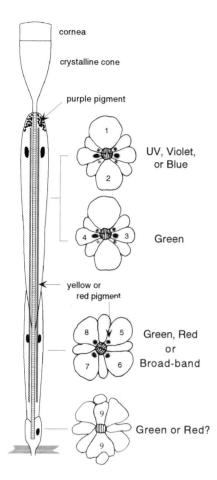

Figure 6.5
Anatomy of a *Papilio* ommatidium, consisting of the dioptric apparatus, the cornea and crystalline cone, and nine photoreceptor cells (1–9) surrounded by pigment cells (not shown). Together, the rhabdomeres of the photoreceptors form the fused rhabdom. The rhabdomeres of the four distal photoreceptors (R1–R4) make up the distal two thirds of the rhabdom; the rhabdomeres of the four proximal photoreceptors (R5–R8) form most of the proximal part of the rhabdom; and the rhabdomere of the basal photoreceptor (R9) occupies the basalmost part. R1 and R2 contain purple pigment granules, and the R3–R8 cells have either yellow or red pigment clustered near the rhabdom. Electrophysiological characterization shows that R1 and R2 are either UV, violet, or blue cells. The spectra of R3 and R4 peak in the green, and R5–R8 are either green, red, or broadband cells. The spectral characteristics of the R9 cells have not yet been clearly determined.

which create a refractive index distinctly higher than that of its watery surroundings. Light that enters the eye through an ommatidia's corneal lens is channeled into the rhabdom and is guided along the rhabdom until it is absorbed by the visual pigment molecules of the rhabdomeric microvilli membranes. The sensitivity to light (i.e., the probability that a photon will be absorbed) is effectively increased by the rhabdom's waveguide properties. In other words, by joining the rhabdomeres into a fused rhabdom, the photoreceptor cells together optimize light sensitivity.

The identification and localization of the spectral receptor types in an ommatidium can be done in a straightforward manner via electrophysiological recording and subsequent marking with dye-filled glass microelectrodes. A second method of localizing a spectral receptor is via polarization. This approach is based on the property that the microvilli of *Papilio's* photoreceptors are more or less parallel. Photoreceptors with parallel microvilli are known to exhibit a selective sensitivity for polarized light (PS), which is maximal in the direction along the longitudinal axis of the microvilli (Moody and Parriss, 1961). So the polarization sensitivity of *Papilio's* R1 photoreceptor is maximal along the insect's dorsoventral axis, and that of the R3 photoreceptor is maximal along the anteroposterior axis.

Hence, the direction of maximal polarization sensitivity can be used as an indicator of the photoreceptor's location. For instance, if a recorded cell turns out to be a UV receptor, and the sensitivity is maximal for vertically polarized light (light parallel to the dorsoventral axis), the photoreceptor must be either an R1 or an R2.

The polarization method has been applied extensively in measurements of the laterally facing eye region of *Papilio xuthus* (Bandai et al., 1992; Arikawa and Uchiyama, 1996). The directional angle of maximal polarization sensitivity, φ_{max}, was measured with respect to the insect's dorsoventral axis (defined as 0 deg). We found that all green receptors, at least in the distal tier, have a polarization sensitivity peaking at about 90 deg, suggesting that all the green receptors are R3 and R4 cells. Furthermore, we found that R1 and R2 cells are either UV, violet, or blue receptors, and that R5–R9 cells are either green or red or broadband receptors (figure 6.5).

The most surprising and important finding was that photoreceptors with anatomically identical positions can be spectrally different. For instance, the two distal photoreceptors, R1 and R2, can be members of three distinct spectral classes: UV, violet, or blue. This means that the ommatidia of the *Papilio* compound eye are not identical building blocks. Rather, the eye is composed of different types of ommatidia, distinguishable by the spectral receptors that they contain.

The next questions to be asked, then, are how many types of ommatidia exist and how the different types are distributed in the retina.

Colors and Pigments in the Butterfly Eye

Heterogeneity of Ommatidia and Pigmentation

The realization that *Papilio's* ommatidia do not form a homogeneous population initiated a series of detailed anatomical studies. We found that the ommatidial heterogeneity can be directly observed in histological sections. Different types of ommatidia can be readily distinguished by the presence of either red or yellow screening pigments surrounding the rhabdoms in the R3–R8 photoreceptor cells (Arikawa and Stavenga, 1997). About 75% of the ommatidia contain the red pigment and the remaining 25% contain yellow pigment. The red and yellow pigmented ommatidia are randomly distributed.

The colored pigments are concentrated in clusters of granules positioned in the cell soma adjacent to the rhabdom. The pigment clusters most probably function as spectral filters (Stavenga, 1979, 1989) because an intrinsic consequence of the waveguide properties of the (slender) rhabdom is that light propagates partly outside of its boundary (Snyder et al., 1973; Nilsson et al., 1988). Light propagating in this so-called boundary wave can be absorbed by the red and yellow pigments.

The hypothesized spectral filtering has been visualized directly by cutting a fresh compound eye with a vibrating microtome at the level of the proximal photoreceptors. In transmitted light, the ommatidia appear either red or yellow (figure 6.6A; plate 8).

Epifluorescence microscopy reveals another element of the ommatidial heterogeneity. When a *Papilio* eye is observed with UV epi-illumination, part of the ommatidia are found to emit a strong whitish fluorescence, shining like stars in a night sky (figure 6.6B). The fluorescing ommatidia correspond to the ommatidia that look whitish or pale red in transmitted light (figure 6.6A), demonstrating that the fluorescing ommatidia have red pigmentation around the rhabdom. Eye-slice preparations show that the fluorescing material is abundantly present only in the distal portion of the ommatidia, beginning immediately below the proximal tip of the crystalline cone and extending over a distance of about 70 µm (figure 6.7) (Arikawa et al., 1999a).

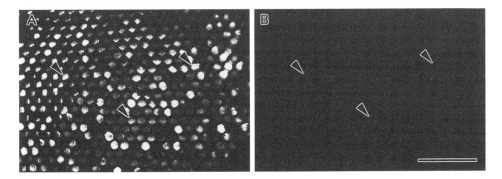

Figure 6.6
(*A*) Ommatidial pigmentation seen in a fresh eye slice observed in transmitted light, i.e., under antidromic illumination. (*B*) Ommatidial fluorescence observed with ultraviolet epi-illumination of the same preparation as in (*A*). The arrowheads indicate identical ommatidia. The fluorescing ommatidia are pale red or pink in transmission. Scale bar = 100 µm. (See plate 8 for color version.)

Furthermore, the number of fluorescing ommatidia is very low in the dorsal eye, indicating the absence of type 2 ommatidia.

Histological and optical microscopic observations have identified three different types of ommatidia in the *Papilio* eye: red pigmented (type 1), red pigmented plus fluorescing (type 2), and yellow pigmented (type 3) (table 6.1).

Further work on the localization of the six types of spectral receptors by intracellular recording and dye injection, combined with optical and histological identification methods, has led to a complete characterization of the three ommatidia types as unique sets of spectral receptors (table 6.1).

Tuning of Spectral Sensitivity by Screening Pigments

What is the functional significance of the spectral filters in the butterfly's ommatidia? An obvious hypothesis is that the spectral filters tune the sensitivity spectra of the photoreceptor cells. The sensitivity spectrum of a photoreceptor cell is in general primarily determined by the absorption spectrum of its visual pigment. However, the sensitivity spectrum is in many cases modified by optical effects, e.g., those due to self-screening of the visual pigment itself and/or to filtering by photostable filter pigments (Neumeyer, 1998). Presumably therefore, the red and yellow filtering pigments as well as the fluorescing pigments function to modify the sensitivity spectra of certain photoreceptors.

Violet Receptor and Fluorescing Pigment

A clear example of the effect of spectral filtering is the strikingly narrow sensitivity spectrum of the violet receptor (figure 6.4). Electrophysiological experiments combined with cell staining and optical identification proved that the violet receptors always reside in the fluorescing ommatidia (table 6.1). Presumably therefore, the fluorescing pigment could play a role in shaping the sensitivity spectrum of the violet receptors.

What, then, is the fluorescing material concentrated in the ommatidia? Seki et al. (1987) reported that the compound eyes of *Papilio* (as well as those of some other butterflies) contain excessive amounts of 3-hydroxyretinol, the alcohol from which the chromophore of butterfly visual pigments, 3-hydroxyretinal, is produced. This finding suggested that 3-hydroxyretinol might be the fluorescing material because its absorption spectrum peaks in the UV range at 330 nm and it is known to highly fluoresce white under UV excitation.

We extracted 3-hydroxyretinol from the *Papilio* eye with high-pressure liquid chromatography (HPLC), measured the fluorescence spectrum, and compared the spectrum with that of the fluorescing ommatidia in the living eye. The two spectra corresponded closely, providing strong evidence that the ommatidial fluorescence originates from 3-hydroxyretinol concentrated in the distal portion of type 2 ommatidia (figure 6.8).

This conclusion immediately suggested a hypothesis for the spectral filter function of the 3-hydroxyretinol. Its strong absorption in the UV range will reduce the

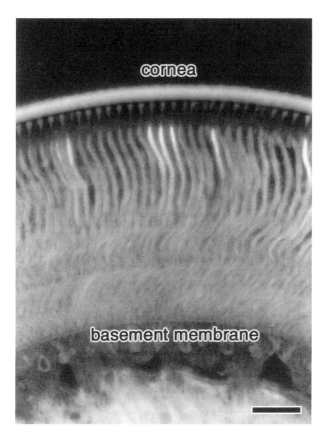

Figure 6.7
Longitudinal section of the eye of *Papilio xuthus* showing selective expression of a fluorescent pigment in a restricted set of ommatidia. The fluorescing pigment (3-hydroxyretinol) is found to be concentrated in the most distal part of the ommatidia over a distance of about 70–100 μm. Scale bar: 100 μm.

Table 6.1
Three types of ommatidia of *Papilio*

Type	%	Fluorescence	Pigment	Photoreceptor spectral sensitivity (opsin mRNA)				
				R1	R2	R3, R4	R5–R8	R9
1	50	–	Red	UV or blue (*PxUV or B*)	Blue or UV (*PxB or UV*)	D-Green (*PxL1 + L2*)	Red (*PxL3*)	? (*PxL1 + L2*)
2	25	+	Red	Violet (*PxUV*)	Violet (*PxUV*)	S-Green (*PxL1 + L2*)	Broadband (*PxL2 + L3*)	
3	25	–	Yellow	Blue (*PxB*)	Blue (*PxB*)	D-Green (*PxL1 + L2*)	D-Green (*PxL2*)	

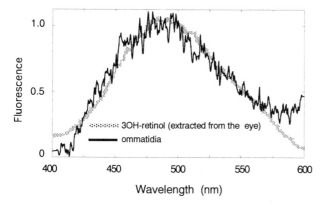

Figure 6.8
Emission spectrum induced by UV excitation measured in the intact eye of *Papilio* (omma-tidia), compared with the fluorescence spectrum of 3-hydroxyretinol extracted from *Papilio* eyes.

absorption of short-wavelength light by the visual pigments and consequently will selectively reduce the spectral sensitivity of the photoreceptors in the UV wavelength range. We tested this hypothesis by using a computational model. The absorption of light in the individual photoreceptors was calculated using the optical waveguide properties of the rhabdom, incorporating all the known anatomical details of the *Papilio* ommatidium (Arikawa et al., 1999a,b).

Briefly, we modeled the rhabdom as a circular cylinder with a diameter of 2.6 μm and a length of 500 μm. In the model, the rhabdomeres of R1–R4 are present in the distal two thirds of the rhabdom, from 0 to 300 μm, and contain various combina-tions of UV, blue, and green visual pigments (Bandai et al., 1992; Kitamoto et al., 1998, 2000). The proximal photoreceptors R5–R8 exist in the proximal one third of the rhabdom, from 300 to 470 μm, and contain either an orange-absorbing or a green-absorbing visual pigment (Arikawa and Uchiyama, 1996). The R9 cell occupies the basal 30 μm of the rhabdom.

The photoreceptors R3–R8 in an ommatidium were assumed to have a constant density of red or yellow screening pigment surrounding the rhabdom. Accordingly, light propagated outside the waveguide is filtered by the screening pigment. Since both R1 and R2 photoreceptors of type 2 ommatidia appear to be violet receptors, we assumed that they contain the same UV-absorbing visual pigment. When the absorp-tion spectrum of the UV visual pigment peaks at a wavelength longer than 330 nm (i.e., above the absorption peak of the 3-hydroxyretinol), spectral filtering by the 3-hydroxyretinol will inevitably shift the sensitivity spectrum of the photoreceptor toward the violet. By taking a peak wavelength of 360 nm for the visual pigment in R1 and R2, and assuming a suitable density of the 3-hydroxyretinol, a sensitivity

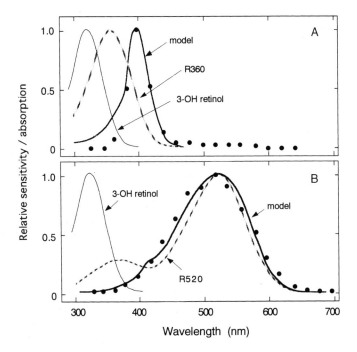

Figure 6.9
(A) Sensitivity spectrum of the violet receptors peaking at 400 nm (solid symbols). Its narrow band is assumed to result from the UV-absorbing (and fluorescing) 3-hydroxyretinol acting as a spectral filter on an ultraviolet-absorbing visual pigment peaking at 360 nm. (B) Sensitivity spectrum of the single-peaked green receptors peaking at 520 nm (solid symbols). The absence of the normally occurring β-band is assumed to result from the UV filter action of the 3-hydroxyretinol.

spectrum was calculated that peaked in the violet range, which is in good correspondence with that measured for violet receptors (figure 6.9A). When the rhodopsin with a 360-nm peak is also present in the R1 or R2 photoreceptors of nonfluorescing ommatidia, the receptors have a sensitivity spectrum similar to the visual pigment's absorption spectrum, a prediction confirmed experimentally (table 6.1).

The 3-hydroxyretinol in the fluorescing (type 2) ommatidia acts as a spectral filter on all photoreceptors present in the type 2 ommatidia. Electrophysiological experiments identified a specific set of green-sensitive receptors, the single-band green (S-green) receptors (figure 6.9B), which have an abnormally shaped (very low) sensitivity spectrum in the UV range. Normally green-absorbing visual pigments have an absorption spectrum with a clear subsidiary band in the UV range, and the sensitivity spectrum of the corresponding photoreceptors should, therefore, exhibit this so-called β-band. It is striking that the S-green receptors are only encountered in what we call the starry (i.e., white-fluorescing) ommatidia. The absence of the β-band in these receptors is now understood; it is filtered out by the 3-hydroxyretinol (Arikawa et al., 1999a).

Red Receptors and Red Pigmentation

Another example of spectral tuning is seen in the red receptors located in the proximal tier of type 1 ommatidia (table 6.1). Their sensitivity spectrum peaks at 600 nm. A peculiar feature of their sensitivity spectrum is its bandwidth. The spectrum is considerably narrower than the absorption spectrum of a visual pigment peaking at 600 nm as predicted by a rhodopsin template (Stavenga et al., 1993). Obviously then, this deviation from the expected may be caused by the red pigmentation around the rhabdom. We also tested this hypothesis with our computational model.

The model allowed a fairly accurate, quantitative description of sensitivity spectra measured from the red-sensitive proximal photoreceptors when a visual pigment with an absorption spectrum peaking at 575 nm was assumed, screened by red pigment with the appropriate density. This resulted in a shift in spectral sensitivity with a peak at 600 nm, which matches the experimental data (figure 6.10).

A similar spectral shift might be thought to occur for the green receptors in the yellow pigmented ommatidia (table 6.1), but the filtering effect of the yellow pigment appears to be minor. A visual pigment peaking at 520 nm filtered by the yellow screening pigment yields a sensitivity spectrum that peaks at 530 nm (Arikawa et al., 1999b).

Localization of Visual Pigments in the *Papilio* Eye by Molecular Biology

Our electrophysiological and optical experiments on *Papilio* suggested that the violet receptors in the fluorescing ommatidia and the UV receptors in the nonfluorescing

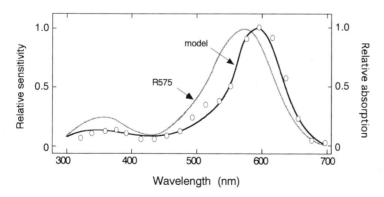

Figure 6.10
Sensitivity spectrum of a subset of R5–R8 cells peaking at 600 nm (open symbols). Its narrow band is assumed to result from red screening pigment acting as a spectral filter on an orange-absorbing visual pigment peaking at 575 nm.

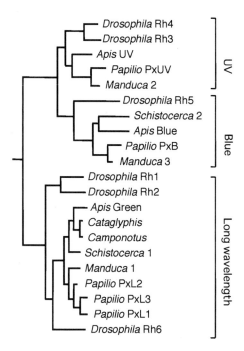

Figure 6.11
Dendrogram of insect visual pigments. The butterfly *Papilio xuthus* has one member in the UV and blue visual pigment classes, but it has three members in the long wavelength class.

ommatidia contain the same visual pigment. We utilized molecular biological methods to investigate the validity of this hypothesis.

We first constructed a cDNA library, starting from mRNA extracted from the *Papilio* retina. Subsequently we cloned five cDNAs from the cDNA library that encode visual pigment opsins. Figure 6.11 shows the phylogenetic relationship of these *Papilio* opsins with other known insect opsins. On the basis of their primary structure, the *Papilio* opsins can be divided into three classes: UV (PxUV), blue (PxB), and long-wavelength-absorbing classes (PxL1, PxL2, and PxL3).

We then identified the photoreceptors that express the opsin mRNAs by performing histological *in situ* hybridization on retinal sections. Figure 6.12 shows a set of sections taken from a single specimen. Figure 6.12A is a fluorescence picture taken under UV epi-illumination.

Labeling PxUV mRNA formed three patterns in R1 and R2 photoreceptors. Either R1 or R2 were labeled; both R1 and R2 was labeled; or neither the R1 nor R2 was labeled. By comparing the labeling pattern with the fluorescence pattern, it appeared that the three patterns corresponded fully with the ommatidia classification we devel-

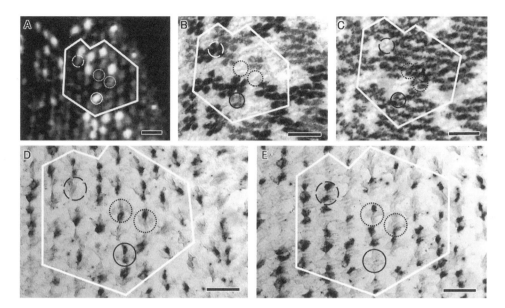

Figure 6.12
Heterogeneous localization of visual pigments in the *Papilio* retina demonstrated by in situ hybridization in serial sections from a set of ommatidia in the same part of the eye. (*A*) Transverse section through the most distal part of the eye showing autofluorescence in the type 2 ommatidia. (*B*) Proximal section labeled by the PxL2 probe. (*C*) Proximal section labeled by the PxL3 probe. (*D*) Distal section labeled by the PxUV probe. (*E*) Distal section labeled by the PxB probe. Circles with solid lines indicate type 1 ommatidia; circles with dashed lines indicate a type 2 ommatidium; and circles with dotted lines indicate a type 1 ommatidium.

oped (table 6.1). The nonfluorescing type 1 ommatidia contain the PxUV mRNA, which codes for a UV-absorbing pigment, yielding the sensitivity spectrum of a UV receptor.

The fluorescing type 2 ommatidia contain PxUV in both R1 and R2 photoreceptors, which have a sensitivity spectrum with a peak in the violet range owing to the filtering action of the 3-hydroxyretinol. Hence our initial assumption appeared to be correct. The UV receptors and violet receptors share the identical UV-absorbing visual pigment.

The PxB probe labeled R1 and R2 receptors in the same three patterns corresponding to ommatidia types. In this case, however, in the type 1 ommatidia, R1 or R2 labeling always differed from the R1 and R2 labeling by the PxUV probe and there was no overlap. The conclusions we drew from electrophysiological recordings, that type 1 ommatidia R1 and R2 photoreceptors act as a UV and a blue receptor, respectively (or vice versa), was confirmed by the in situ hybridization experiments.

The PxB probe never labeled the R1 and R2 photoreceptors of the fluorescing type 2 ommatidia, but it did label both R1 and R2 photoreceptors in type 3 ommatidia. The latter confirmed that R1 and R2 are blue photoreceptors (table 6.1). Modeling suggests that the absorption spectra of the UV and blue visual pigments peak at 360 and 440 nm, respectively.

The PxL1-3 probes appear to label several, partly overlapping classes of photoreceptors. The PxL1 probe labels both R3 and R4 photoreceptors in the ventral two thirds of the eye.

The PxL2 probe labels the R3 and R4 in all ommatidia throughout the whole eye. Since the sensitivity spectra of all R3 and R4 photoreceptors have a clear band in the green (figure 6.4), both PxL1 and PxL2 must be opsins of green-absorbing visual pigments.

Since the dorsal R3 and R4 cells are green receptors that contain only the PxL2, this opsin must constitute a green-absorbing visual pigment. Modeling indicates that its absorption peak wavelength is ca. 520 nm. The ventral R3 and R4 photoreceptors have a similar peak wavelength. If both PxL1 and PxL2 are expressed, the two visual pigments present must together determine the sensitivity spectrum with a green peak. Because the sensitivity spectrum approximates the absorption spectrum of the PxL2 visual pigment, it means that the peak wavelength of the PxL1 visual pigment must be rather similar; i.e., that the ventral R3 and R4 photoreceptors contain two similar, but definitely not identical, green-absorbing visual pigments. The PxL2 probe also labels the R5–R8 photoreceptors in both type 2 and type 3 ommatidia.

The PxL3 probe labels the R5–R8 photoreceptors of both type 1 and type 2 ommatidia. The sensitivity spectra of the red-sensitive R5–R8 photoreceptors of type 1 ommatidia, which are only labeled by PxL3, were thought to be a product of visual pigment absorbing maximally at 575 nm. The PxL3 opsin must belong to this visual pigment.

The labeling of the R5–R8 photoreceptors in type 2 ommatidia by both PxL2 and PxL3 probes shows that these photoreceptors contain both PxL2 and PxL3 opsins. As noted earlier, the PxL2 opsin belongs to a green-absorbing visual pigment. The combined expression of the green (PxL2) and red (PxL3) visual pigments in type 2 ommatidia R5–R8 photoreceptors must determine these receptors' sensitivity spectrum, a broadband spectrum without a β-band (figure 6.4). The absence of the β-band can be readily explained from the strong UV filtering of the 3-hydroxyretinol in the type 2 ommatidia.

Both PxL1 and PxL2 label the basal, R9 photoreceptor throughout the *Papilio's* retina. In this case, however, no reliable electrophysiologically determined sensitivity spectra are available that would allow speculation about the relative expression levels of both opsins.

Ommatidial Heterogeneity and Color Vision

Heterogeneity in the Eyes of Butterflies

An analysis of the eye of *Papilio* has revealed the bewildering complexity of its retinal organization. Different types of ommatidia are randomly arranged. There are arrangement variations between eye regions. The ommatidia contain several visual pigments and photoreceptors are filtered by a number of screening pigments. The butterfly's striking eye regionalization and retinal heterogeneity is by no means a feature unique to *Papilio xuthus*. Such regionalization (Stavenga, 1992) and heterogeneity (Arikawa and Stavenga, 1997) are widespread among insects and are probably a relatively basic design component of compound eyes.

An example is the small white, *Pieris rapae*, another butterfly species whose ommatidia have been well studied. The basic structure of the *Pieris* ommatidia is similar to that of *Papilio* (figure 6.13). There are nine photoreceptors in each ommatidium. Four distal photoreceptors contribute rhabdomeres to the distal two thirds of the rhabdom; four proximal photoreceptors add rhabdomeres in the proximal third; and the rhabdomere of the ninth cell is restricted to the basalmost portion of the rhabdom.

The ommatidial heterogeneity can be visualized by the same methods used in *Papilio*. Histological examination reveals three types of ommatidia based on the pigmentation around the rhabdom (Qiu et al., 2002). The pigment granules occur in four clusters, but the distribution pattern around the rhabdom is different among ommatidia. The arrangement of the clusters is trapezoidal (type 1), square (type 2), or rectangular (type 3). Epifluorescence microscopy shows that type 2 ommatidia fluoresce under blue-violet and UV.

A third approach to identifying ommatidia types is to utilize the tapetal reflection method. Tapetal reflection differs systematically between ommatidial types; types 1 and 3 reflect red (610 nm) light, whereas type 2 reflects deep red (670 nm) light. This difference is probably due to structural and pigmentation dimorphism of the tapetum and the rhabdom. As explained earlier, the fluorescent and screening pigments probably affect the sensitivity spectra of the ommatidial photoreceptors. In fact, in this insect, the different types of ommatidia contain different sets of spectral receptors, at least in the distal tier (Qiu and Arikawa, 2003). Apparently *Pieris rapae* has at least five spectral receptor types (Shimohigashi and Tominaga, 1991), but an analysis of the optical components determining their sensitivity spectra has yet to be performed.

Electrophysiological recordings on two nymphalid species, *Sasakia charonda* and *Polygonia c-aureum*, also revealed the presence of five or more spectral receptor types (Kinoshita et al., 1997). The long-wavelength receptors of *Polygonia*, a flower nectar feeder, have an increased sensitivity in the red wavelength region compared with those in *Sasakia*, a nonflower visitor. Consequently, the increased sensitivity in the red of *Polygonia* may be related to flower detection. This hypothesis has been amply discussed for other butterflies by Briscoe and Chittka (2001), who have compiled an extensive list of spectral receptors, including the peak wavelength sensitivity, of lepidopterans and other insect species (Briscoe and Chittka, 2001).

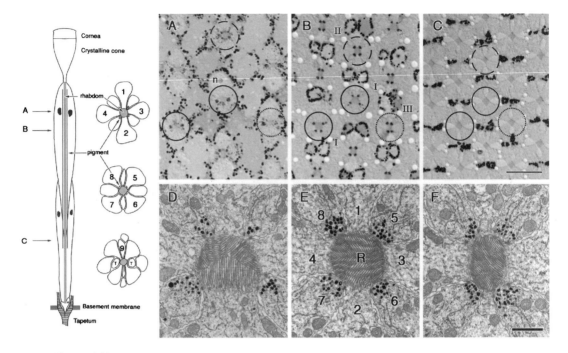

Figure 6.13
Structure and heterogeneity of the ommatidia of the small white *Pieris rapae crucivora*. Four distal photoreceptors (R1–R4) and four proximal photoreceptors (R5–R8) together make up virtually the complete rhabdom. Cell R9 adds only the basalmost part. The rhabdom is surrounded by clusters of R5–R8 pigment over most of its length, except for a short distal and proximal part. Sections at depths of 140 μm (*A*), 300 μm (*B*), and 360 μm (*C*) show that the retina is composed of three types of ommatidia, which are distinguishable from the shape of the rhabdom and the pigment clusters surrounding it, being roughly trapezoidal (*D*), square (*E*), and rectangular (*F*). The pigment clusters are either red or deep-red colored. A tapetum, created by tracheoles, exists proximal to the rhabdom.

Spectral Shifts Induced by Red Photoreceptor Pigment and Function of Red Sensitivity

The sensitivity spectrum of a photoreceptor cell that receives light filtered by red screening pigment depends on the absorption spectrum of the visual and screening pigments and its effective density. A distinct red sensitivity, with spectra peaking at or above 600 nm, has been noted in several butterfly species (S. L. Swihart and Gordon, 1971; Bernard, 1979; Scherer and Kolb, 1987a; Steiner et al., 1987). In principle this could be exclusively based on red-absorbing rhodopsins. However, the longest peak wavelength of an insect rhodopsin determined so far is 600 nm (Bernard, 1979; Bernard et al., 1988), and the often aberrant spectral shape of the sensitivity spectra indicates that red pigment filters play a key role in the red sensitivity of butterflies. A red filter can shift the sensitivity spectrum of a photoreceptor that would otherwise peak in the green or orange toward longer wavelengths; i.e., into the red range.

Shifting the sensitivity spectrum of a photoreceptor with a short-wavelength-absorbing filter is a well-known phenomenon—for instance, the effects of oil droplets in bird cones (Govardovskii, 1983) and the carotenoid filters in stomatopod rhabdoms (Marshall et al., 1991b). Filtering inevitably causes a reduction in absolute sensitivity, but this cost can be reduced by the reflective tapetum and offset by the benefit of enhanced discrimination of color contrast (Govardovskii, 1983).

The red receptors of butterflies may be of special importance during oviposition for discriminating leaves suitable for the larvae (Bernard and Remington, 1991; Chittka, 1996; Kelber, 1999a). The extremely dense red pigmentation in the Pieridae and the apparently dual system for enhancing red sensitivity strongly suggest that spectral discrimination in the red is especially well developed in this family (Kolb and Scherer, 1982; Scherer and Kolb, 1987a). However, red sensitivity is probably common among butterflies and may serve several functions, including feeding and mate recognition (Bernard, 1979; Scherer and Kolb, 1987a; Kinoshita et al., 1999).

The creation of red receptors via selective red filtering by photoreceptor screening pigments is not restricted to butterflies. Sphecid wasps apply the same principle (Ribi, 1978a). It is intriguing that sphecids, like butterflies, also arrange the red pigments in four clusters in one class of ommatidia, and that this class is randomly distributed within a rather crystalline ordered ommatidial lattice (Ribi, 1978b).

Butterfly Eye Shine

Butterflies, except the Papilionidae, exhibit a colorful eye shine that is due to a reflecting tapetum present in each ommatidium proximal to the rhabdom. The tapetum is formed by a tracheole folded into a stack of layers, alternately consisting of air and cytoplasm, which creates an interference reflection filter. Incident light that has passed through the rhabdom without being absorbed is reflected by the tapetum. The consequent eye shine is due to that reflection. Bernard and Miller (1970) observed that the differences in the characteristics of the eye shine in a number of butterfly species indicated both clear regionalization and ommatidial heterogeneity (W. H. Miller, 1979).

We surveyed the eye shine of twenty-seven butterfly species belonging to the families Lycaenidae, Satyridae, Pieridae, Nymphalidae, and Danaidae (Stavenga et al., 2001). We focused on four areas of the compound eyes: frontal (the forward-looking position); dorsal and ventral (oriented 70 ± 20 deg upward and downward, respectively, in the near midsaggittal plane); and medial (oriented toward the horizontal plane, approximately 30 deg lateral to the midline).

We found that more ommatidia contribute to the eye shine in the frontal eye region than in other regions, suggesting that butterflies have the highest spatial acuity frontally (Stavenga et al., 2001) (figure 6.14; plate 9). The pattern of eye shine also indicated regionalization and local heterogeneity of the compound eyes. The ommatidia in the dorsal eye regions tend to reflect light of a shorter wavelength than the frontal and the ventral regions. This is most likely related to some specialized function of the dorsal eye region, but further details are not known. The eye shine color is usually not unique, even within a restricted eye region, indicating that there are locally at least two types of ommatidia.

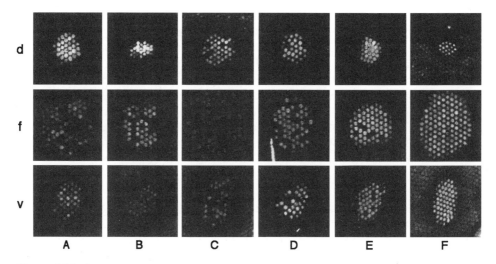

Figure 6.14
Epi-illumination microscopy showing ommatidial heterogeneity via eye shine in the eyes of various butterfly species: (A) *Hypolimnas bolina*, (B) *Cyrestis thyodamas*, (C) *Argyreus hyperbius*, (D) *Euploea mulciber*, (E)*Parantica aglea*, and (F)*Precis almana* [(A)–(C), (F) are Nymphalidae; (D) and (E), Danaidae. Dorsal (d), frontal (f), and ventral (v) eye regions were all photographed with the same microscope objective. Because eye shine is observable only in ommatidia that have their visual field coincident with the aperture of the microscope, the density of visual fields (i.e., their spatial acuity) is highest frontally. The eye shine color depends on the species, and the different colors reflect strong heterogeneity. Each figure is $400 \times 400 \, \mu m^2$. (See plate 9 for color version.)

Normal epi-illumination reflection microscopy does not allow observation of butterfly eye shine with large-aperture objectives because of severe background reflections. However, a special epi-illumination microscope has recently been developed, so that the regionalization and local heterogeneity of butterfly eyes can be readily visualized in a large area of the eye. This has allowed us to extend the findings of our previous work (Stavenga, 2002b).

Again, we found that a specialized dorsal eye region is very common (figure 6.15; plate 10). The extent of the dorsal region can be large, as in *Bicyclus anynana* (figure 6.15A), rather small as in *Pieris rapae* (figure 6.15C), or even virtually absent, as in *Heliconius melpomene* (figure 6.15B). Local heterogeneity is the rule, especially in the middle and the ventral regions of the eye.

Heterogeneity in the Eyes of Insects

Ommatidial heterogeneity has been previously reported in flies (Franceschini et al., 1981; Hardie et al., 1981), digger wasps (Ribi, 1978b), moths (Meinecke and Langer, 1984), backswimmers (Schwind and Langer, 1984), and butterflies (Bernard and Miller,

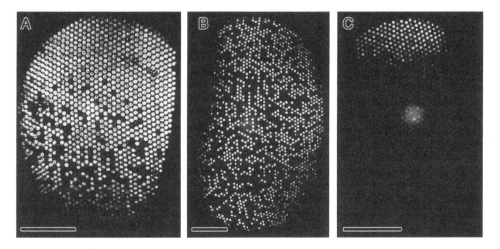

Figure 6.15
The eye shine pattern in the eyes of (*A*) the satyrine *Bicyclus anynana*, (*B*) the heliconian *Heliconius melpomene*, and (*C*) the small white, *Pieris rapae* observed with a large-aperture optical setup. The ommatidia in the three species reflect either predominantly yellow or red light. The red reflection is absent in a large dorsal area in the eye of *Bicyclus anynana* and in a small dorsal area of *Pieris rapae*. In *Heliconius melpomene*, both reflection types coexist throughout the eye. The central hot spot is due to reflection on the lens surfaces of the microscope objective. The dark areas in (*A*) and (*B*) are due to dust specks; the dark facets in (*C*) have a strong deep-red reflection. Scale bars: 300 μm. (See plate 10 for color version.)

1970; Arikawa and Stavenga, 1997). The evidence has been mainly anatomical and optical and only a little physiological, except in the case of flies. In the latter, the spectral sensitivities of the two central photoreceptors, R7 and R8, vary among ommatidia (Hardie, 1986). This has been underscored by molecular analyses in *Drosophila* (Chou et al., 1999; Salcedo et al., 1999).

We have recently demonstrated that the distribution of UV and blue receptors in the honeybee, *Apis mellifera*, has similarities to that of *Papilio* (M. Kurasawa et al., 2002). A honeybee ommatidium contains nine photoreceptors, eight large cells (R1–R8) stretching most of the length of the ommatidium, and one small, basal photoreceptor (R9) (Gribakin, 1975). Probes developed for the three honeybee opsins have now been successfully used to identify the photoreceptors expressing the various rhodopsins. The probe that hybridizes specifically to the mRNA encoding the green opsin labels six of the nine photoreceptors in all ommatidia (R2–R4, R6–R8). The two other probes, for the two short wavelength receptors (UV and blue), appear to exhibit a labeling pattern similar to that in *Papilio*. In some ommatidia, the UV probe labels photoreceptors R1 and R5. The blue probe labels both these receptors in a separate set of ommatidia, and the UV and blue probes each label either one of these photoreceptors in a third set of ommatidia.

Our finding that the honeybee retina, like that of *Papilio*, is heterogeneously organized, reinforces our hypothesis that retinal heterogeneity is related to color processing (Arikawa and Stavenga, 1997). For instance, the heterogeneity seen in the eyes of flies is restricted to the central photoreceptors, which mediate color vision (Fukushi, 1990; Troje, 1993). Furthermore, it is well established that moths rely heavily on color vision for flower feeding (Kelber and Henique, 1999). So, as expected, recent anatomical and molecular biological work on the moth *Manduca sexta* (White et al., 2003) shows a heterogeneous organization of the spectral receptor types in their ommatidial lattice very similar to that of diurnal butterflies (e.g., the papilionid *P. xuthus*; Arikawa and Stavenga, 1997; Kitamoto et al., 2000), and the nymphalid *Vanessa cardui* (Briscoe et al., 2003). The accumulating evidence from an increasing number of species suggests that common organizational principles underlie insect color vision.

Butterflies in a Colorful World

The extremely richly endowed visual system of butterflies evidently provides these animals with a versatile information-processing apparatus. Research has taught us that the functional capacities of the butterfly's compound eyes are strongly regionalized and locally heterogeneous. The regionalization can often be easily recognized in the intact eye by the eye shine. Because the dorsal eye is usually directed upward toward the blue sky, it may be presumed that short-wavelength discrimination is optimized there. Clear retinal specializations for detecting the polarization of sky light have been described (Kolb, 1986; Perez et al., 1997). On the other hand, color discrimination is probably most diverse in the ventral eye regions, as indicated by electrophysiological recordings on *Papilio xuthus* (Arikawa et al., 1987), microspectrophotometry on lycaenids (Bernard and Remington, 1991), and the heterogeneity in eye shine (Stavenga et al., 2001; Stavenga, 2002a,b). This may be related to the presence of flowers in the portions of the visual field observed by the ventral eye.

Whether ultraviolet light plays a role in color discrimination is still unclear, but it is unquestionably a major factor in detection of objects. For example, males of the Japanese small white, *Pieris rapae crucivora*, utilize UV for mate discrimination (Obara and Majerus, 2000), and the UV patterns in flowers (the so-called "nectar guides") serve to lure butterflies to their hosts (Wehner, 1981). Perhaps the same basic principles are used in the detection of red objects. Certain butterflies detect their partners by their red wing coloring (Silberglied, 1984), and subtle changes in the spectral content in the long-wavelength range of leaves may be detected with the aid of the red receptors (Kelber, 1999a).

Many aspects of these spectral discrimination strategies have yet to be discovered, so there may be quite a few surprises in store. For research on their visual capacities, the colorful butterflies will undoubtedly be a rich and rewarding source.

7 Seasonal Variation in the Visual World of Crayfish
Takahiko Hariyama

Crayfish are a part of the order Decapoda, and live mainly in shallow, fresh water throughout the world except in polar regions. There are over 500 species (Barnes, 1987) living in streams, ponds, lakes, and caves (Cooper et al., 1998).

The crayfish body is composed of fourteen segments and the telson. The first eight segments form the thorax, which is covered by a carapace. The last six segments form the abdomen. All the segments bear appendages. The first three pairs of thoracic appendages are modified as maxillipeds. The remaining five pairs of thoracic appendages are legs, and the first pair is enlarged and chelate.

The abdominal appendages, called pleopods, are biramous. In males, the first pair of pleopods is modified into copulatory organs, or gonopods. The gonopods extend forward on the underside of the carapace between the thorax and the abdomen, i.e., on the eighth thoracic segment. The length and shape of the tips on these paired gonopods are sometimes quite different in different species of crayfish. The female gonopores are located on the sixth thoracic segment.

At the head of crayfish under the rostrum there is a pair of compound eyes with movable stalks, and there are two pairs of antennae between the eyes. The first pair of antennae possess two short filaments, and the second pair have a long sensory filament. The second set of antennae consist of a number of short basal joints bearing a long flexible flagellum. The basal joints are equipped with flexor and extensor muscles, while the flagella are made up of a large number of annuli and contain only sensory receptors. The carapace is conspicuously roughened and is separated by lengthwise grooves in the middle.

Adults of *Procambarus clarkii* are about 5 to 7 cm in length from the tip of the rostrum to the tip of the telson. Adults of this species are colored dark red and have a wedge-shaped black stripe on the abdomen. Juveniles are a uniform gray, sometimes possessing granular black spots. The chelae are large and long in adults.

Feeding Behavior

Crayfish are omnivorous scavenger-predators that feed on a variety of animals and plants. Crayfish prey on small, live fish by using hydrodynamic orientation (Breithaupt et al., 1995). In fact, they can use their second pair of antennae to find a moving object when blinded (Sandeman, 1985; Varju, 1989; Breithaupt et al., 1995). Sometimes crayfish fight each other (Huber and Delago, 1998), and if they are hungry enough, display cannibalism.

Food is caught or picked up with the chelipeds and passed to the maxillipeds. The food is shredded by two pairs of maxillas and three pairs of maxillipeds. The third segment above the first maxilla bears toothed jaws (or mandibles) used for crushing food. Before it enters the mouth, the shredded food is crushed by the jaws. The digestive tract of a crayfish consists of three main regions: the foregut, midgut, and hindgut.

Crayfish are an important food for many other animals, including people.

Locomotion

Crayfish walk slowly, both backward and forward, along the substrate (Davis, 1971), primarily using their four pairs of thoracic walking legs. The first two pairs of walking legs end in small chelae. The walking movements of the legs move the gills and create convection in the carapace.

Generally, crayfish move by walking slowly, but when startled, they make rapid flips of their abdomen and telson by suddenly contracting the abdominal muscles. The result is rapid backward swimming (D. H. Edwards et al., 1999). Wiersma(1938) established that the giant axons of the crayfish nerve cord drive the tail-flip escape responses.

Ecology

Crayfish live beneath stones, in holes, or within debris, especially in muddy places. They excavate burrows in the mud, which they use for overwintering and retreats. Because they live in shallow, fresh water, the temperature of their habitats is easily affected by the sun's radiation and the air temperature.

The water of their environment during mating season contains a lot of mud, and this affects the spectrum of down-welling light. Muddy water absorbs more of the shorter than the longer wavelengths. Hence the transmission spectrum is biased toward red (figure 7.1a; plate 11).

Procambarus clarkii (Girard) was brought to Japan from North America about 70 years ago and naturalized. It is now one of the more widely distributed crustaceans in Japan. There is a commonly accepted story that only about sixty *P. clarkii* were brought to Japan as food for the bullfrog, *Rana catesbeiana* in June 1930 at Ohfuna, Kanagawa Prefecture. However, there is an old article (Mitaku, 1951) written in Japanese concerning *P. clarkii* and *Procambarus acutus*, and it emphasizes that the two species were imported several times from North America to Japan. The number of imported animals was not clear, but the original *P. clarkii*, but not *P. acutus*, spread all over Japan. Their main habitat is rice fields covered by fresh water.

Mating Behavior

Sexual Dimorphism of the Chelae
The chelae of crayfish are dark red and prominently studded with bright red knobs. The shapes of the chelae in females and males are quite different. The female has a wide space at the center of a chela, but the male does not have a space when it closes

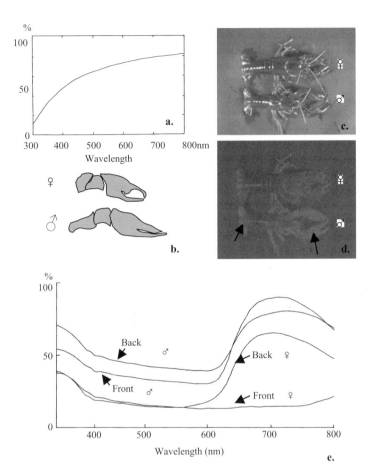

Figure 7.1
(*a*) The relative spectral transmittance of the water where the crayfish normally live. (*b*) The shape of the chelae. The female chela (top) leaves a space when it is closed. (*c*) Dorsal view of female and male crayfish. (*d*) Dorsal view of female and male crayfish through a red cutoff (>640 nm) filter. The arrows indicate the bright area in the chelae and telson. (*e*) Spectral reflection curve of the chela from the front and back sides. (See plate 11 for color version.)

its chela (figure 7.1b). The male crayfish holds the female's chelae with his larger chelae throughout copulation.

During the mating season, the color of male chelae appear to become brighter red compared with other times. Figure 7.1c shows a dorsal view of female and male crayfish. When the chelae and the telson of males are observed through a red filter, the reflected color is brighter than that reflected from a female (figure 7.1d, arrows). We measured the spectral reflection of the chelae with a Shimazu MPS-500, using MgO_2 as a white standard. The spectra of male and female chelae obtained from the front and back sides are shown in figure 7.1e. They show peaks in the red and UV regions, except for the reflection from the female front side. The reflectance intensity of the red region measured from the female front side is apparently lower than the others. The reflectance of male chelae on the back and front sides was higher than that of the female's throughout the whole spectrum from 300 to 800 nm.

Sex-Specific Behaviors and Sexual Signaling with the Chelae
Dunham (1978, p. 565) offered this description of sexual signaling in his review article: "Initial contact between male and female crayfish during the breeding season typically elicits a series of aggressive interactions. If the male establishes dominance, and the female exhibits submissive postures, the male will invert the female and mount her." It is difficult to determine whether the active interactions between male and female crayfish are fighting or not; however, it is true that the male crayfish moves his chelae in front of the female during the so-called fighting and/or mating behavior.

Behavioral observations in the laboratory or field reveal that when crayfish meet each other, the male pursues the female (figure 7.2). The male crayfish stands in front of the female and moves his chelae at the initial step of mating behavior. The female responds to the movement, sometimes by fighting the male and sometimes by exhibiting submissive postures. In other words, visual assessment of the male's signaling is of key importance in crayfish mating. This is also true for the semiterrestrial fiddler crab, *Uca*. In this case, the male fiddler crab attracts a female by waving the large pincer in a semaphore fashion (Zeil and Hofmann, 2001).

If the female is receptive, the male crayfish moves toward the female from the back or front side and holds her chelae. Obviously, then, the crayfish's chelae are very important throughout the entire mating ritual.

Sexual Pheromones
A sexual pheromone is a substance released by an organism that influences the sexual behavior of another individual of the same species. For instance, male crabs are attracted to premolt females and exhibit characteristic display and search behaviors when they are near. However, when females are prevented from releasing urine, there is no evidence of male attraction to them (Ryan, 1966). Chemical signals, such as pheromones, between males and females play important roles in recognition of sexual partners (Dunham, 1988). Male crayfish show different behavior toward males and

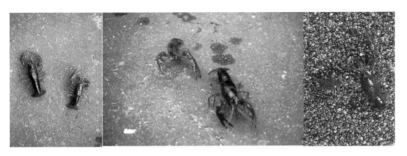

a.

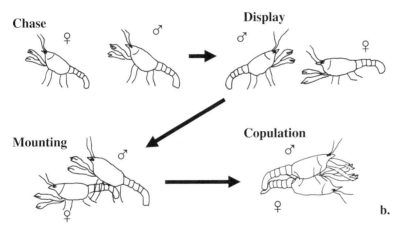

b.

Figure 7.2
The ethogram of crayfish mating behavior.

females. Behavioral and neurophysiological tests demonstrated the existence of sex pheromones that apparently play a role in eliciting the appropriate response. (Ameyaw-Akumfi and Hazlett, 1975; Dunham, 1978, 1988).

Copulation

In most copulations, the male crayfish holds the female's chelae from the back or front side and mounts her (figure 7.2b). At the last step of mating behavior, the male crayfish inverts the female. The gonopods are locked into position and inserted into the gonopores. The male then straightens his abdomen while depositing his spermatophores, which pass from the gonopore to the copulatory pleopods, or gonopods. In most aquatic decapods, mating occurs shortly after molting (Ryan, 1966). However, there is no correlation between mating and molting in *P. clarkii*.

Caring for Eggs and Juveniles

The fertilized eggs are attached to the female's pleopods on the underside of her jointed abdomen. Thus the pleopods are used for carrying eggs and are sometimes fanned to move water over the eggs. The eggs hatch on the pleopods. Although the young can move by themselves, they cling to their mother's pleopods until the third larval instar, at which time they are big enough to manage on their own. When the broods are removed from their mother, they can collect around her in the absence of visual or physical contact with her, suggesting that larval discrimination is based on a chemical stimulus released into the water by the brooding females (Little, 1975).

The Crayfish Visual System

General Organization

The crayfish's two stalked compound eyes are located under the rostrum and are normally held horizontally. Each adult compound eye possesses about 3000 ommatidia, the number of which increases at every molting (Hafner and Tokarski, 1998). Investigations of postembryonic eye growth in crustaceans show that crustacean compound eyes grow neither isometrically nor allometrically, but certain eye components may follow their own separate growth patterns (Keskinen et al., 2002).

The structure of the dioptric apparatus is characteristic of superposition eyes (Nilsson, 1983), which have a clear zone between the cornea and deeper-lying retina. There is a pigment cell in the clear zone, and pigment granule migration can be elicited by a brief exposure to light (Olivo and Larsen, 1978).

Structure of the Ommatidia

Each ommatidium consists of a dioptric apparatus and associated retinula cells. The dioptric apparatus has three clear areas: the cornea, the crystalline cone, and the crystalline thread. The surface of the cornea is rather flat, which is seemingly an adaptation to living in shallow water. The photoreceptive area, the rhabdom, consists of eight retinula cells (Bernhards, 1916), seven of which contribute to the rhabdomere. The rhabdomere is a spindle-shaped structure with alternating layers; that is, the axial portion of a rhabdom has a cross-banded appearance. The microvilli in one layer of the rhabdomere are oriented perpendicular to those in the next layer.

One apical retinular cell (R8) is situated distally just below the crystalline tract (P. Kunze and Boschek, 1968; Krebs and Lietz, 1982) and has a λ_{max} of 430 nm (Cummins and Goldsmith, 1981). The rest of the seven retinula cells (R1–R7) have a high sensitivity around the green portion of the spectrum, as described later. The microvillar membranes that make up the rhabdomere contain numerous visual pigments.

Characteristics of the Visual Pigments

The visual pigment rhodopsin consists of an integral membrane protein, an opsin, and a chromophore. Opsins and chromophores themselves absorb shorter wavelengths of light. Rhodopsin absorbs longer wavelengths. The spectral absorbance characteristic of rhodopsin is determined by the interaction between the opsin and the chromophore. The first chromophore to be identified in any visual pigment was retinal (Wald, 1953). Subsequent studies on visual pigment showed that three additional chromophores are present in nature: 3-dehydroretinal (Bridges, 1972), 3-hydroxyretinal (Vogt, 1983), and 4-hydroxyretinal (Matsui et al., 1988). Visual pigments with 11-*cis*-3-dehydroretinal as their chromophore absorb light at longer wavelengths than retinal-based pigments and occur in many freshwater vertebrates (Bridges, 1972; Knowles and Dartnall, 1977).

The ratio between 3-dehydroretinal-based and retinal-based visual pigments changes, depending on environmental factors such as temperature and light (Bridges, 1972; Knowles and Dartnall, 1977; Tsin and Beatty, 1979). The compound eye of the crayfish possesses two kinds of chromophores, retinal and 3-dehydroretinal, and we have found that there is a seasonal variation in the 3-dehydroretinal content. It is definitely lower in summer than during the rest of the year (Suzuki et al., 1984, 1985).

Seasonal Differences in Spectral Sensitivity

Early Studies Inconclusive

Since the first investigations using electroretinography (ERG) (D. Kennedy and Bruno, 1961), there have been many papers dealing with the spectral sensitivity of the crayfish eye. The spectral properties of crayfish visual systems have been studied using five technical approaches: electroretinography of intact eyes, mass response from the sustaining fibers of the visual nerve, spectrophotometry of the extracted pigment, microspectrophotometry of individual photoreceptors, and single-cell recordings of retinular cells. However, these studies reported a wide variation in the maximum sensitivity, or λ_{max}, ranging from 530 to 640 nm (table 7.1).

The seasonal variation in the spectral sensitivity curves was measured from intracellular recordings by Nosaki (1969), who found a λ_{max} of about 560 nm in winter and about 600 nm in summer. Waterman and Fernandez (1970) reported the maximum sensitivity of the same animal to be 538–634 nm in winter. However, these differences are thought to have arisen from absorption by the pigment granules (Bryceson, 1986). At that time, Suzuki et al. (1984, 1985) reported that the compound eye of the crayfish possesses two kinds of chromophores—retinal and 3-dehydroretinal—and that there is a seasonal variation in the 3-dehydroretinal content; the 3-dehydroretinal content in summer being lower than during the rest of year.

Discovery of Seasonal Variation in Spectral Sensitivity

We reexamined the relationship between the spectral sensitivity of single retinula cells and their chromophore content. We used adult male and female crayfish (*Procambarus clarkii*) collected locally in Japan and kept at 25°C under a 12 : 12-hr light-dark cycle for at least a week. These were the summer-type crayfish in which the eye contains only retinal (see figure 7.3a, top). We simulated conditions for the winter-type

Table 7.1
The wide variation in the reported maximum sensitivity of crayfish eyes

Study method	λ_{max} (nm)	Species	Author(s)
Electroretinography	575	*Procambarus*	Kennedy and Bruno (1961)
	560	*Procambarus*	Wald (1968)
	570	*Orconectes*	
	565	*Orconectes*	Goldsmith and Fernandez (1968)
	546–560	*Procambarus*	Kong and Goldsmith (1977)
	570–600	*Procambarus*	Fujimoto et al. (1966)
	560 (10)	*Procambarus*	Meyer-Rochow and Eguchi (1984)
	580 (30)		
Mass response from sustaining fibers	560–570	*Procambarus*	Woodcock and Goldsmith (1970)
	570–575	*Procambarus*	Trevino and Larimer (1970)
Extracted pigment	510 and 562	*Orconectes*	Wald (1967)
	525 and 556	*Procambarus*	
	530	*Orconectes* and *Procambarus*	Goldsmith and Wehner (1977)
Microspectrophotometry of single rhabdom	565	*Orconectes*	Goldsmith and Fernandez (1968)
	565	*Orconectes* and *Procambarus*	Goldsmith (1978)
	535	*Orconectes*	Cronin and Goldsmith (1982)
	530	*Astacus*	Hamacher and Stieve (1984)
Intracellular recording	560	*Procambarus*	Nosaki (1969)
	600		
	538–634	*Procambarus*	Waterman and Fernandez (1970)
	572	*Cherax*	Bryceson (1986)
	590–600		
	540–640	*Procambarus*	Hariyama and Tsukahara (1988)

crayfish, which have both retinal and 3-dehydroretinal, by maintaining them at 5°C in continuous darkness for at least a month (see figure 7.3a, bottom).

We then used high pressure liquid chromatography (HPLC) to examine the chromophore content of the animals. The eyes were removed from the end of the eyestalks, and the retinae removed. The amounts of different chromophores in the retina were estimated by measuring the amount of oxime forms (Suzuki et al., 1983). Examples of chromatograms of animals reared in each condition are shown in figure 7.3a. The chromophore contents of the experimental animals are equivalent to crayfish caught during the corresponding seasons.

We measured the spectral sensitivities of our animals using standard intracellular recording techniques. Although retinula cells can be penetrated with an electrode from 300 μm below the surface of the cornea, it is preferable to continue penetration to

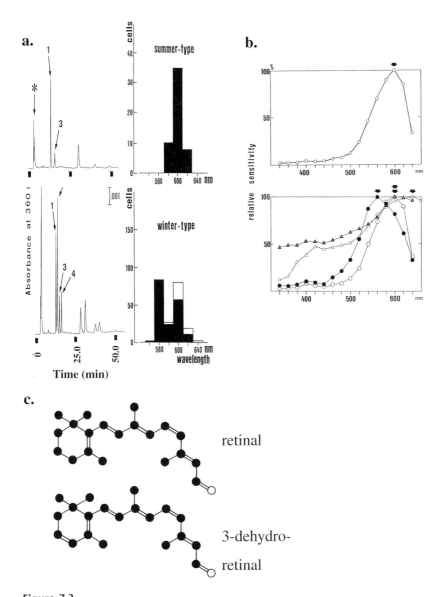

Figure 7.3
(a) Examples of chromatograms of high pressure liquid chromatography and the distribution of the wavelength of maximum sensitivity (λ_{max}) of a retinula cell. The eye of the summer-type crayfish had only retinal and most of the λ_{max} were at 600 nm. However, the eye of the winter-type crayfish had both retinal and 3-dehydroretinal and the distribution of the winter-type λ_{max} was more scattered than that of the summer type. Solid bans indicate narrower spectral sensitivity, open bars indicate broader spectral sensitivity. The asterisk is the solvent effect; 1 is 11-*cis*-retinal; 2 is 11-*cis*-3-dehydroretinal; 3 is all-*trans*-retinal; and 4 is all-*trans*-3-dehydroretinal. (b) The mean spectral sensitivity curve from 20 cells of summer-type crayfish (*upper*) and the curve obtained from 62 cells of wintertype-crayfish (*lower*). Four different sensitivity curves were distinguished in winter-type crayfish. (c) Molecular structure of 11-*cis*-retinal and 11-*cis*-3-dehydroretinal. (*a* and *c* are reproduced from Hariyama and Tsukahara, 1988, with the kind permission of Pergamon Press.)

about 1000 µm into the eye so that recordings are obtained from an area of the retina served by retinula cells that have not been damaged by the preparatory surgical treatment. These cells usually have high sensitivity and an apparently normal receptive field. In order to eliminate the effect of migration of screening pigments, the experimental animal was fully dark adapted for 1 hr or more before the experiment. The duration of light stimulation was 150 ms and the interval of each stimulation was 45 s. The stimulating light was irradiated through the "on axis."

The right side of figure 7.3a shows the distribution of the wavelength of the λ_{max} of each retinula cell. We found four types of spectral sensitivity curves, and the curves of each retinula cell were classified according to their λ_{max} and the shape of the curve.

The eyes of summer-type crayfish have a λ_{max} of 600 nm (figure 7.3b, top). The distribution of λ_{max} for the winter-type eye was more scattered than that for the summer type (figure 7.3b, bottom). There was no apparent seasonal difference in the spectral sensitivity of the R8 (apical) cells, all of which had a λ_{max} at about 440 nm.

Chromophores and Absorption Spectrum of Visual Pigments

The eyes of the summer crayfish contained only retinal and showed just one class of spectral sensitivity curve (λ_{max}, 600 nm). However, the eyes of the winter-type crayfish contained both retinal and 3-dehydroretinal and showed four patterns of spectral sensitivity. From the results, we speculated that the variation was caused by a seasonal change in the chromophore contents. However, a group of cells appear with λ_{max} at a shorter wavelength (about 560 nm) when 3-dehydroretinal is present in the winter-type eye. Two possible working hypotheses can explain this phenomenon. One is that the visual pigment with 3-dehydroretinal absorbs shorter wavelengths than retinal does. However, this hypothesis contradicts the generally accepted theory (Bridges, 1972). The other hypothesis is that the retinal pigment absorbs shorter wavelengths than 3-dehydroretinal, as is commonly accepted, and the difference in the spectral sensitivity is caused by the synthesis of an additional opsin.

To test these two hypotheses, we performed some selective light adaptation experiments. To avoid any artifacts caused by light absorption by the pigment granules, the light adaptation experiments were performed with a crude rhabdom preparation, rather than the whole eye. Rhabdoms were detached from a surgically separated retina by placing the retina in von Harreveld's solution and rotating it slowly. The crude rhabdom fraction was separated by centrifugation in a sucrose gradient and resuspended in saline. Light microscopic observation revealed that the fraction included mainly detached rhabdoms without soma or pigment granules (figure 7.4a). The procedure was performed using a night viewer.

Two tubes of suspensions were exposed to either 540- or 640-nm light (7.0×10^{15} quanta/cm^2/s) for 10 s, respectively. The suspensions were treated by the oxime method for HPLC analysis (figure 7.4b). The longer wavelength (640 nm) caused 11-*cis*-3-dehydroretinal to isomerize to the all-*trans* form, while the shorter wavelength (540 nm) isomerized 11-*cis*-retinal. The visual pigment that contained 11-*cis*-retinal as

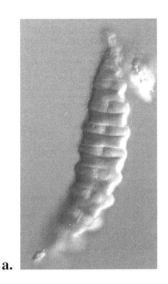

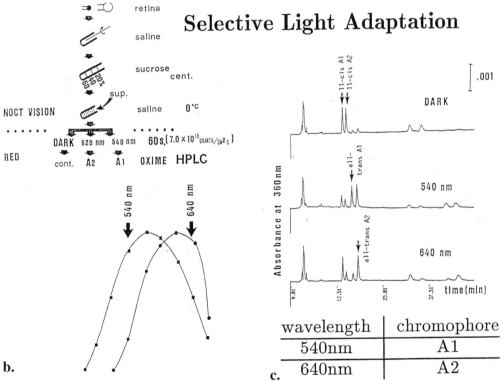

Figure 7.4
(*a*) The detached rhabdom in a crude rhabdom preparation. (*b*) The procedure of selective light adaptation. The crude rhabdom preparations were irradiated by 540 and 640 nm, respectively. (*c*) Chromatograms from the selective light adaptation with dark adaptation as a control. The visual pigment containing retinal as a chromophore absorbs more at a shorter wavelength than that containing 3-dehydroretinal. (The top part of *c* is reproduced from Hariyama and Tsukahara, 1988, with the kind permission of Pergamon Press.)

the chromophore absorbed shorter wavelengths than that which contained 11-*cis*-3-dehydroretinal (figure 7.4c). These results indicate the presence of a newly synthesized opsin in winter.

Differences between "Winter" and "Summer" Eyes

Retinula cells were classified according to their λ_{max} and the shape of their sensitivity curve. The λ_{max} of the narrower curves were at 560 and 600 nm, and those of the broader curves were at 600 and 640 nm (figure 7.3b). All of the four winter-type curves were found in a single eye (figure 7.3b, bottom). Because the summer-type crayfish have only one type of spectral sensitivity curve, it is strange that four kinds of spectral sensitivity curves were obtained from the eye of a winter-type crayfish, which contains only two kinds of chromophores. The results of superimposing the hypothetical absorption spectra, computed from Ebrey's (1977) nomogram, on the spectral sensitivity curves (figure 7.3b) are shown in figure 7.5. The spectral sensitivity curves obtained from the eye of summer-type crayfish fit the hypothetical absorption spectrum of retinal (figure 7.5a). In the winter-type eye, the two narrower curves (figure 7.5b) fit the hypothetical absorption spectra of retinal, while the two broader curves (figure 7.5c,d) fit the hypothetical absorption spectra of 3-dehydroretinal.

The close fit of the hypothetical absorption spectrum for retinal and 3-dehydroretinal indicates that at least two types of opsins must have been induced in the winter-type eye. If the winter-type opsin binds with retinal, the λ_{max} of the resulting pigment is 560 nm. If the winter-type opsin binds with the 3-dehydroretinal, the λ_{max} would be 600 nm and the spectral sensitivity curve should be broader. If the summer-type opsin conjugates with the 3-dehydroretinal, the λ_{max} may shift toward longer wavelengths (640 nm). The other conjugation, summer-type opsin with retinal, may reveal no difference between the summer and winter types. All of these possibilities were satisfied by our experimental results.

Much has been said about the λ_{max} of the spectral sensitivity curves of crayfish (table 7.1). As described earlier, it has been widely considered that the variation of the λ_{max} is due to absorption by pigment granules (Bryceson, 1986). If this alone were a sufficient explanation, it is strange that such large variations would be found in the crayfish eye. Nosaki (1969) was the first to report a seasonal change in crayfish spectral sensitivity. The following year, Waterman and Fernandez (1970) noticed this phenomenon and reported, in addition, that there is a change of λ_{max} in the winter. However, in the latter paper, the light stimuli were not restricted to the "on axis" during intracellular recordings. Hence the observed variation might have arisen from oblique stimuli. In 1984, Meyer-Rochow and Eguchi reported that the eye of *P. clarkii* reared under low (10°C) and high temperatures (30°C) showed different spectral sensitivities, peaking at 560 and 580 nm, respectively. However, the ERG method used cannot reveal the actual spectral sensitivity curves of individual retinula cells. The difference in the spectral sensitivity curves between the summer-type and the winter-type eye, however, demonstrates clearly that a visual pigment based on retinal and 3-dehydroretinal exists in the crayfish retinula cells at certain times of the year.

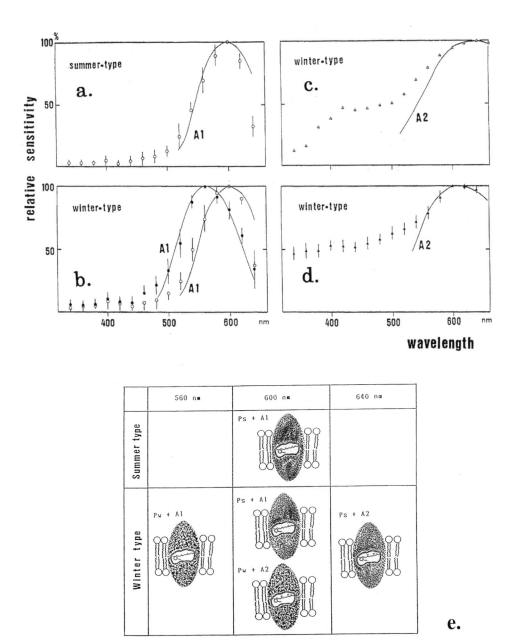

Figure 7.5
Comparison of hypothetical absorption spectra. (*a*) The spectral sensitivity curves from the eye of summer-type crayfish fit the hypothetical absorption spectra of retinal. (*b*) The two types of spectral sensitivity curves from the eye of winter-type crayfish fit that of retinal. (*c*), (*d*) The two types of spectral sensitivity curves of winter-type crayfish fit that of 3-dehydroretinal. The vertical lines indicate the standard deviation of each recording from twenty cells. A1, retinal pigment; A2, 3-dehydroretinal pigment. (*e*) Explanation of the existence of four different types of visual pigment. (Reproduced from Hariyama and Tsukahara, 1988, with the kind permission of Pergamon Press.)

Chromophores and Visual Pigments

Visual pigment consists of an apoprotein, opsin, bound by Schiff base coupling to a retinoid chromophore. Spectral sensitivity depends on the interaction between these two components. As described earlier, intracellular recordings from individual retinular cells confirm the presence of two different chromophores, but four different spectral sensitivity curves. Since a complex between a given chromophore and an opsin is expected to produce only one type of spectral sensitivity curve, it has been proposed that there are two different types of opsin (figure 7.5e). In order to test this hypothesis, we tried to produce monoclonal antibodies to the opsin content of the eye of winter-type crayfish. To generate antibodies to crayfish rhodopsin, the eyes of ten crayfish were removed and the retinae homogenized on ice in 0.5 ml of 2% Ammonex in phosphate-buffered physiological saline. After 30 min, the solution was centrifuged at 1500 rpm for 5 min and the supernatant mixed thoroughly with an equal volume (0.5 ml) of Freund's complete adjuvant. This mixture was then injected intraperitoneally into BALB/c mice. After the common procedure for monoclonal antibody production, we obtained several monoclonal antibodies against the crayfish retina, lamina, and medulla. To test whether the antibodies bound to the rhabdom were anticrayfish rhodopsin, the molecular weights of bound antigens were estimated by western blotting. Four antibodies were bound to the band at 35 kDa, which is in agreement with the estimated molecular weight of rhodopsin found in previous work (de Couet and Sigmund, 1985). This agreed also with measurements taken using the retinyle opsin techniques applied to the sodium dodecylsulfate–polyacrylanide gel electrophoresis (SDS-PAGE) slab gel track. These results are strong evidence that these four monoclonal antibodies are indeed anticrayfish rhodopsins.

The antigen sites of all four antibodies were observed by immunohistochemistry. Two were found in all rhabdomeres, including the apical retinula cell, R8. Another was localized to cells R1–R7, and the fourth was confined to only a few retinula cells. As it were, the rhabdomeres were stained singly, so that in some instances the staining pattern resembled the teeth of a comb. This reflects the crustacean layered rhabdom structure of the crayfish retina and suggests the existence of different types of opsin in the individual retinula cells (Hariyama et al., 1989).

Relationship between Vision and the Environment

Reproductive Cycles

A pioneering study by Suko (1958) showed that crayfish reproductive behavior is cyclical. In the laboratory, we found that the copulation frequency of *P. clarkii* is higher in spring and autumn than in the other seasons. In order to confirm this observation, we collected crayfish in the field to count the frequency of copulations and ovipositions (figure 7.6). Crayfish did indeed become sexually mature and copulate in the spring or autumn. Furthermore, egg laying usually peaked just after peak copulation times. The frequency of both copulation and oviposition was higher in autumn than in spring and was the lowest in summer. In the winter, crayfish crawl into their burrow and do not move. Hence winter is not a reproductive season.

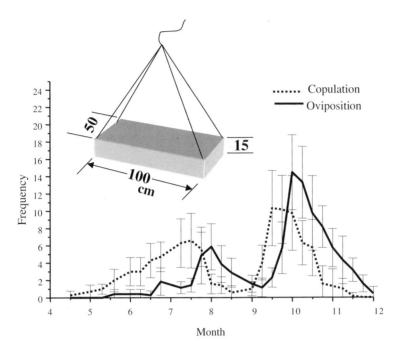

Figure 7.6
Annual copulation and oviposition frequency.

Environment during Mating Season

It has been suggested that the spectral sensitivity of the eye adapts to environmental light conditions. Freshwater fishes with a light environment biased toward red have 3-dehydroretinal as a chromophore, which absorbs light in the longer wavelength region. During winter, the water where the crayfish live is clean. However, during mating season it may contain many particles of mud and other debris so that the light environment becomes biased toward red (figure 7.1a).

Seasonal Differences in the Subjective Perceptual Worlds of Crayfish

Seasons of Black and White

In the summer, the crayfish possesses at least two chromatic channels: blue (440 nm) and red (600 nm). There is a possibility that they have color vision using those two channels. However, sensitivity in the blue region might be ineffective in the reddish environment of the hot season. Hence the crayfish may lose its color vision in summer.

The Colorful Season

Color vision can provide information for the detection of borders and objects that is not available to a black-and-white visual system. For example, consider the problem of detecting chelae against a background of reddish-brownish sand in a stream. When the chelae have about the same luminance as the sand or the crayfish's body, the task of discriminating the chelae from the background would be difficult at best for an achromatic system. This would be particularly true given that the water where the crayfish live normally absorbs light in the short-wavelength region, biasing the environmental light toward red (figure 7.1a). Hence some variation in illumination would be necessary to change the relative luminances of the chelae and background. Without such a change, it is very difficult to distinguish the chelae or even a potential mate's body in a strictly black-and-white world.

As noted, during the mating season, *P. clarkii* produces four different visual pigments and shows the four associated spectral response curves by combining two different chromophores with two different opsins. Those results suggest that the crayfish may be using this system to provide better contrast in a muddy environment with poor visibility for color discrimination. This system may provide better contrast characteristics through the presence of a new winter-type opsin, and the sharpening of each visual channel by the use of units responding broadly at wavelengths offset by the presence of the different chromophore.

Behavioral Experiments in the Colorful Season

Crayfish display a reproductive cycle (figure 7.6) and experience a comparatively colorful perceptual world during the mating season (figure 7.5). The spectral reflectance characteristics of the crayfish's chelae (figure 7.1) and the results of various behavioral experiments (figure 7.2) suggest that the chelae play an important role in mating.

To investigate the specific role of chelae color, we documented copulation frequency in the laboratory. Field-collected male and female crayfish were randomly chosen and released into an aquarium filled with sand and the water from their natural environment. Both sides of male and female chelae were painted with several colors (figure 7.7a). Copulation frequency was counted over a 2-hr period. The copulation frequency associated with reflectances in the red region (VI and VII) was the same as that for control animals (figure 7.7b). This indicates that chelae color plays an important role in copulation and that the most important spectral parameter is in the red range.

Evolution of the Crayfish Visual System

Animals that belong to the arthropod phylum are the most diverse and abundant on the earth. They represent about three-fourths of all known animal species. Arthropods have relatively small brains yet have become well adapted behaviorally to a wide range of environments. Behavioral adaptation to environmental changes, with a relatively small number of neurons, seems to be accomplished by changing the properties of the peripheral, rather than the central nervous system itself.

The enormous evolutionary success of arthropods in terms of species richness and diversity has depended to a great extent on the sophistication of their eyes. Based on the structure of their compound eyes, we can classify them into several categories.

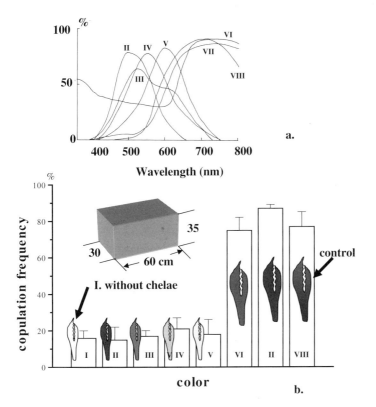

Figure 7.7
(*a*) Spectral reflection of several paints (II is blue, III is geen, IV is yellow-green, V is yellow, VI is orange, VII is red). (*b*) The copulation frequency for 2 hr in a 60-cm aquarium. The mean values and the standard deviations were obtained from twenty-five couples in each column. In I the chelae were removed and there was no significant difference from I to V. If the reflections of chelae included the red region (VI and VII), the copulation frequency was the same as that for the control.

There are several types of dioptric apparatus (Nilsson, 1989) and many types of rhabdoms (Meinertzhagen, 1991). This diversity of eye type may be a product of the limited information-processing capacity of the relatively small arthropod brain. That is, although the arthropod groups have very small brains, they live in the same complex environment as we humans do. However, in order to survive in this complex world, arthropods need to acquire and process a considerable amount of specific information. Hence, given the limited information-processing capacity of their small brains, their peripheral sensory systems need to be finely adapted to their environment in order to do the necessary prefiltering. That seems to be why small animals display a wide morphological diversity in their peripheral sensory organs.

8 The Unique Visual World of Mantis Shrimps
Thomas W. Cronin and Justin Marshall

General Characteristics

Of all the diverse creatures that make up the modern Crustacea, the mantis shrimps—properly known as stomatopod crustaceans (order Hoplocarida)—are among the oddest (figure 8.1; plate 12). More than 400 species of modern stomatopods are recognized, although the actual number is probably much higher. They are committed predators, hunting cryptically from burrows or roaming coral reefs in search of prey, which consist of small to moderate-sized invertebrates and fishes. Their ancestors diverged from the main line of crustacean evolution in the Devonian, some 400 million years ago, and they have followed a strange and unique path of their own to the present. Because of this ancient separation, mantis shrimps express a number of characteristics found in no other animals, and their visual systems may be the most unusual feature of all.

Stomatopod behavior is complex, and most species occupy rich visual environments, so good vision is critically important to their survival. As crustaceans, however, their central nervous systems are relatively small and simple. Hence, the fundamental complexity of visual stimuli presents major challenges to the analytical capacity of the stomatopod brain. These challenges are met by the use of an elegant, modular, retinal design combined with extensive preprocessing of parallel streams of visual information flowing toward the brain. The modular, hierarchical organization simplifies the categorization of visual data and facilitates quick decision making in the central nervous system. How the mantis shrimps do this is the subject of this chapter.

Spearing and Smashing
All stomatopods are armed with a powerful prey-capture device formed from their second maxillipeds (figure 8.2; plate 13). This subchelate raptorial appendage is powerfully muscled and heavily armored. It strikes with an impact that in some species approaches that of a small bullet (Burrows, 1969). Stomatopods are conventionally separated into "spearers" and "smashers" (Caldwell and Dingle, 1975, 1976), depending on the design and use of their raptorial appendages. In spearers, the terminal segment (the dactyl) is armed with a series of spines. The strike is launched with the dactyl extended, and the spines either pass through the prey like a harpoon or rapidly snip it in two as the appendage closes like a jackknife. The attack of a smasher is less elegant but generally more destructive. Here, the heel of the raptorial appendage is solidly armored (as in figure 8.2), and the strike is initiated with the dactyl flexed, so that the heel hits the target. Such a strike can shatter a crab or small snail to bits. To

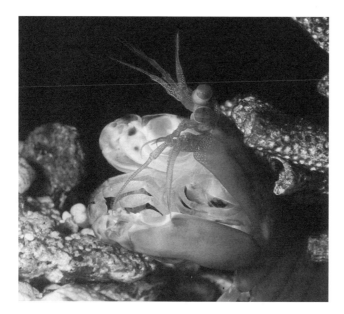

Figure 8.1
The stomatopod, *Gonodactylaceus glabrous*, which is found in the Indo-Pacific. This species is a typical smasher, living on coral reefs. Note how colorful the animal is (particularly the yellow meral spots used in signaling), and the prominent compound eyes at the front end of the cephalothorax. (Photograph by R. L. Caldwell.) (See plate 12 for color version.)

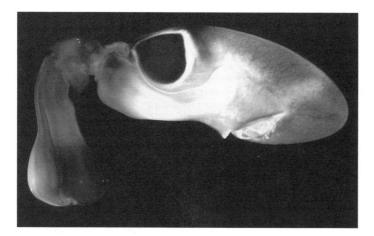

Figure 8.2
Medial view of the raptorial appendage of *Gonodactylus smithii*, a smasher. Note that the dactyl (the terminal segment) is folded back and that its "heel" is both expanded and armored for hitting prey. The purple meral spot, which is characteristic of this species, is very prominent. (See plate 13 for color version.)

attack soft-bodied prey (or a human finger), the smasher extends its daggerlike dactyl, piercing the target deeply.

Stomatopods rely on their raptorial appendages to obtain food and to defend themselves; damage to these appendages places their owner's survival in doubt. It is thus crucial that a stomatopod know the precise location, distance, and identity of any object or animal under attack. While several sensory systems contribute, vision clearly plays the critical role in this task. Stomatopod compound eyes are of the apposition type, with each set of receptors in a given ommatidium (the unit of a compound eye) forming a single rhabdom served by its own separate optical apparatus. In most crustaceans, ommatidia throughout a single compound eye are nearly identical, and together, one-by-one, they map the visual field. The apposition design lends itself to great flexibility because each ommatidium may be individually oriented within the overall array and specialized for a particular task. Stomatopods have taken this flexibility to new limits, however, using their eyes for unique analytical combinations of the spatial, spectral, and polarizational distributions of light in their underwater habitats.

Design Features of Stomatopod Eyes

In species of all three major superfamilies of stomatopods, each eye is a monocular range finder (see Ahyong and Harling, 2000 for a recent account of stomatopod phylogeny). The ability to skew the structure of the apposition compound eye is exploited by stomatopods, producing overlapping visual fields in ommatidia of the dorsal and ventral halves of the eye. Range (i.e., distance) to an object in view is, therefore, a simple function of the particular sets of ommatidia that simultaneously image it, a potential that was recognized in the first published account of mantis shrimp eyes (Exner, 1891; see also Horridge, 1978). In species of the superfamilies Squilloidea and Lysiosquilloidea, the eye is dorsoventrally elongated, extending the baseline for monocular stereopsis (Manning et al., 1984; Cronin, 1986; Marshall and Land, 1993a; Harling, 2000) (see figure 8.3; plate 14). About 70% of all ommatidia in the eye inspect a strip of space roughly 10 deg high (Marshall and Land, 1993a). Within this space, one patch of ommatidia forms an acute zone, functionally like the fovea of vertebrate eyes, where objects are seen with unusually high resolution.

Being able to range targets monocularly frees the eyes for independent movement, a strange stomatopod behavior that will be explored later in this chapter. It also permits an individual to survive following the loss of, or serious damage to one of its eyes. Furthermore, it circumvents the necessity for extremely fine motor control and proprioceptive monitoring of the visual angle between the two eyes, a particular benefit because crustaceans do not appear to be capable of fine-scale determination of eye position. A less obvious consequence of this eye design is that the skewing of ommatidial axes in the eye halves liberates other ommatidia nearer the equator for exotic specializations that provide special analysis of the spectrum and polarization of light. Before discussing these aspects of stomatopod vision, we turn to a consideration of the photic properties of the habitats of stomatopods and the objects they view.

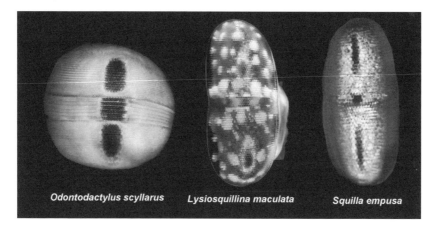

Figure 8.3
Eyes of the gonodactyloid stomatopod *Odontodactylus scyllarus*, the lysiosquilloid *Lysiosquillina maculata*, and the squilloid *Squilla empusa*. Gonodactyloids and lysiosquilloids have six-row midbands, while squilloids have only two ommatidial rows here. Note also the three pseudopupils in each eye (the dark spots in particular groups of ommatidia), which indicate the eye regions looking directly at the camera. Three pseudopupils indicate that each eye has trinocular vision. (See plate 14 for color version.)

The Coral Reef and Its Photic Environment

Almost all modern stomatopod species inhabit shallow, tropical marine waters, rarely living below depths of a few dozen meters. Many live in coral reefs, which offer an abundance of cracks, crevices, and holes to serve as refuges and home burrows. Such reefs can be dazzlingly colorful places, with profuse, spectrally distinct details and shifting patterns of polarized light (Cronin and Shashar, 2001). Other species hunt from burrows they construct in soft sand or silt. The water in which stomatopods live and hunt is generally transparent and clear, favoring the evolutionary development of their vision. But water can provide a difficult visual environment, especially when the depth and consequent filtering of downwelling light increases (figure 8.4). Many stomatopods inhabit brilliantly illuminated surface waters, but those that are found only slightly deeper must contend with a world that is lit by increasingly dimmer, bluer light. At all depths, the scattering and absorptive properties of water make for a low-contrast, hazy visual environment that obscures the visibility of distant objects. Many special features of mantis shrimp vision operate to enhance this inherently poor contrast and to maintain reliable visual function in the photically unpredictable submarine world.

Mantis shrimps are not only interested in the visually rich environment of the coral reef and its inhabitants, both predators and prey. They, themselves, are frequently beautifully colored animals. The reef-dwellers (primarily members of the

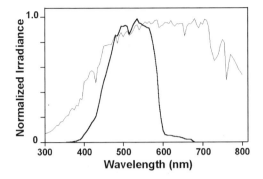

Figure 8.4
Normalized spectra of downwelling irradiance at the surface of the water (thin line) and at a depth of 20 m (thick line). In the deeper water, the spectrum becomes much narrower, limiting the options for color vision in the stomatopod species found there. The data were acquired in stomatopod habitat on the Great Barrier Reef, Australia.

superfamily Gonodactyloidea) are the most stunning of all (figure 8.1) (Caldwell and Dingle, 1975, 1976; Cronin et al., 1994c; Marshall et al., 1994; Manning, 1995). Their markings are neither arbitrary nor pointless. The most prominent markings are employed in signaling, primarily to other stomatopods, and must therefore be coevolved with vision for discriminability and rapid recognition.

Whenever aggressive competence is high, evolution favors those who can quickly evaluate risk in encounters with conspecifics. Mantis shrimps can dispatch a conspecific, or another similarly sized stomatopod, with a single strike. So a critical sensory task is to know who and what the shrimp is facing. Likewise, mating must occur between these samurailike creatures. So signals indicating readiness to mate or readiness to fight must be sent and interpreted clearly and unambiguously. Such decisions are best made quickly and from a safe distance, which favors the evolution of signals that can be detected visually. As will become clear later, these signals are not restricted to the visual spectrum that we know, nor even to colors alone.

Eye Design, Data Streams, and Central Processing
Stomatopod behavior is complex. Their communication systems are sophisticated and flexible, and their visual systems provide a wealth of information about the spatial distribution of light and motion that surrounds them, including fine analyses of color and light polarization. As in most arthropods, incoming visual information is extensively preprocessed by the primary visual centers in the ganglia within the eyestalks. In mantis shrimps these are the lamina and the three layers of the medulla which are homologous to the lamina, medulla, lobula, and lobula plate in insects. However, stomatopods may be unusual in that much of the processing probably occurs at the earliest stages of vision, as a direct consequence of the design of the eye and its

constituent ommatidia. For instance, in the case of monocular range-finding, mentioned earlier, depth measurement automatically proceeds from ommatidial visual field overlap (see Schiff and Candone, 1986, for a conception of how this might work). Likewise, polarization, ultraviolet, and spectral stimulus parameters are segregated into parallel data streams that flow into the central nervous system already having been preprocessed at the level of individual ommatidia (Cronin and Marshall, 2001). In fact, the stomatopod visual system is a model for how incoming sensory information can be simplified by the fundamentals of anatomical organization so that only the critical aspects of incoming stimuli are conveyed to the central nervous system for decision-making processing.

Mantis Shrimp Eyes and Visual Circuitry

Ocular and Ommatidial Anatomy
The stomatopod eye is divided into three distinct regions, with the dorsal and ventral halves separated by a specialized region called the midband. This consists, with rare exception, of either two (superfamily Squilloidea) or six rows (superfamilies Lysiosquilloidea and Gonodactyloidea) of ommatidia (Manning et al., 1984; Harling, 2000) (see figure 8.3).

The fields of view of all the midband ommatidia cover an essentially planar slice of visual space that extends through the center of the overlapping regions of the peripheral ommatidial arrays (see Marshall, 1988; Marshall et al., 1994; Marshall and Land, 1993a,b). The existence of the midband region proceeds directly from the geometry of the whole eye. If there is to be overlap between ommatidia that are spatially separated on the eye's surface, there will necessarily be at least a few about midway between these that also point in the same direction. These allow the animal to perform a more detailed analysis of a strip of space extending through the center of the overlapping visual fields.

Midband Ommatidia
Ommatidia in the relatively simple, two-row midband in the eyes of squilloid species are structurally like those in the rest of the eye (Schönenberger, 1977; Marshall et al., 1991a; Cronin et al., 1993). Their photoreceptive units, or rhabdoms, are constructed on the plan used by most decapod crustaceans (shrimps, lobsters, and crabs; see Eguchi and Waterman, 1966). There is a main rhabdom assembled from the microvilli of seven retinular (photoreceptor) cells arranged in a circular pattern, usually topped by a much smaller eighth receptive cell. Squilloid eyes are probably derived from more complex ancestral designs (Ahyong and Harling, 2000; Harling, 2000). Their simpler ommatidial layout enhances vision in the murky, nocturnal waters in which they hunt. In contrast, six-row midbands always contain highly specialized sets of ommatidia, with every row expressing specific design features (Marshall, 1988; Marshall et al., 1991a,b) (see figure 8.5; plate 15). Fortunately, only minor variations occur in these specializations in most species, making their description relatively straightforward.

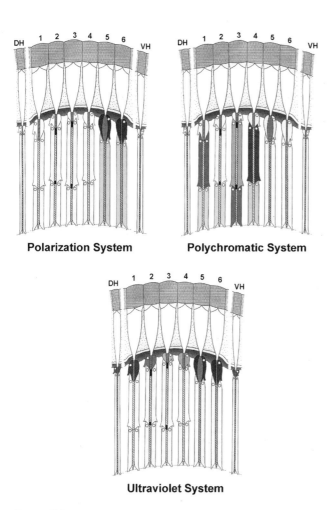

Figure 8.5
Three schematic views of ommatidia from typical six-row midbands, showing the polarization system (left), the polychromatic system (right), and the ultraviolet system (bottom), using the Caribbean species *Neogonodactylus oerstedii* as a model. The midband rows are numbered 1–6 from dorsal to ventral; DH, dorsal hemisphere of the compound eye; VH, ventral hemisphere. In the polarization system, blue indicates the eighth (UV sensitive) retinular cells; green indicates the cells of the main rhabdom. In the polychromatic system, each color suggests the wavelength range (seen by humans) to which the corresponding receptor class is most sensitive, from violet to red. The bottom schematic shows the ultraviolet receptors of the midband and peripheral retina, in which different colors suggest ultraviolet-sensitive cells operating in different spectral regions (the color indicated for R8 cells of row 3 is putative, as these have not yet been characterized). (See plate 15 for color version.)

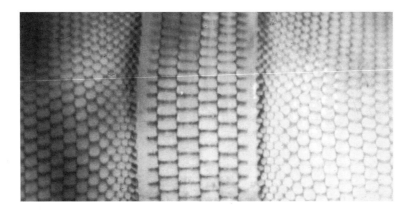

Figure 8.6
The corneal surface of ommatidia in the six-row midband of *Odontodactylus scyllarus*. Here
the corneal facets are rectangular to allow the ommatidia to be packed into rows (unlike the
hexagonal lattice of the peripheral regions, seen on each side). Dorsal is on the left in this
image. The facets in midband row 4 (the fourth from the left) contain a yellow pigment,
which is probably used to tune receptor spectral sensitivity in underlying photoreceptors.

Ommatidial rows in the midband are numbered from 1 (dorsal) to 6 (ventral) (figure
8.5).

The ommatidia in all midband rows have conventional apposition optics. Each
has an overlying, rectangular cornea (figure 8.6) and a crystalline cone that focuses
rays of light onto the rhabdom tip. It is common for the cornea in row 4 to contain
a yellow pigment, which may be significant in tuning color receptors, as explained
later. The rhabdoms of midband ommatidia undergo the greatest modifications from
the typical crustacean plan.

The two most ventral midband rows, rows 5 and 6, are similar in structure
and superficially like those in the peripheral regions of the eye. Their large, main
rhabdoms are built by seven retinular cells. Here, however, the overlying eighth
cell's rhabdomere is much longer than usual (i.e., 20% or more of the length of
the entire rhabdom; Marshall et al., 1991a), and all of its microvilli are aligned parallel to each other. In contrast, in other crustaceans, the microvilli of the (homologous) eighth retinular cell are mutually orthogonal (Waterman, 1981). This atypical
organization is associated with polarization vision, which we will discuss later in the
chapter.

The main rhabdoms in rows 5 and 6 are nearly square in cross-section, and have
very thinly layered sets of perpendicular microvilli contributed in successive layers by
different subsets of retinular cells (Marshall 1988; Marshall et al., 1991a). Again, these
are structural adaptations that improve polarization vision (see Nilsson et al., 1987).
In addition, the ommatidia in rows 5 and 6 are rotated 90 deg to each other, enhancing their role in the analysis of polarized light.

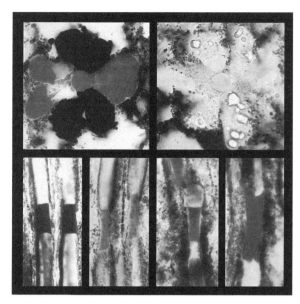

Figure 8.7
Filter pigments occurring in midband photoreceptors (rows 1–4) of various stomatopods, to illustrate the spectral diversity as seen in fresh-frozen cryosections. The top two panels are cross-sections, while the lower four panels are filters sectioned longitudinally. (See plate 16 for color version.)

In the dorsal four rows of six-row midbands, the rhabdom is divided into three tiered photoreceptive regions. The topmost tier is homologous to that in the rest of the eye and consists of microvilli provided by the eighth retinular cell. Here, microvillar orientations are like those of typical crustacean R8 cells. They are mutually orthogonal and polarization-insensitive. The underlying main rhabdom is quite unusual, however. It is split into two functional tiers placed in series, each containing microvilli from a different subset of the seven ommatidial retinular cells; three retinular cells contribute to one tier and four contribute to the other. Microvilli in each tier are arrayed in a nonparallel arrangement, eliminating any differential sensitivity to polarized light (Marshall et al., 1991b). This part of the stomatopod eye is devoted purely to the spectral analysis of light.

The junctions of the tiers in rows 2 and 3 contain photostable, colored filter pigments (figure 8.7; plate 16) (see Marshall et al., 1991a,b; Cronin et al., 1994a; Cronin and Marshall, 2001), up to four classes of which are found in each eye. The filters are paired with specific visual pigments for precise tuning of spectral sensitivity in underlying photoreceptor tiers. The interactions of tiers, visual pigments, and filters are potentially very complex and produce a bewildering variety of spectral receptor classes in each retina. An understanding of receptor cooperation amid this diversity is critical to a full understanding of stomatopod vision.

Specializations for Polarization Vision

Polarization analysis requires the presence of at least two input streams, each representing different polarization responses. This can be achieved with a single polarization-responsive receptor class if the eye rotates over time, providing what might be called temporal polarization vision. This is certainly possible given the very mobile eyes of mantis shrimps. Much more common, however, in mantis shrimps as elsewhere, is the presence of two or more spectrally identical receptor classes with differential polarization sensitivity. (A full analysis of linearly polarized light actually requires three sets of polarization receptors, but this ideal case is rarely, if ever, seen in animal vision.)

Microvillous photoreceptors naturally respond differently to polarized light because of the nonrandom arrangements of the visual pigments (see Waterman et al., 1969; A. S. Snyder and Laughlin, 1975; Goldsmith and Wehner, 1977; Waterman, 1981). However, their natural dichroism presents some difficulties when the visual system must disentangle spectral from polarizational components of a stimulus (see Wehner and Bernard, 1993). Here, two general rules apply. First, receptor systems devoted to polarization vision should all have identical spectral sensitivities. In particular, they should all contain the same rhodopsin class. Or, second, receptor systems devoted to color vision should be polarization insensitive (i.e., by abolishing their inherent sensitivity), either by having mutually orthogonal microvilli produced by each receptor cell, by pooling inputs from cells with microvilli of different orientations, or by having the microvilli of any single cell be nonparallel (via splaying or rotating the receptors). Stomatopods religiously follow the second rule, but they flagrantly violate the first by producing many spectral sensitivity types of polarization receptors. However, the receptors are grouped into classes that function in parallel, avoiding information transfer between spectral classes and preserving the purity of polarization analysis in each.

Specializations of Peripheral Ommatidia   Rhabdoms throughout the peripheral regions of the eye are all identical and similar in structure to those of other crustaceans. The uppermost R8 rhabdomere is polarization insensitive because of its orthogonal microvilli. The main rhabdom consists of successive perpendicularly oriented microvillar layers that are contributed by different sets of retinular cells, all with the same visual pigment (see Cronin and Marshall, 1989a,b; Marshall et al., 1991a). Hence, light arriving from each ommatidium's receptive field is given a two-axis polarization analysis, as is typical of most insects and arthropods. This is done by opponent processing of receptor output from the two classes (Yamaguchi et al., 1976; Glantz, 2001). Furthermore, ommatidia in the dorsal and ventral hemispheres are twisted 45 deg to each other, which, since their visual fields overlap, may provide a four-axis polarization analysis (Marshall et al., 1991a).

Specializations in Ommatidia of Rows 5 and 6   The main rhabdoms in rows 5 and 6 normally contain a visual pigment that is different from that of the peripheral recep-

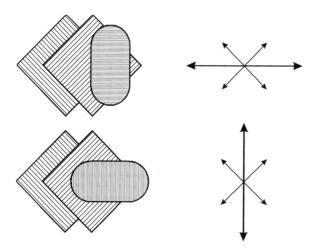

Figure 8.8
Schematic illustration of microvillar orientations (and hence preferred *e*-vector orientations) in receptors of rows 5 and 6 ommatidia. The directions of cross-hatching in the square forms indicate orthogonal orientations in successive layers of microvilli in retinular cells 1 to 7 in the main rhabdoms, while vertical hatching in the ovals represents the orientations of the microvilli of eighth retinular cells. The arrows to the right of each schematic show the preferred *e*-vectors of the various receptor classes. Each long arrow indicates that of the ultraviolet-sensitive, eighth retinular cells.

tors, but all species examined so far have very similar visual pigments, with maximum absorbance near 500 nm (Cronin et al., 2000). The main rhabdoms here are layered, providing two-axis polarization analysis (figure 8.8). Axons from row 5 and 6 receptors contribute to a unique visual pathway that serves to isolate their polarization information from that of peripheral receptors.

In these two midband rows, the parallel microvilli of the eighth-cell rhabdomeres are rotated 90 deg between rows, so microvilli of R8 rhabdomeres in row 5 run horizontally (parallel to the plane of the midband), while those of row 6 are oriented vertically (figure 8.8). The eighth retinular cells are short-wavelength receptors, described in detail later in this chapter; so if input from those of row 5 can be compared with row 6 input, mantis shrimp eyes may possess ultraviolet polarization vision.

Sensitivity to Circularly Polarized Light   The presence of the oriented eighth-cell rhabdomeres above the main rhabdoms of row 5 and 6 ommatidia could produce sensitivity to circular polarization in the receptors of the main rhabdoms. In circular polarization, the plane of polarization, or *e*-vector angle, rotates through 360 deg with the passage of each wavelength of incoming light. Circular polarization is much rarer in nature than linear polarization, but it can be produced by reflection from some biological materials (including crustacean cuticle; see Neville and Luke, 1971), or by passage through the correct thickness of a birefringent material (i.e., one in which the refractive index varies with the plane of polarization of the light passing through it). Circular polarization can be converted back to linear polarization when it transits an appropriately thick birefringent plate that retards the light polarized on one axis by a quarter wavelength relative to light polarized on the perpendicular axis. Such a structure is known as a quarter-wave retarder.

As it happens, crustacean rhabdomeres are naturally birefringent because of their arrays of parallel lipid membranes. So the eighth-cell rhabdomeres in rows 5 and 6 may act as quarter-wave retarders. If this is the case, they would convert circularly polarized light back to linearly polarized light, which could in turn be analyzed by the underlying receptors of the main rhabdom, the receptors of which are arrayed at plus and minus 45 deg, the correct angles for analysis of right and left circularly polarized light.

We do not know at present whether stomatopods really do recognize circularly polarized light, but if they do, the R8 rhabdomeres in rows 5 and 6 could have the dual function of polarization sensitivity at short wavelengths and quarter-wave delay in the wavelength region analyzed by the main rhabdom. The function of polarization vision is considered later in the chapter, but for now, the observation that stomatopods may analyze circular polarization has prompted a search for such polarization in their signals and in the habitats they occupy.

Specializations for Polychromatic Vision

The color vision systems of animals are commonly categorized by the number of primary spectral channels that contribute to them. Thus, human color vision is said to be trichromatic because it is based on three cone classes. Similarly, color vision in most birds and some fishes involves four cone types and is therefore tetrachromatic. When referring to stomatopod color vision, we prefer to use the term *polychromatic*, emphasizing the fact that many spectral channels are involved, with no particular implication concerning how these channels are combined for the central representation of color (Cronin, 1994). Stomatopods with two-row midbands have spectrally simple retinas (Cronin, 1985; Cronin et al., 1993), but in species with six-row midbands, spectral analysis of light is very unusual and probably unique among all modern animals. It is rigidly controlled both by the systems of visual and filter pigments and by the geometric arrangements of receptors and tiers.

Visual pigment diversity in single species of stomatopods is truly extreme. In midband rows 1–4, each tier of each main rhabdom contains a different visual pigment (rhodopsin), for a total of eight different rhodopsins. Their wavelengths of maximum absorption range from about 400 to 550 nm (varying with species; Cronin and Marshall, 1989a,b; Cronin et al., 1993, 1994b,d, 1996, 2000). The rhodopsins of the eighth (UV-sensitive) cells are thought to vary as well (Marshall and Oberwinkler, 1999). So there are twelve different visual pigments in just these four rows of ommatidia! There are two more classes of rhodopsins, UV sensitive and middle-wavelength sensitive, throughout all ommatidia of the peripheral retina. The eighth retinular cells and main rhabdoms in rows 5 and 6 add yet another two (the same in both rows). The grand total, then, is sixteen rhodopsins per species, one for each morphologically distinct retinal region. The next largest number of different rhodopsins occurs in adult butterflies, which have six opsins in their retina (Kinoshita and Arikawa, 2000; Briscoe, 2000). Recall that humans have only four rhodopsin classes in their eyes, three in cones and another in the rods. Clearly, stomatopods with six-row midbands have the potential for extraordinary color vision.

Theory suggests that a total of three visual pigments is the maximum useful for color vision in the human spectral range, or perhaps four if vision is extended to include the ultraviolet or far-red range (Barlow, 1982; Bowmaker, 1983). This is because the naturally broad absorbance spectra of typical visual pigments (~60 nm halfband-width) normally provide redundancy in a limited spectral range owing to absorption overlap. Mantis shrimps have avoided these theoretical constraints by using photoreceptors with very narrow spectral sensitivity functions (halfbandwidths of about 20 nm). This is achieved by the control of light maintained by tiered receptors in conjunction with filter pigments between some sets of tiers.

Figure 8.9 illustrates how tiering and filtering produce the receptor classes that mantis shrimps use to analyze color. The example shows row 2 receptors in the main rhabdoms of the Indo-Pacific gonodactyloid species *Haptosquilla trispinosa*. The top panels illustrate normalized absorbance spectra of the intrarhabdomal filters (left) and the visual pigments (right). Note that there is quite a bit of overlap of the absorbance spectra of the filters and the visual pigments, providing the potential for trimming short-wavelength sensitivity of the underlying photoreceptors.

Using the measured filter spectra and idealized visual pigment spectra (functions developed by Stavenga et al., 1993), as well as the actual dimensions of the retina, it is straightforward to compute the sensitivity spectra of the photoreceptors and the effects of filtering by any overlying retinal structures such as filters or photoreceptor tiers. In this case, the calculations ignore absorption by the optics or the eighth cell's rhabdomere, which act only at very short wavelengths. (However, absorption by these elements can affect the sensitivity functions of other midband receptors.) The results of this modeling are illustrated in the three lower panels of the figure.

First, sensitivity functions are computed assuming that the photoreceptors are unaffected by any sort of filtering; the resulting sensitivities are spectrally broad and show considerable overlap, as they do in typical photoreceptor cells. In the middle panel, the effects of retinal tiering are included. Sensitivity in the distal tier remains unchanged, but absorption by its visual pigments sharpens the underlying proximal tier's spectral sensitivity and pushes it to longer wavelengths. The bottom panel reveals the great benefit provided by the retinal filters, which give both tiers of the main rhabdom very narrow, sharp sensitivity profiles. Such filtering tunes sensitivity spectra both by narrowing the spectral range and by shifting the spectral location of photosensitivity. These effects enable the mantis shrimps to expand the numbers of potential receptor classes from four to twelve within the spectral range of 300 to 700 nm.

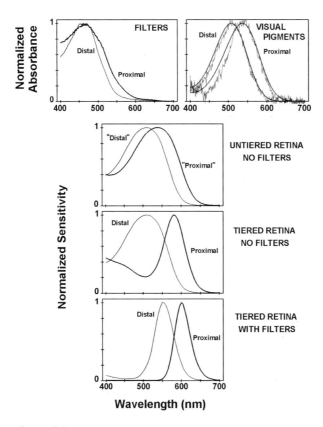

Figure 8.9
Analysis of the effects of retinal tiering and filtering in row 2 ommatidia of the Indo-Pacific species, *Haptosquilla trispinosa*. The top two panels show the absorption spectra of filter pigments (left) and visual pigments (right) measured microspectrophotometrically in intact, fresh-frozen retinae. The jagged curves represent raw data and the smooth curves represent idealized visual pigment spectra fitted to these data. The lower three panels show the effects of retinal tiering and filtering, as explained in the text.

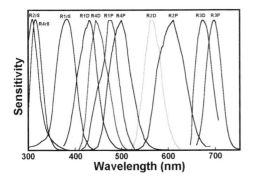

Figure 8.10
Spectral classes of all described receptor cell types in midband rows 1–4 of the Caribbean stomatopod species, *Neogonodactylus oerstedii*. These results were obtained from single-cell electrophysiological recordings. The upper-case R refers to the row number in the midband; the lower-case r8 refers to the sensitivities of eighth retinular cells. Row 3 is still undescribed. D, distal tier; P, proximal tier.

The eight tiers in the main rhabdoms of midband rows 1–4 are obviously specialized for spectral analysis, and their overlying eighth-cell rhabdomeres may also contribute to this system, for a potential total of up to twelve primary color classes. Eleven of these twelve classes have actually been measured electrophysiologically in *Neogonodactylus oerstedii*, a Caribbean species. In this species, each spectral function is extremely sharp; the functions are arrayed quite evenly across the entire visual spectrum, from near 300 to beyond 700 nm (figure 8.10). *Neogonodactylus oerstedii*, like other shallow-water species, smothers the full spectrum of visible light with multiple receptor classes. The functional significance of this design is considered later.

The spectral range for color vision displayed by *N. oerstedii* is the greatest measured in any animal. Such range is useful only in bright, white-light environments which, in marine habitats, would only be in waters that are very shallow and clear. The extreme short- and long-wavelength spectral classes would be blind in mantis shrimps living deeper or in murky water, where ultraviolet or far-red photons are absent. Species living in the latter habitats tend to express visual pigments more in keeping with the spectral range of available light (Cronin et al., 1994d, 2000).

More significantly, the pigments used in the intrarhabdomal filters are different from those of shallow-water species. Specifically, the filter pigments used to tune the very long-wavelength receptor classes (those peaking beyond 650 nm in figure 8.10) are significantly blue shifted in species living more than a few meters deep (see Cronin et al., 1994b,d, 2001, 2002; Cronin and Caldwell, 2002), and the spectral position of the longest-wavelength receptors peaks near 600 nm. In some low-light species, only

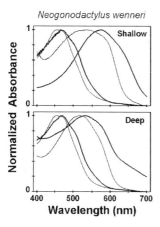

Figure 8.11
Absorbance spectra of filters in ommatidia of the Caribbean species, *Neogonodactylus wenneri*, collected in shallow water (3 m, top panel) and deep water (30 m, bottom panel). Distal filters and proximal filter classes are plotted in thin and thick lines, respectively. The spectra of both row 2 filters are found to the left in both panels. Note that while row 2 filters are similar or identical in both shallow- and deep-living animals, the filters in row 3 are strongly blue shifted in the deep-living set.

two or three filter classes exist (Cronin et al., 1993, 1994a), presumably to increase retinal illumination.

A recent, unexpected finding is that the ensemble of filter pigments in the retina can be altered adaptively within a single species when individuals are exposed to new lighting environments (Cronin et al., 2001). Both gonodactyloid and lysiosquilloid species have such variable filters, invariably found in row 3 ommatidia (which always include the longest-wavelength receptor types). An example is seen in figure 8.11, which shows the absorbance spectra of filters of the gonodactyloid species *Neogonodactylus wenneri*, collected in shallow (2 m) or deep (30 m) water in the Florida Keys of the United States. Row 3 filters, placed at longer wavelengths, are blue shifted in the deep-living animal, while the row 2 filters are identical in animals from both habitats.

The Ultraviolet Visual System
We have noted the short-wavelength sensitivity in the eighth retinular cell class a number of times. Rhabdomeres of these cells are always found at the top level of the rhabdom, immediately below the crystalline cones (Cronin et al., 1994e; Marshall and Oberwinkler, 1999) (see figure 8.5). The axons from these cells project through the lamina (normally the first synaptic layer in the crustacean visual system) to the medulla externa, the second layer of interneurons (discussed in the next section). This implies that ultraviolet stimuli may be processed separately from stimuli coming from

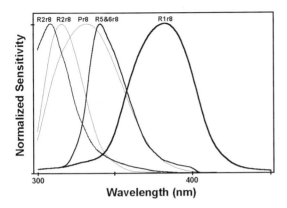

Figure 8.12
The sensitivity spectra, characterized by single-cell electrophysiological recording, in eighth retinular cells (r8) of all classes (except those of row 3) in *Neogonodactylus oerstedii*. Note the broad spectral range covered by these receptors and the narrowness of the sensitivity spectra of some classes, probably produced by filtering in the overlying cornea or crystalline cones. The upper-case R refers to the row number in the midband; the lower-case r8 refers to the sensitivities of eighth retinular cells. P refers to the peripheral retina (dorsal and ventral hemispheres, both of which contain identical eighth-cell types).

the main rhabdoms, although the precise neural wiring of the UV system is yet to be clarified.

Ultraviolet vision in stomatopods with six-row midbands follows the organizational themes already described: functional diversity and liberal use of filtering. In *Neogonodactylus oerstedii*, spectral sensitivities of the eighth retinular cells have been determined for all classes except those of row 3 (figure 8.12) (Marshall and Oberwinkler, 1999). Like the polychromatic system, these receptors cover an extended spectral range (peaking at wavelengths from 310 to 380 nm), using an unequaled diversity of UV-absorbing visual pigments. The sensitivity functions are invariably narrower than those that would be produced by a UV-rhodopsin acting alone, which implies that components in the cornea or crystalline cone act as ultraviolet long-pass filters, tuning the receptors and incidentally reducing short-wavelength sensitivity in the main rhabdoms as well.

Modeling suggests that the visual pigments required to form the observed sensitivity classes have spectral maxima as short as 290 nm (Marshall and Oberwinkler, 1999). These spectral positions are located 50–60 nm toward shorter wavelengths than other ultraviolet visual pigments. The molecular mechanisms that might tune such extremely short-wave receptor molecules are not known. Also unknown at present is whether the functional diversity contributes to ultraviolet color vision or has some other, unanticipated function.

Neural Circuitry of the Visual System

The polychromatic midband, multiple UV receptors, and complex polarization sense of mantis shrimps, together with the unusual way in which spatial information is sampled in the retina, prompt the obvious next question: How is all this information processed? What messages finally reach the relatively small brain of the mantis shrimp? As already hinted, we suspect that much of the signal processing is done peripherally, which is the strategy of many invertebrates (Wehner, 1987). However, work within this area of the stomatopod visual system has only just begun.

The eyestalks of stomatopods contain four levels of neural interaction: the lamina ganglionaris, medulla externa (ME), medulla interna (MI), and medulla terminalis (MT). Thereafter, visual information leaves each eyestalk via the optic nerve and travels to the brain (figure 8.13).

In these respects, stomatopods are much like other arthropods (Strausfeld and Nassel, 1981), and an analysis of the structure of these nerve plexi has revealed a number of facts. First, streams of information from the peripheral retina, midband color vision rows 1–4, and the midband polarization rows appear to remain separate at least to the medulla interna. For instance, color information encoded by midband rows 1–4 is wired to discrete portions of the lamina, medulla externa, and medulla interna. This organization of information streams is clear from an examination of sections of the eyestalk (e.g., figure 8.13).

Second, each ommatidium in the retina sends axons (eight in total, one from each of the retinular cells) to a single laminar cartridge. That is, even within a single retinal region, there is no crosstalk between adjacent ommatidia at this level. Again, this is very much like the organization in other arthropods (Strausfeld and Nassel, 1981). What is interesting here, however, is that laminar cartridges from the peripheral retina, midband rows 5 and 6, and midband rows 1–4 look quite different, even in sections examined with a light microscope (figure 8.13c) (Marshall et al., 1994).

Third, the construction of the laminar cartridges is said to be insectlike (Strausfeld and Nassel, 1981). Each contains four monopolar cells whose job it is to receive information from the photoreceptor axons terminating in the lamina. In common with insects and other crustaceans, the R8 cell axon does not terminate in the lamina, but passes through the cartridge to the medulla externa. Its close association with the lamina cartridge suggests that it may supply information to monopolar cells at this stage, but this has yet to be demonstrated clearly.

Finally, two discrete termination layers exist in all lamina cartridges. One layer receives information from three of the R1–R7 cells, and the other receives information from the remaining four R1–R7 cells. A similar pattern exists in crabs (Stowe, 1977) and crayfish (Sabra and Glantz, 1985), and has been linked to polarization opponency. Apparently the former set of three cells samples the e-vector of light orthogonal to the latter set of four cells. This has important implications for both polarization and color opponency in stomatopods.

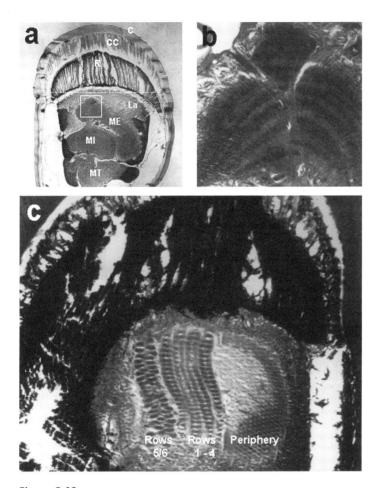

Figure 8.13
Neural wiring beneath the stomatopod eye. (*a*) Longitudinal section through the eyestalk
of *Neogonodactylus oerstedii*, the optic nerve exiting the bottom of the photograph. C,
cornea; CC, crystalline cones; R, retina; La, lamina; ME, medulla externa; MI, medulla
interna; MT, medulla terminalis. The dotted line is the level of the section shown in (*c*),
and the square is enlarged in (*b*). (*b*) Enlarged portion of the ME from (*a*), showing a wedge-
shaped portion that receives input from the midband ommatidia only. (*c*) Transverse
section through the eyestalk at the level of the dotted line in (*a*). Owing to the curvature
of the eye, the cornea and crystalline cones can be seen on the very edge of the top. The
black retina is visible below them, within which the six midband rows are visible. The
lamina is the more lightly stained structure in the bottom center of the photograph.
The lamina cartridges of ommatidia from the different eye regions are easily visible as
distinct structures (the dark blobs most readily seen in the neatly organized ommatidial
rows of the midband.).

Seeing the World through the Mantis Shrimp's Eyes

Stomatopods display a variety of unique eye movements that are functionally related to their remarkable and unusual optical arrangements (Cronin et al., 1988; M. F. Land, 1995; M. F. Land et al., 1990; Marshall and Land, 1993a,b). Even compared with the eye movements of other crustaceans, they seem most strange. Before describing the eye movements in detail, however, it is worth reiterating the specific optical adaptations that are behind them.

Each stomatopod eye is monocularly trinocular; that is, all midband photoreceptors and as many as 70% of the photoreceptors within the two hemispheres examine a 10-deg strip in visual space (Exner 1891; Horridge, 1978; Marshall and Land, 1993a,b). Second, stomatopods from two superfamilies (the Gonodactyloidea and Lysiosquilloidea) possess areas of especially high acuity embedded within this strip (Horridge, 1978; Marshall and Land, 1993a,b). This acute zone is functionally analogous to the vertebrate fovea. Stomatopods from the superfamily Squilloidea do not have acute zones but still display monocular trinocularity (Marshall and Land, 1993a,b). Third, the overall extent of the visual field in many species is less panoramic than in many crustaceans, and is generally weighted frontally. This is probably a direct result of the animal's propensity to view the world from within the safety of its home burrow.

Stomatopod eye movements fall into four categories: optokinetic stabilization, scanning, saccadic acquisition, and tracking. One notable feature of stomatopods is that each eye can perform any of these eye movements independently, and the often large, independent eye movements can be quite unnerving when first seen (figure 8.14a). How visual information related to eye movements is encoded or even unscrambled by the stomatopod's brain is not yet known.

A second general feature of their eye movements is that they appear to switch tasks or time-share according to what is (apparently) required of them (M. F. Land et al., 1990). For instance, an object of interest may be acquired within the acute zone of one or both eyes and then either tracked or scanned, depending on what the object is doing. In either of these two cases, there is some apparent coherence between right and left eye movements, although the coherence may be illusory because both eyes are doing the same thing. The situation actually may be more like two people watching the same tennis match. At any time during such apparently coherent eye movements, however, one of the shrimp's eyes may wander off to fixate or scan some other interesting object.

The Eye Movements

Optokinetic stabilization is an important feature of any visual system and is a class of eye movements driven by large-field or panoramic movements, such as the view out of the window of a train. In this instance, our eyes are drawn to follow the passing scene and then flick forward as the part of the scene we were following disappears from view. Such a system stabilizes a visual scene on the retina relative to the viewer

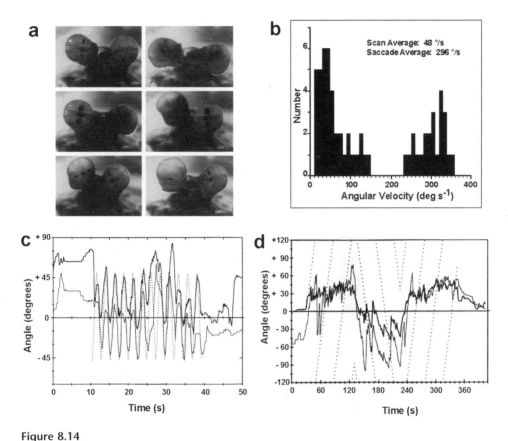

Figure 8.14

Stomatopod eye movements. (*a*) Video frames of spontaneous eye movements made by *Odontodactylus scyllarus*. Note the independence of the movements, the position of the midband (showing the rotational component of eye movements, possibly important for polarization vision), the triple pseudopupil visible in some eye positions, and the extra-large triple pseudopupil in the middle two photos, which indicates that the animal is looking at the camera with its acute zone. (*b*) Summary of angular velocities of eye movements made over a 5-min period by *O. scyllarus*. The speeds of the eye movements were calculated using a computer tracking technique described in M. F. Land et al. (1990), binned in 10 deg/s lots, and plotted as a bar chart. Note the two populations of eye movement types: slow, averaging about 48 deg/s, represent scans; fast, averaging about 300 deg/s, are saccades. (*c*) Plot of the horizontal component of eye movements for both eyes of *Neogonodactylus oerstedii* while tracking a moving stimulus (dotted line). The thick and thin lines indicate movements of the right and left eyes, respectively. Note the saccade to the position of the target made by the right eye as the target begins to move, and also that in this case each eye tends to track the target when it crosses to its own side. See Cronin et al. (1988) for details. (*d*) Optokinetic stabilization movements in stomatopods are disorganized compared with those seen in other crustaceans, such as crabs (Sandeman et al., 1975), because other eye movements (saccades, scans) often usurp control of eye function.

(Carpenter, 1988). A mantis shrimp that found itself looking out of a train window (presumably from an aquarium) would do the same thing.

In the laboratory, an analogous but simpler large-field visual stimulus can be presented by rotating a striped or patterned drum around a tethered animal (Sandeman et al., 1975). When viewing such a stimulus, the mantis shrimp's eye movements are independent and, compared with other animals, are rather lazy and often distracted (figure 8.14d) (Cronin et al., 1991). This may reflect the task-switching behavior referred to earlier. Long, slow drum-following movements alternate with fast flicks as the eyes reach their physical limits. However, optokinesis is often interrupted by other eye movements, making it appear that the shrimp is satisfied that its world remains where it was the last time it looked.

Scanning eye movements are seen only in stomatopods and a few other invertebrates, including jumping spiders and heteropod mollusks (M. F. Land, 1995). All of these creatures possess linear, one-dimensional retinae, so the animal must move its photoreceptors over an object of interest in order to sample the relevant information. For scanning eye movements to work for a mantis shrimp, they must be made perpendicular to the plane of the midband and be performed sufficiently slowly to allow the photoreceptors to take in the available information. For *Odontodactylus scyllarus*, this is about 40 deg/s, which is ideal for the photoreceptor's internal physiology (M. F. Land et al., 1990). Such slow, deliberate movements fall into a very different category compared with the rapid, saccadic, acquisitional eye movements of which the shrimps are also capable (figure 8.14b) (Cronin et al., 1988). Also, because many of the peripheral ommatidia view the narrow strip sampled by the midband photoreceptors, such slow scanning may enhance range-finding (i.e., distance estimation).

Saccadic, acquisitional movements are rapid relocations of gaze made in order to place an object's image in the acute zone, where the optical axes of the ommatidia are tightly packed, enhancing spatial resolution. Most animals with acute zones, including humans, make such gaze shifts. However, stomatopods, chameleons (Ott et al., 1998), and sand-lance fish (Pettigrew and Collin, 1995) are in a small group of animals whose eyes can make saccades independently (figure 8.14c). The speeds of such eye movements vary among species and are roughly correlated with eye size and distance to be moved. However, they are generally several hundreds of degrees per second. During the saccade, visual input is presumably turned off (as it is in humans; see Carpenter, 1988) to prevent retinal slip from disorienting or confusing the animals.

Visual tracking also requires an acute zone and generally follows what is called foveal acquisition (i.e., the initial placement of the object's image within the acute zone). After foveal acquisition, the eye may moved in order to keep the object's image within the acute zone. Again, no other crustacean makes such precise eye movements. [Although crayfish may keep objects toward the frontal visual field, and crabs make apparent saccades when orienting visually to the local horizon (Zeil, 1989).]

Figure 8.14c shows the horizontal eye movements of a stomatopod tracking an object that is wiggled backward and forward in front of it. Here, the eyes may work independently or, if the object is interesting, both may make the same movements simultaneously.

Objects can be tracked up to quite a high velocity. Eye placement and movement during tracking is controlled by afferent input from the peripheral ommatidia only (Cronin et al., 1992). This makes sense because the striplike visual field of midband ommatidia provides little or no information about the actual location of an object in extended space.

Saccadic and tracking eye movements can give stomatopods an air of primatelike awareness (M. F. Land et al., 1990). However, unexpected interruptions and/or changes in eye movements remove such an impression. The stomatopod's hunting strategy often is to launch attacks from the stable, well-known base of its home burrow. This environmental stability may be a clue to how they manage to sort out all of the assumedly confusing information that they receive when their eyes are doing different things.

Color Vision

It may seem unnecessary to prove that an animal with twelve or more photoreceptor types, each with a different spectral preference, possesses color vision. However, anatomical or physiological demonstrations of polychromacy say nothing about how photoreceptors are used, and behavioral experiments are needed to fully examine color vision in any animal (Neumeyer, 1991). Von Frisch was one of the first to recognize this and developed a series of experiments with bees that exploited their readiness to feed from artificial, colored "flowers." The basic paradigm was to train a bee to feed from, say, a yellow container and then test it with the yellow container placed amid an assortment of variously shaded gray containers. Without color vision, a bee would perceive yellow as a shade of gray and confuse one of the gray containers with the yellow one (K. von Frisch, 1914). However, bees did not confuse yellow and gray, and neither do stomatopods when confronted with similar tests. Hence, both possess color vision.

In the case of stomatopods, the feeding task is modified to take advantage of their curious but violent nature. The large gonodactyloid, *Odontodactylus scyllarus*, is very inquisitive about any object placed in front of its burrow and will rush out, manipulate the object, and bash it with the heel of its raptorial appendage. *O. scyllarus* is a smasher capable of breaking aquarium glass, and had no trouble breaking into the food containers with glass coverslip sides that we devised to test its color vision (figure 8.15). During training, one side of a glass, cube-shaped food container was covered with colored plastic. During testing, the shrimp was presented with an empty colored cube and two other empty gray cubes, chosen from a series of seven shades of gray.

In the test, the stomatopods easily learned to discriminate red-, green-, and yellow-colored cubes from gray cubes, although they never succeeded in discriminating the blue shade that we used (figure 8.15) (Marshall et al., 1996). That failure is interesting,

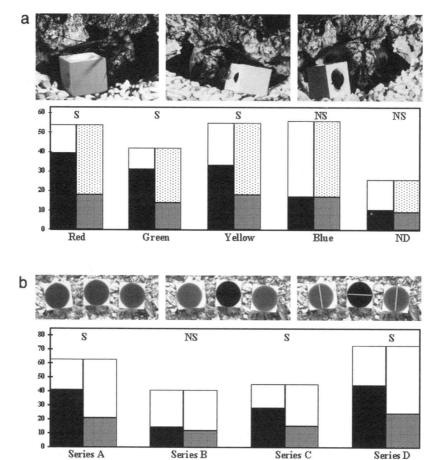

Figure 8.15

Behavioral tests of color and polarization vision. (*a*) Colored feeding cubes used with stomatopods in tests. The empty sides of the cubes are covered with glass coverslips and food is placed in the middle of the cube. The results of the tests are given for each of the colored cubes as well as for an attempt to train the animals to a specific neutral density (ND). For each color, the expected choice ratios are shown by the dotted gray bars on the right and the observed ratios by the black-and-white bars. S, significant difference between observed and expected choices (*P* > 0.001 in chi-squared test); NS, not significantly different. Further details are given in the text and in Marshall et al. (1996). (*b*) The front surface of "polaroid" feeding cubes similar to those in (*a*) are shown in the row of three photographs. (*Left*) The cubes photographed in the positions they would be seen by the stomatopod during choice tests. (*Center*) The same cubes photographed through a vertically oriented polarizing filter to show the orientation of the "polaroid" film on the cubes. (*Right*) Lines on cubes drawn to emphasize the direction of the "polaroid" film on each cube. The graphs show the results from three-way choice tests and follow the same principles as in (*a*). Series A, C, and D are three experimental series choice tests with *Odontodactylus scyllarus* and *Gonodactylus chiragra*, respectively. These different types of tests were devised to overcome possible edge effects and unwanted patterning in the cubes (see Marshall et al., 1999). In series B we also tried to train animals to discriminate cubes that differed only in neutral density.

especially since the blue is clearly distinguishable to us. However, it gives us some insight into the stomatopod's color vision capabilities.

Of the colors we chose, the blue plastic turned out to be the least saturated (Endler, 1990). Later, we found that the blue cubes appear most like the gray cubes, especially to a set of dichromatic systems (see Marshall et al., 1996, for more details). This implies a threshold for stomatopods in their ability to discriminate colors that is related to the saturation (or intensity) of the color. It also implies that at least in some ways their color vision is inferior to ours. A better understanding of stomatopod color vision will require more behavioral tests.

Polychromatic Vision and Color Constancy   A number of other animals use filtering mechanisms to sharpen the spectral sensitivities of their photoreceptors. Birds (Bowmaker, 1980; Partridge, 1989), reptiles, and a few fish and marsupials possess colored oil droplets that are analogous to the filter pigments seen in rows 2 and 3 of the stomatopod midband (even down to their construction from carotenoids). In birds, these filters perform exactly the same function that they do in stomatopods, and the result is a set of four sharply tuned, well-spaced color photoreceptor classes that are essentially ideal for discriminating any of the colors available to birds (Govardovskii, 1983; Vorobyev et al., 1998).

Such sharp, slightly overlapping sensitivities not only enhance discrimination, they may also give their owners a greater sense of color constancy. Color constancy is the ability to perceive a color as the same, despite changes in illumination. This would be especially beneficial in environments with changing lighting conditions (Maloney and Wandell, 1986). For us, color constancy works well if we move from sunlight to fluorescent room lights (and, indeed, room lighting is designed with this in mind). However, it fails under the yellow illumination of street lamps, where red objects look a sickly green. Birds flying from open sunlight into forest shade may face the same problem, and it has been suggested that their steep-sided overlapping color sensitivities may improve color constancy for them (Govardovskii, 1983).

Stomatopods, and indeed all aquatic animals, face greater variations in illumination than do any land animals because water absorbance changes the available light from broad-spectrum sunlight to essentially blue-green over just a few meters (figure 8.4).

We have discussed how the sharp color sensitivities of stomatopods may help them overcome this challenge (Osorio et al., 1997). A single species may live at depths that differ by more than 10 m. Because of their very broad visual spectral range (300–710 nm in some species) and their reliance on colors for signaling (see Caldwell and Dingle, 1976; Chiao et al., 2000), color constancy may be of particular importance to them. The fact that spectral sensitivities change within and between species over various water depths is certainly related to this problem. It is interesting that only under extreme duress, as is the case for species living in very deep waters, are the very red sensitivities actually discarded. We currently do not know the fate of UV photoreceptors in such animals.

Stomatopod sensitivities can be readily modeled (as 18-nm-wide Gaussian curves) and their performance at natural visual tasks compared with broadband, humanlike sensitivities (nonfiltered visual systems, approximated by 50-nm-wide Gaussians). We did such a comparison by examining measured colors from reef fish and stomatopods, under illumination, at depths of 0 and 5 m in both coastal and oceanic water types (Osorio et al., 1997). Our main findings were first, that sharp spectral sensitivities greatly improve color constancy. Second, we found that that the photoreceptor spectral spacing required for such constancy is that actually seen in stomatopods. That is, the spectral tuning curves not only facilitate color constancy, but their positioning in the spectrum is almost exactly what one would predict to optimize signal constancy (Osorio et al., 1997, and references therein).

Polarization Vision

The perception or use of polarized light is foreign to us. We do make use of polarizing filters in photography, and in sunglasses polarizers reduce reflections from water and other shiny surfaces. Many invertebrates (A. W. Snyder, 1973; Waterman, 1981; Wehner, 1987) and some vertebrates (Hawryshyn, 1992; see Browman and Hawryshyn, 2001), make use of polarized light in a variety of tasks, such as navigating (Wehner and Lanfranconi, 1981), reducing scatter and reflection (Lythgoe, 1979), breaking silvery camouflage, and signaling (Marshall et al., 1999; Shashar et al., 1996). The underwater world, especially in shallow waters, is full of polarized light (Ivanoff and Waterman, 1958; Cronin and Shashar, 2001), and stomatopods are, of course, sensitive to different e-vectors in rows 5 and 6 of the midband and possibly in the peripheral retina (Marshall et al., 1991a).

As with color vision, behavioral tests are needed to determine exactly how polarized light might be used (Wehner, 2001). However, we have recently shown that stomatopods are capable of learning e-vector orientation (Marshall et al., 1999) using an adaptation of the feeding-cube test described earlier. We did this by replacing the colored plastic with polaroid dichroic linear polarizing film set at different angles (figure 8.14b).

Our finding that stomatopods can discriminate such cubes was surprising in that many animals display rather hard-wired responses to polarized light (analogous to the wavelength-specific behaviors described later). Stomatopods and cephalopods are the only animals known to respond to polarization cues in a way that implies that the perception of them is analogous to the perceptual experiences provided by normal color vision (Bernard and Wehner, 1977), and both groups probably use polarized signals from various body regions to communicate (Shashar et al., 1996; Marshall et al., 1999). Stomatopod antennal scales and uropod paddles are particularly striking in this respect, and both of these body areas are brandished during combat or meetings between stomatopods (Caldwell and Dingle, 1975). As with many other aspects of stomatopod biology, however, there is much to learn before these ideas can be substantiated.

Evolution of an Integrated Sensory World in Mantis Shrimps

Is the Mantis Shrimp's Eye an "Ear"?

It is very hard to imagine what the colored world of stomatopods might be like subjectively, or what specific information might be sent to the mantis shrimp's brain to affect its behaviors. Although it is possible to speculate about color constancy (e.g., Osorio et al., 1997) and fun, for some persons, to try to conceptualize twelve-dimensional color space, what is almost certain is that the stomatopod's polychromatic retina must simplify the spectral stimuli that it receives. This, after all, is the job of any sensory system. Some animals, notably the relatively polychromatic butterflies (Arikawa et al., 1987; Kelber, 1997), perform behaviors that are hard-wired responses to certain colors; these are known as wavelength-specific behaviors. In these cases, the underlying neural system, from photoreceptor to brain, discriminates colors per se. It need only respond in a fixed way to a specific wavelength of light.

In principle, this sort of perception could help explain the complexity of stomatopod color vision. A fixed response to a specific meral color spot, for instance, could be useful. There is, however, no evidence for such a simple color sense, and the color vision tasks that we have described show that stomatopods are capable of learning and discriminating different hues. Furthermore, butterflies show true color vision in addition to wavelength-specific behaviors, so the two types of color vision can coexist (Kelber, 1999b; Scherer and Kolb, 1987a,b).

Currently we are investigating two nonmutually exclusive hypotheses to explain the overdeveloped color sense of stomatopods. The first is that this is a system based on multiple dichromatic channels. The second is that it is a color system that examines color space in a way similar to that in which the cochlea examines auditory space. We review the evidence for the latter hypothesis first.

Stomatopod color space stretches from 300 to just over 700 nm in *Neogonodactylus oerstedii*, and the photoreceptor sensitivity curves are arrayed evenly within this range (figure 8.10). This is reminiscent of the cochlea, in which the hair cells (in humans) are sensitive to an array of frequencies from about 20 Hz to 20 kHz. As the stomatopod eye looks at colors, they may not be coded by an opponent comparison of overlapping spectral sensitivities, but rather by the pattern of stimulation across the various sensitivities (Marshall et al., 1996; Neumeyer, 1991). This method of color vision is not known to exist anywhere else in the animal kingdom. For such a system to function, information from each of the spectral channels would have to remain separate, as it does in the vertebrate auditory nerve. The potential for the separation of color data streams is structurally present in stomatopods, at least to the level of the lamina ganglionaris (see earlier discussion), and beyond this stage the overall pattern of stimulation may be analyzed by comparing ommatidial types.

In the alternative multiple dichromacy hypothesis (Marshall et al., 1996; Chiao et al., 2000), each of the four midband rows 1–4 examines a relatively narrow window in the spectrum and discriminates colors using an opponent mechanism, with potentially very fine spectral detail and constancy that is due to the sharp, steep spectral sensitivity curves within this window. The idea has come from a consideration of the R1–R7 cells of rows 1–4 in the midband only; its extension to UV sensitivity requires between-row comparisons of R8 cell signals. Such hypothetical comparisons would be processed in one of the medullae, rather than in the lamina ganglionaris.

Persuasive but as yet unsubstantiated evidence for multiple dichromacy of R1–R7 cells in midband rows 1–4 is twofold. First, the separation of R1–R7 cells into two tiers, each with its own sensitivity, both of which project to a discrete laminar cartridge beneath the retina, suggests that interaction between these cell subsets could occur within that cartridge. Close examination of the anatomical identity of the cell subsets suggests that such a color opponency could have been borrowed from an older polarization opponency, which is present in many crustaceans (Marshall et al., 1991a; Sabra and Glantz, 1985; Glantz, 2001).

Typically, cells numbered 1, 4, and 5 possess microvilli orthogonal to those in cells numbered 2, 3, 6, and 7. So, between them, the cell sets possess the potential to discriminate e-vectors by opponency. There is evidence from laminar cartridge structure that such comparisons are made here (Marshall et al., 1991a; Sabra and Glantz, 1985). In stomatopod rows 1–4, the very same cell sets, 1, 4, and 5 versus 2, 3, 6, and 7, are those which have become reorganized to construct separate rhabdom tiers (figure 8.5), and, therefore, with no reorganization of subretinal wiring, polarization opponency could be swapped for color opponency. Second, the actual spectral separation of the sensitivities of the upper and lower tiers of each row is ideal for individual dichromatic systems, with overlap between curves at around the 50% sensitivity level (Osorio et al., 1997).

Finally, in the debate between the two hypotheses, additional indirect support for the cochlealike method of color vision comes from the unusual way that stomatopods examine visual space. Since all the midband and many of the peripheral photoreceptors look into the same narrow strip of visual space to examine the colors of objects (and perhaps their polarization and spatial characteristics), the eyes perform their rather slow scanning movements perpendicular to the plane of the midband (figure 8.15). In this way, spectral detail is almost literally painted in, and some form of temporal memory must exist for what has just been scanned. Performing several color opponency calculations as the midband is swept over objects is perhaps difficult, and the simpler option of reading out the output of the whole system to encode color may be easier. This dividing up of color space into a series of segments and monitoring their relative output is more akin to a digital form of color vision. Many line-scan cameras and remote-sensing devices such as "push-broom" cameras work on exactly this principle (Brooke, 1975). The astute reader will have noted by now that the real answer to the questions raised by all of these exciting possibilities is that we still do not know what color information reaches the stomatopod brain.

Combining Spatial, Chromatic, and Polarization Cues

The central processing of the emergent features of a visual scene, including its spatial, chromatic, and polarizational organization, is poorly understood for any animal group, including the mantis shrimps. Nevertheless, the neat, almost crystalline structural design, combined with some knowledge of photoreceptor specializations, eye movements, and shrimp visual behavior, provides an entry point into understanding how mantis shrimps see. Once again, the inference is that function follows structure and that behavior relies on function.

Mantis shrimps inhabit a contrast-limited world in which absorption and scattering of light obscure the visual scene, a situation analogous to looking into a dense fog. Multiple color and polarizational channels offer a way to penetrate that fog. Scattering varies with wavelength, and polarization provides an independent way to make faint objects stand out (Shashar et al., 1996). As already noted, the presumably opponent, dichromatic spectral systems of midband ommatidia in rows 1–4 repeat the opponencies of the polarizational receptors of rows 5 and 6. The implication is that spectral and polarizational comparisons are analogous in mantis shrimp vision, and that variation in the spectral or polarizational domain provides similar modes of seeing. If this is true, both color and polarization are aspects of vision that enhance visibility and contrast underwater, and are blended together in central perception at each point in visual space.

Of course, all these receptor types are restricted to midband ommatidia, and their shared visual fields occupy just a strip of space. As noted earlier, mantis shrimps must somehow get the chromatico-polarizational aspects of a stimulus located properly in the extended visual field. This is where the slow visual scans become important. By sliding the eye over a scene, passing the planar view of midband ommatidia past some sort of central registration of space (or at least some point in space), the scene becomes colored and polarized. This sort of vision requires the alternate use of ocular stabilization to register form and motion, and scanning to add midband sensations. Here we see an ultimate biological example of what is called sensor fusion in military and remote-sensing parlance. It is the combination of separate, parallel (in space), or serial (in time) channels to produce a unified sensory representation of the visual world.

Complexity and Simplicity in the Visual System

As we have noted throughout, mantis shrimp eyes are very complex organs. Many unique features add to this complexity, including triply overlapping optical sampling within much of the visual field, tiered rhabdoms of many types containing an unequaled diversity of visual pigments, and multiple levels of filtering (by the cornea, the tiered receptors, and the intrarhabdomal filters). The product of all of this evolutionary bioengineering is a retina that sends multiple, parallel streams of sensory data incorporating information about space, motion, spectrum, and polarization. Spectral information is sorted into at least twelve channels (e.g., figures 8.10 and 8.12), with polarization allotted a similar number (figure 8.8) (see also Marshall et al., 1991a).

One's initial impression is of a hopelessly complex jumble of data streams leaving the retina. However, this is probably misleading. The ability of the retina to do so much information sorting at the first step of vision eliminates much of the need for subsequent disentanglement of information. Whether the eye acts like a visual ear or like a series of chromatic and polarizational opponent processing systems, the processing and interpretation of sensory information that is normally relegated to higher visual centers is apparently handled automatically by the mantis shrimp's photoreceptors or by second-stage processing at the level of their target interneurons. Hence, we may view the anatomical complexity of this shrimp's eyes as an elegant precursor to an analytical simplicity that reduces the function of the brain to simply initiating the appropriate response to the presorted sensory information with which it is provided. In the end, a relatively simple nervous system (compared with that of vertebrates, at least) is perhaps given great analytical flexibility in that it need deal only with incoming data that have already been sorted, preprocessed, and encoded.

The Octopus's Garden: The Visual World of Cephalopods

Ian G. Gleadall and Nadav Shashar

To construct a picture of the world of an octopus, it is important first to appreciate what an octopus is, the kinds of senses that it has, and the kind of life that it leads.

Octopuses (figure 9.1a; plate 17) belong to the class of mollusks called Cephalopoda, which includes squids, cuttlefishes, and nautiluses (Norman, 2000; Nixon and Young, 2003). For most people, the term *mollusk* brings to mind herbivorous garden snails and filter-feeding shellfish. The typical modern cephalopod, however, is a relatively large, highly mobile predator, equipped with a sophisticated brain that coordinates complex behavior patterns for pursuing and capturing prey, escaping from predators, and mating. Unlike most of their more familiar relatives, modern cephalopods (except the nautiluses) have rid themselves of or greatly modified their ancestral molluscan shell. On the one hand, this allows them to move quickly and freely, but on the other hand they no longer enjoy the protection that a hard shell provides. Hence their final defense is to attempt an escape after producing a cloud of ink that may be either a discrete "decoy cloud" (a pseudomorph about the same size as their own body), or a larger "smoke screen" (Hanlon and Messenger, 1996).

Modern cephalopods (figure 9.1a–c) have also modified the ancestral molluscan foot into a number of dexterous arms with numerous suckers (figures 9.1a,e and 9.2) (Schmidtberg, 1999) to capture and hold prey. They have also acquired the ability to swim rapidly by a form of jet propulsion in which water is ejected from the mantle cavity (a large pocket covering the abdomen and enclosing the gills) through a muscular funnel (Trueman, 1980; Otis and Gilly, 1990). Octopuses generally have relatively large arms, which they use to walk over the seabed, and rarely use their jet propulsion system. In contrast, squid and cuttlefish generally have much shorter arms that are never used for walking. They have a much more streamlined body and have fins for sustained swimming at lower speeds. Their jet propulsion system is more highly developed, enabling some species to leave the water and glide some 40 to 50 m through the air (Young, 1971; M. J. Wells and O'Dor, 1991; Hanlon and Messenger, 1996; Nixon and Young, 2003).

It is surprising, for such sophisticated animals, that most species mature, mate, and die within 1 or 2 years. So the life of cephalopods is very much a race against time, during which they are balanced on a knife edge between their need to capture enough prey to fuel the high energy demands of rapid growth and development and their need to avoid being captured themselves.

Apart from large mammals such as whales, dolphins, and seals, the main predators of cephalopods are fish. In fact, fishes and modern cephalopods have been competing for a range of similar ecological niches for about 200 million years (Packard,

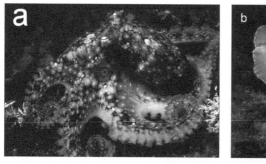
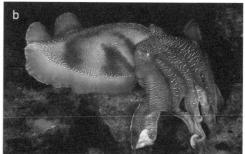
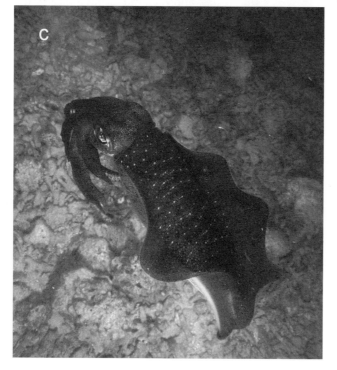

Figure 9.1
Representatives of modern cephalopods to illustrate some of the main features of these animals. (*a*) *Octopus bimaculatus*, viewed from the left side, with skin color and pattern providing good camouflage against a rocky seabed. The blue and red "bulls-eye" near the center of the picture is an ocellus ("false eye-spot"); the animal's left eye is above this ocellus. Note the lightly coiled arms with many pale-colored suckers. (*b*) A giant cuttlefish (*Sepia apama*, which reaches a body length close to 1 m when fully grown) seen from the right side, hovering just above the seabed. Note the undulating fins (not present in octopuses) and the dark blotches on its back, which are waves of expanding chromatophores moving like the shadows of passing clouds over the otherwise pale body. Note also the arm extending toward the bottom of the picture. Its flattened appearance and different coloring from the other arms are part of a courtship display. (*c*) The loliginid squid *Sepioteuthis lessoniana*. Note its more slender, tubular shape compared with the cuttlefish, the relatively small and slender arms, and the metallic greens and reds of iridescent coloration, particularly on the head.

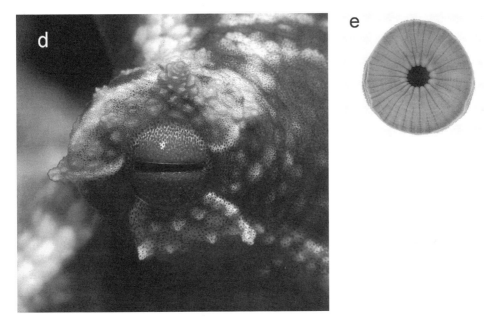

Figure 9.1 (continued)
(*d*) Closeup of an octopus's eye with its rectangular, slit-shaped pupil. (*e*) A sucker, 3 cm in diameter, from the arm of *Octopus conspadiceus*. (Photos *a–d* reprinted with permission from M. Norman, *Cephalopods, A World Guide*: *a*, courtesy of Roger Hanlon, and Conchbooks, Germany; *b–d*, Courtesy of Mark Norman, Aquanautica.) (See plate 17 for color version.)

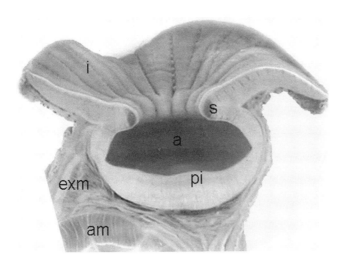

Figure 9.2
Section through the sucker shown in figure 9.1*e*. This shows the basic structure of the funnel-like disk, the infundibulum (i), atop a cup-shaped cavity, the acetabulum (a), and a portion of the arm's sophisticated musculature (am). exm, extrinsic muscle; pi, piston; s, sphincter muscle.

1972; Aronson, 1991), and they show many similarities in the ways that they have evolved (Packard, 1969a, 1972; Aronson, 1991; Budelmann, 1994, 1996). The next sections explain the neurophysiological apparatus that equips cephalopods to compete against rivals such as the fishes. We then discuss how cephalopods use this apparatus to see their world.

Information Input: The Senses

Octopuses and their relatives have the well-developed set of sensory organs that one would expect of such vulnerable, tasty, soft-bodied animals. Of these, vision seems to be the most important both for octopuses, which are typically loners, and squids, which usually swim in schools and interact socially. They also have sophisticated mechanoreceptors used in balance and vibration detection. Chemoreception is also important to cephalopods. In fact, octopuses have a special area of the brain not present in squid or cuttlefish (the subfrontal and inferior frontal lobes) that is involved with the chemotactile memory system (M. J. Wells et al., 1965; M. J. Wells, 1978; J. Z. Young, 1989b, 1995; Hanlon and Messenger, 1996).

The Chemical Senses

In the octopus, the distinction between taste and olfaction is difficult to make, particularly since the functions of its olfactory organ are obscure. Gustation (taste) is a direct contact sense for checking the quality of food about to be eaten (B. Lindemann, 2001), so the stimulant is present in high concentrations and typically involves high threshold responses (probably in the micromolar range; see Bardach and Villars, 1974). In contrast, olfaction (smell) is a distance sense typically involving low-threshold responses to perhaps only a few molecules of stimulant.

Gustation In a highly alert octopus, the suckers are moving constantly, touching and tasting whatever they contact. They are tough enough, though, to bear the octopus's weight when it is on the seabed (figure 9.1a), and each has a coating of cuticle that is shed and regularly replaced. The suckers are also able to adhere to objects by muscular vacuum-generated suction and, when coordinated with the arm musculature, can create forces strong enough to subdue a large, sharp-pincered crab or to force open tightly closed clam shells.

Octopuses have some 10,000 chemoreceptors per sucker arranged in budlike groups of 8–10 (Graziadei and Gagne, 1976a), compared with only about 300 per sucker in cuttlefish and squid (Budelmann et al., 1997). There are also taste receptors in the "lips" that enclose the mouth parts at the center of the arms (Graziadei, 1964). The physiology of these taste receptors has yet to be investigated.

Olfaction The octopus olfactory organ is a small, inconspicuous pouch located behind each eye, just inside the edge of the mantle where it is attached to the head. In squids, the edge of the mantle is free and the olfactory organ is located on the skin just behind each eye. The olfactory nerves project to areas of the brain involved with controlling gonadotropin release (M. J. Wells and Wells, 1959; Messenger, 1971; J. Z. Young, 1971; M. J. Wells, 1978). In squids there is also a projection to the lower motor areas of the brain that mediate fast escape responses (Messenger, 1979a).

The respiratory movements of the octopus's mantle open and close the olfactory organ cyclically (I. G. Gleadall, unpublished results). Such pulsate exposure of the olfactory organ probably minimizes the effects of habituation and is ideal for monitoring the quality of water entering the mantle cavity (Atema, 1985). In squids, a classical jetting escape response can be elicited if a dilute solution of their own ink is introduced into the water flowing over the organ. Electrophysiological patch studies of individual olfactory receptor cells confirm that the effective stimuli include levo-3,4-dihydroxyphenylalanine (L-DOPA, a precursor of an alarm substance in the ink) and various potassium channel blockers which, when placed near the olfactory organ, can also elicit an escape response (Lucero et al., 1992, 1994; Lucero and Gilly, 1995). Experiments with cuttlefish have demonstrated that a variety of stimuli elicit increases in breathing movements of the mantle, including water previously containing sea turtles (predators), food, or another cuttlefish (Boal and Golden, 1999).

Woodhams and Messenger (1974) have suggested that the olfactory organ also detects prospective pheromones, and Messenger (1979a) has suggested its involvement in synchronizing sexual maturation or spawning. Pheromone detection in mammals is mostly the domain of the vomeronasal organ, the receptor organ of the accessory olfactory system. Whether the cephalopod olfactory organ has distinct primary olfactory and secondary pheromone-detecting functions remains to be determined.

Mechanoreception

Touch and Proprioception   The suckers are the main organs of touch and they contain a number of cells that have the morphological characteristics of mechanoreceptors (Graziadei and Gagne, 1976b). The muscles of the arms and mantle contain a large number of presumptive proprioceptors (Boyle, 1977). In addition, squids have large epidermal hair cells on their neck that form a proprioceptive neck receptor to provide information on head position (Preuss and Budelmann, 1995b).

The Lateral Line System   Lines of epidermal hair cells on the head and arms of octopod hatchlings, cuttlefish, and squid are analogues of the fish lateral line system and are able to detect water movements as small as 0.06 μm (Budelmann and Bleckmann, 1988; Budelmann et al., 1991). Experiments in complete darkness have shown that this system enables cuttlefish to catch small shrimps (Budelmann et al., 1991) and that squids, like fish, use both vision and lateral line reception in their schooling behavior (Lima et al., 1995).

The Statocysts   The statocysts, a pair of spherical sacs embedded in the cartilage of the head just beneath the central brain, are sophisticated organs of balance (figure 9.3)

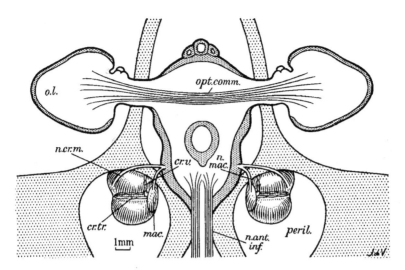

Figure 9.3
Diagram of a transverse section through the cranial region of *Octopus vulgaris* to illustrate the statocysts in relation to the central nervous system (eyes and optic nerves omitted). The paired statocysts are each suspended in a perilymph-filled cavity in the cranial cartilage (dotted region) close to the subesophageal lobes of the central brain (the esophagus is the central round profile). Note the optic commissure passing through the supraesophageal part of the central brain, connecting the optic lobes. cr.tr., transverse crista of statocyst; cr.v., vertical crista; mac., macula; n.cr.m., median crista nerve; n.ant.inf., inferior antorbital nerve; n.mac., macula nerve; opt. comm., optic commissure; o.l., optic lobe; peril., perilymph. (Reprinted with permission from figure 1 in J. Z. Young, The statocysts of *Octopus vulgaris. Proceedings of the Royal Society, London* 152: 3–29, 1960, Royal Society of London.)

(J. Z. Young, 1960a, 1989b). They are important for correct posture during swimming and walking and include structural and functional analogues of the semicircular canals of the vertebrate inner ear (Williamson, 1995a,b). As in the vertebrate system, cephalopod statocysts are intimately involved in the control of eye muscles (Williamson and Budelmann, 1991; Budelmann and Young, 1993). They also maintain countershading, keeping the most dorsal surface darkly colored and the most ventral surface pale, even if the animal is held in an unnatural position (Ferguson et al., 1994; Preuss and Budelmann, 1995a).

In octopuses, there are two types of statocyst receptor cell, each with a different level of sensitivity (Williamson and Budelmann, 1985; J. Z. Young, 1989a,b; Budelmann and Williamson, 1994), apparently to provide information for balance during walking and jet-propelled swimming.

The mechanoreceptors in the statocysts, the neck proprioceptor system, and the lateral line system have been examined in detail, but little is known about the touch

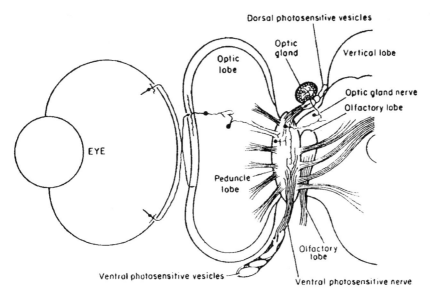

Figure 9.4
Diagram showing the well-developed photosensitive vesicles of the squid, *Todarodes pacificus*, and their connections with the central nervous system. (Reprinted from F. Baumann, A. Mauro, R. Milecchia, S. Nightingale, and J. Z. Young, The extra-ocular light receptors of the squids *Todarodes* and *Illex*. *Brain Research* 21: 275–279, Copyright 1970, with permission from Elsevier.)

and muscle proprioceptors (Budelmann and Young, 1984; Budelmann et al., 1987, 1997; cf. Gillespie and Walker, 2001).

Extraocular Photoreception
Most cephalopods have extra-ocular photoreceptors, or photosensitive vesicles (figure 9.4), which, in octopuses, are typically small organs on the stellate ganglion (Baumann et al., 1970; Messenger, 1991; Cobb et al., 1995b). In squids, they are intimately associated with the optic lobes and their afferents innervate the peduncle lobe of the optic tract (Baumann et al., 1970), although their exact function is unknown. In enoploteuthid squids (which live in the twilight mesopelagic zone of the ocean depths) the photosensitive vesicles are greatly enlarged and there is strong evidence that they are used to measure the intensity of down-welling light (R. E. Young, 1972; Seidou et al., 1990). Hence they may also be involved in circadian and/or circalunar rhythms and migratory behavior (cf. Baumann et al., 1970; Cobb et al., 1995a).

Vision
Image-forming vision is undoubtedly the most important of the cephalopod senses. In some sepiolids (bobtail squids) the eyes, together, can account for half of the

brightness

size

orientation

form

plane of polarization

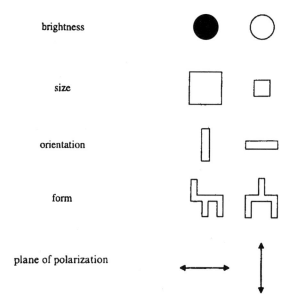

Figure 9.5
Diagram summarizing and illustrating the five classes of information that octopuses can extract from their visual world. (Reprinted from J. B. Messenger, The eyes and skin of Octopus. *Endeavour* 3: 92–98. Copyright 1979, with permission from Elsevier.)

animal's weight, and in some squids the volume of the optic lobes can be more than four times that of the rest of the brain (Messenger, 1981). Learning and memory experiments have revealed that octopuses can make fine discriminations between pairs of objects differing in brightness, size, orientation, form, or plane of polarization (figure 9.5) (Messenger, 1991).

General Morphology of the Eye Superficially, cephalopod eyes are astoundingly similar to those of marine vertebrates (Pumphrey, 1961; Levine, 1980; Messenger, 1981; for detailed reviews, see Messenger, 1981, 1991; Budelmann et al., 1997). They are fluid filled, with well-defined retina, lens, and pupil. Their transparent lens crystallins are derived by recruiting detoxification stress proteins such as glutathione S-transferase (Tomarev et al., 1991). In cephalopods, the lens is suspended by ciliary muscles and interrupted by a connective that partitions the eye into anterior and posterior chambers. There is almost no spherical aberration in the lens, and its very short focal length conforms to the Matthiessen ratio of 2.5 times the lens radius, as it does in fishes. This allows a depth of focus from a few centimeters to infinity (Pumphrey, 1961; Muntz, 1977a; Sivak, 1991; Sivak et al., 1994).

Visual stimuli can be resolved at up to 100 Hz at high stimulus intensities, which is comparable to the retina of diurnal vertebrates (Hamasaki, 1968a), and the rate of dark adaptation is about the same as that of the nocturnal owl monkey (Hamasaki, 1968a). The rod-only eye of the cartilaginous (sharklike) fish provides the closest parallel to the cephalopod eye (Packard, 1972).

The octopus pupil (figure 9.1d) is a horizontal rectangular aperture in low light, and contracts to a horizontal slit in response to bright light (Muntz, 1977a). The movements of the pupil appear to be correlated with the degree of adaptation of the retina. In dim light, after exposure to a bright flash of light, the pupil first expands and then contracts as the retina regains its sensitivity and the screening pigment is retracted to expose more photoreceptive membrane (Muntz, 1977a; Gleadall et al., 1993).

The photoreceptor outer segments are typically much longer in cephalopod than in vertebrate eyes: some 200–400 μm in octopuses, and as long as 600 μm in the firefly squid. Combined with a high density of visual pigment, which produces a surprisingly broad spectral sensitivity (Hamasaki, 1968b), the cephalopod retina is a superb photon-capturing apparatus. This is particularly the case in the firefly squid.

Photoreceptors

The basic component of the cephalopod retina is a long, slim, rod-shaped photoreceptor cell (figure 9.6a). The visual pigment is contained in the folded cell membrane, which forms an orderly array of fingerlike processes called microvilli (Moody and Parriss, 1961; Tonosaki, 1965; T. Yamamoto et al., 1965, 1976; Goldsmith, 1991). Tight packing of the microvilli gives them each a hexagonal profile *in vivo* (Hamanaka et al., 1994). The microvilli all lie in the retina's tangential plane, protruding laterally as two blocks (called rhabdomeres) on opposite sides of the outer segment of the cell, so that all the microvilli of a given cell are aligned in one direction only (Moody and Parriss, 1961; Tonosaki, 1965; T. Yamamoto et al., 1965, 1976). The alignment of molecules of visual pigment within the microvillar membrane is such that the photoreceptor cell absorbs light most efficiently in one orientation of polarization (figure 9.6b) (J. Z. Young, 1971; Goldsmith, 1991).

Afferent information from the photoreceptors travels via axons (approximately 1 μm in diameter) through the optic nerves to the adjacent optic lobe (Tonosaki, 1965), where they form acetylcholinergic synapses (Lam et al., 1974; K. Tasaki et al., 1982; Silver et al., 1983). Within the retina, collaterals (approximately 0.1 μm in diameter) arise from a specialized region at the base of the photoreceptor cell body and ramify in the tangential plane of the eye, in the plexiform layer (Tonosaki, 1965; T. Yamamoto et al., 1965, 1976; J. Z. Young, 1971; A. I. Cohen, 1973). These collaterals communicate with the collaterals and cell bodies of other photoreceptor cells via structures characteristic of electrotonic junctions (M. Yamamoto, 1984; M. Yamamoto and Takasu, 1984), and are thought to be involved in lateral inhibition. Similar (but much longer) junctions have also been reported to occur between the photoreceptors themselves, along the portion of the outer segment beneath the rhabdomeres, distal to the basement lamina (Norton et al., 1965; Cohen, 1973), and are presumed to be responsible for opponent interactions that enhance the retina's polarization sensitivity.

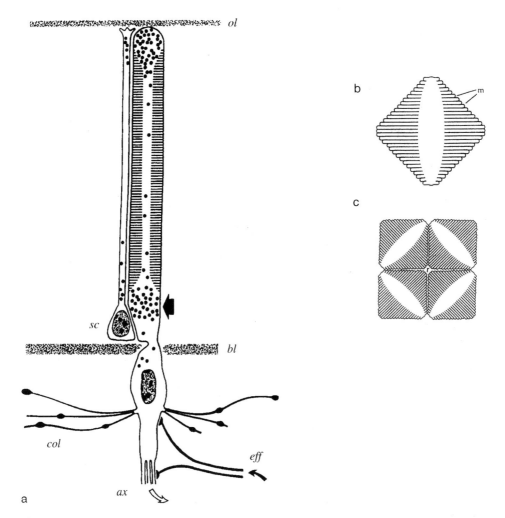

Figure 9.6

(*a*) Diagram of the main components of the octopus retina (the distal surface of the retina is at the top of the diagram). The photoreceptive pigment (rhodopsin) is located in tightly packed microvilli lying perpendicular to the main axis of the cell in two blocks or rhabdomeres. The collaterals (col) are very fine processes arising near the base of the photoreceptor cell body. The varicosities on the collaterals represent synapses onto other photoreceptor cells. Axonlike processes (ax) project to the optic lobes (open curved arrow). The black dots represent screening-pigment granules (the proximal aggregation of screening pigment just distal to the basement lamina does not migrate; black arrowhead). bl, basement lamina; ol, outer lamina (in contact with the cameral liquid); eff, efferent nerves from the optic lobe arriving (filled curved arrow) to synapse with the photoreceptor cell; sc, supporting (glial) cell. (*b*) Diagram of a photoreceptor cell in tangential section showing its two rhabdomeres and the unidirectional arrangement of their microvilli (m). (*c*) Diagram of a tangential section through a single rhabdom showing the arrangement of microvilli along the two orthogonal planes corresponding to the vertical and horizontal directions in the visual field. The space at the center of the rhabdom (r) contains the slender process of a supporting cell (omitted from this diagram). (Drawing *a* reprinted with permission from Gleadall et al., 1993; *b* and *c* reprinted from Gleadall, 1994.)

The photoreceptors show rapid mechanical contraction in response to light (J. Z. Young, 1963; I. Tasaki and Nakaye, 1984), a phenomenon also seen in vertebrates (Besharse and Iuvone, 1992). Screening pigment is present within each photoreceptor as immobile granules at the base of the outer segment (figure 9.6a). These probably block stray light that enters the retina from behind the eye. Mobile pigment granules migrate within the main axis of the cell as part of the light adaptation process (Gleadall et al., 1993).

Retina Morphology

The octopus retina is composed almost entirely of a tightly packed matrix of photoreceptors, with the microvilli held in a tightly organized lattice by a network of protein filaments (Saibil and Hewat, 1987). There are no interneurons in the retina. Glia is the only other cell type. The photoreceptors are arranged with each cell's microvilli aligned along one of two orthogonal planes, with a rhabdomere from one side of each of four adjacent cells forming a rectangular structure called a fused rhabdom (figure 9.6c) (A. W. Snyder et al., 1973). The spacing between rhabdoms is about 7 μm in *Octopus vulgaris* and remains constant during growth. Hence the number of rhabdoms increases as the eye grows, from approximately 10,000 in young animals weighing about 0.4 g, to 870,000 in animals weighing 20 g, and approximately 5 million (i.e., 20 million cells) in an octopus weighing 1 kg (Packard and Sanders, 1969; Packard, 1969b; J. Z. Young, 1971).

Polarization Sensitivity

Polarization sensitivity is the capacity to respond differentially either to *e*-vector orientation or to the degree of polarization of a light stimulus. Partial linear polarization is a prominent attribute of scattered, refracted, and reflected light in nature (Waterman, 1984). The light-guiding properties of the fused rhabdom (A. W. Snyder, 1973; A. W. Snyder et al., 1973) ensure that the absorption of photons travelling down it proceeds efficiently. As light moves down the rhabdom, each of the cells contributing to it most efficiently absorbs photons with the *e*-vector parallel to the orientation of its rhodopsin molecules. However, since the cephalopod photoreceptor cell is so long, polarization sensitivity might be thought to be poor in dim light, because all of the relatively few available photons (whatever their *e*-vectors) could be absorbed by a given cell as they pass through the massive stack of microvilli (see Stowe, 1983). In practice, though, polarization sensitivity is very high in the octopus retina, even in dim light, because of the opponent interactions between cells with peak sensitivities to different *e*-vectors (see later discussion).

Information Processing: The Octopus Nervous System

Arms on Auto

In addition to an impressive inventory of sense organs, and in order to analyze the information coming from them, cephalopods have a sophisticated nervous system

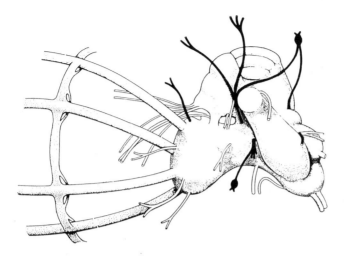

Figure 9.7
Diagram of the octopus central brain, from the left side. Note four of the eight large arm nerves on the left (anterior), joined by an interbrachial connective that helps in the coordination of arm movements. The oculomotor and ophthalmic nerves (which coordinate eye movements) are in black. The central circular profile represents the optic tract, lying just superior to the obliquely oriented magnocellular lobe (which coordinates the "escape response"). (Reprinted in modified form from J. Z. Young, 1971 by permission of Oxford University Press.)

(figures 9.7 and 9.8). In octopuses in particular, much of the nerve tissue is in the arms because each of the hundreds of suckers along the arms is controlled by its own ganglion (a cluster of functionally related nerve cells). In *Octopus vulgaris* there are an estimated 350 million neurons in the arms, compared with 92 million in the optic lobes and 42 million in the central brain (J. Z. Young, 1988).

Each sucker ganglion controls the local reflexes, receiving thousands of inputs from the touch and taste organs in the corresponding sucker, and sending motor neuron efferents to the muscles controlling the sucker's movements. This explains the oft-observed phenomenon in which octopus arms can move and react to touch and taste stimuli for several hours after amputation. Each sucker ganglion also communicates directly with the ganglia of other nearby suckers, and with the brain, by way of the large arm nerves (Graziadei, 1962, 1971).

However, the arm and sucker functions are thought to be largely autonomous. The octopus's central nervous system probably suppresses the large amount of sensory information available from the arms (Hanlon and Messenger, 1996), except when the octopus focuses its attention on any increased activity in the sucker afferents when an arm contacts a biologically important stimulus.

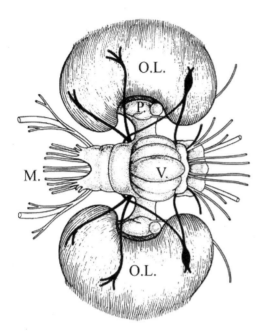

Figure 9.8
Diagram of the central nervous system as seen from above, showing the relatively large size of the optic lobes (O.L.). The vertical lobe (V.) is an important memory center (see figure 9.9) containing five gyri occupying the top and sides of the supraesophageal part of the central brain. M. indicates a set of nerves involved mostly with the mouth parts (the two larger diameter nerves are two of the eight arm nerves; see figure 9.7). (Reprinted in modified form from J. Z. Young, 1971 by permission of Oxford University Press.)

Memory Lanes

The memory system of the octopus's brain is partitioned into different regions concerned with vision and tactile input, although there is some overlap between regions. The vertical lobe appears to be the most essential part of the brain for visual learning and memory, and the median inferior frontal lobe for tactile learning and memory (figure 9.9) (Bradley and Young, 1975; J. Z. Young, 1991).

The Visuomotor System

The visuomotor system includes the optic lobes, central brain, and motor nerves involved in behaviors in which vision plays a central role (feeding, walking, and swimming; figures 9.7 and 9.8).

The retina projects retinotopically to the optic lobe. Within the optic lobes, there are layers of cells with their dendritic fields oriented either vertically or horizontally (J. Z. Young, 1960b). This suggests that the octopus visual system has feature-selective

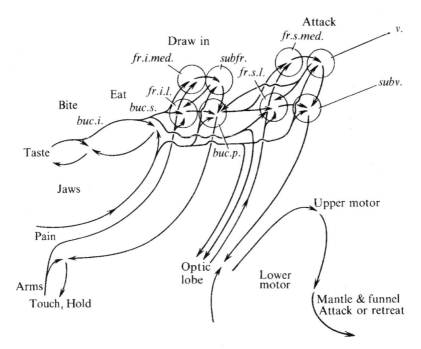

Figure 9.9
Diagram summarizing the visual and chemotactile memory systems of the octopus brain. Although not entirely independent, each system basically consists of four lobes within the supraesophageal central brain. The lateral and median inferior frontal, posterior buccal, and subfrontal lobes form the chemotactile system; and the visual system consists of (together with the optic lobes) the lateral and median superior frontal, subvertical, and vertical lobes. buc., buccal; i, inferior; l., lateral; med., median; p., posterior; s, superior; subfr., subfrontal; subv., subvertical; v., vertical. (Reprinted from J. Z. Young, 1971 by permission of Oxford University Press.)

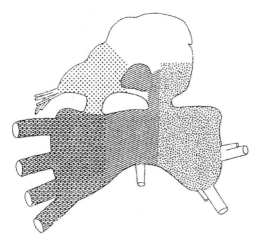

Figure 9.10
Diagrammatic sagittal section illustrating the distribution of brain regions governing the movements of the limbs of an octopus: armlike, manipulative (dots); and leglike, ambulatory (diagonal hatch). The overlap of shading in the anterior subesophageal brain (to the left) indicates regions using common pathways for both manipulative and ambulatory functions. The posterior (flecked) region is concerned mostly with swimming and breathing movements; the unshaded part of the supraesophageal brain governs visual learning and memory.

cells similar in function to those in mammals (J. Z. Young, 1973). The orderly organization of dendritic fields also fulfills the criterion for the orderly representation of the visual world that allows enhanced detection of an object's contours via contrast mechanisms such as polarization vision.

The octopus uses its eight limbs as legs for walking and as arms for capturing and manipulating prey. Hence the brain includes motor centers devoted to these tasks separately and together (figure 9.10). In addition to the basic eight, squid and cuttlefish have two very long tentacles that are shot forward to capture prey. Hence they need coordinated binocular vision, whereas octopuses usually watch their prey with only one eye (Budelmann and Young, 1984).

Complex Behavior
A wide variety of behaviors have been recorded in cephalopods (Hanlon and Messenger, 1996). Courtship and mating, for example, can be complex and elaborate, especially in shoaling and schooling species of squid and cuttlefish (figure 9.1b). Sophisticated reproductive behavior has been documented in several species, including elaborate courtships and sneak matings by smaller males. This behavior involves an elaborate repertoire of body postures and changes in skin texture, color, and polarization motifs (Sauer et al., 1997; Hanlon et al., 1999b).

The Skin: Control of Color and Texture

One of the most outstanding features of octopuses is their remarkable repertoire of body colors (figure 9.1a). What makes them so attractive and interesting is that the colors are not static or uniform, but change dynamically from moment to moment, as does the posture and skin texture in an active animal (Hanlon et al., 1999a,b). The skin contains a complex battery of elements that contribute various effects to its colors and polarization patterns. The major elements are the chromatophores, which are bags of melanin-based yellow, orange, red, or black pigment, depending on their age (Packard, 1995; Messenger, 2001). The chromatophores are under direct nervous control via an assortment of neurotransmitters acting on muscles that expand the bags to darken the skin (Loi et al., 1996). When relaxed, the bags shrink to reveal lighter, reflective layers of iridophores and white leucophores deeper in the skin. Because the chromatophore muscles are directly innervated by the central nervous system, cephalopods can change color very rapidly, and by looking at the skin, one gets the impression that one can see what an octopus is "thinking," so to speak (Packard and Hochberg, 1977).

Iridescent spectral reflections from iridophores give to the octopus's appearance a series of metallic colors ranging from blue to pink (figure 9.1c). Such colors are common in shallow-water squid and cuttlefish (Mathger and Denton, 2001), and in spot or stripe markings in shallow-water octopuses (figure 9.1a) (Roper and Hochberg, 1988). Polarization patterns also are created mostly by light reflected from stacks of platelets within the iridophores (Denton and Land, 1971; Mathger and Denton, 2001). The arms of many shallow-water squids have a special population of innervated iridophores in which rapid changes in platelet position produce dynamic changes in patterns of partially linearly polarized light (implicated in communication; see later discussion).

Cephalopods are masters at cryptically matching their body appearance to the background against which they might be seen. This matching involves body posture, texture, and coloration, and complex body patterns (Hanlon and Messenger, 1996); it requires not only sensing the external environment but also being aware of one's body size and the patterns being generated (Hanlon and Messenger, 1988). One species of octopus can even mimic the shape and movements of other animals (Norman, 2000; Norman et al., 2001). In deciding which patterns to produce, it has been shown for cuttlefish that the relative sizes of bright objects (such as pebbles and stones) and the proportion of the background occupied by these objects somehow are assessed in selecting between a disruptive or uniform body pattern (Hanlon and Messenger, 1988; Chiao and Hanlon, 2001).

What Cephalopods See: The General Picture

To live a long and successful life, it is critical that an octopus be able to visually identify a nearby animal as potential mate, prey item, or predator. Hence the visual system must have the means to clearly distinguish an object from background luminance, despite low light intensities and/or contrast-reducing murky water. In this regard, cephalopods apparently use their polarization sensitivity to enhance the contrast of an object.

The Colorblind Octopus in a World of Color

Amazingly, octopuses are blind to the beauty of their own colors. Except for the firefly squid (see later disscussion), cephalopods possess only one visual pigment based on the chromophore retinal (Muntz and Johnson, 1978; Seidou et al., 1990). The spectral sensitivity of the electroretinogram (ERG) mirrors that of the visual pigment and is not altered by adapting the retina to different-colored lights (Hamdorf et al., 1968; Hamasaki, 1968b). Also, there are no known filtering structures that might alter the spectral sensitivity of any of the photoreceptor cells, for example, as do the oil droplets in some turtle and bird cone cells (Bennett and Cuthill, 1994; Okano et al., 1995), the carotenoid-based filters of some stomatopods (Marshall et al., 1991b), or the screening pigments in certain grasshoppers (Kong et al., 1980).

Associative learning experiments have shown that hues matched for brightness cannot be discriminated by *Octopus vulgaris* (Messenger et al., 1973; Messenger, 1977), *Enteroctopus dofleini* ("*Octopus apollyon*"; Roffe, 1975), or by the squid *Todarodes pacificus* (Flores, 1983). Also, octopuses and cuttlefishes will display appropriate disruptive skin patterns when they are on a seabed of stones of mixed brightness, but the patterns do not appear if the stones reflect similar degrees of brightness, even if they differ markedly in color (e.g., green versus yellow; Marshall and Messenger, 1996; Messenger, 1997).

So, to hide from a predator with color vision by matching the background as closely as possible, the octopus has to rely solely on its ability to match the brightness of light reflected from the substrate with that reflected from its own body. The mechanism of brightness matching appears to depend upon the ratio of light received by the ventral retina (from down-welling surface light) to that received by the dorsal retina (reflected from the surface of the substrate; Packard, 1995). It is intriguing that the octopus's skin color system produces astonishingly close cryptic matches to the substrate (Hanlon et al., 1999a) despite the absence of pigments that can directly produce shades of green, cyan, blue, or violet (Hanlon and Messenger, 1996).

In darker conditions, the chromatophores are expanded by contraction of the chromatophore muscles, producing body coloration in shades of red and brown. At higher light intensities where color discrimination by predatory fish is at its most effective, the chromatophores are relaxed, contracting to pinpoints and revealing leucophores deeper in the skin. The leucophores reflect light at a brightness similar to that reaching the octopus from the nearby substrate, and with similar wavelengths. This provides sufficient color matching to hide the octopus effectively from predators with color vision (Messenger, 1974, 2001).

Polarization Sensitivity and Its Uses

Stimulating an isolated octopus or squid retina with a source of polarized light produces an ERG response of uniform magnitude, regardless of the angle of polarization with respect to the retina (K. Tasaki and Karita, 1966a,b). A similar result is obtained after preadapting the retina with light polarized at 45 or 135 deg to the horizontal and vertical axes of the retina. However, adapting the retina with light polarized in either the vertical or horizontal orientation results in a sinusoidal response to stimuli of uniform intensity as the polarizer is rotated stepwise through 360 deg (figure 9.11). The peaks coincide with the orientation orthogonal to the adapting angle of polarization (Tasaki and Karita, 1966a,b; Messenger, 1981).

These data indicate the existence of two physiological channels of polarization detection in the cephalopod retina. The requirement for different levels of adaptation in these channels, in order to obtain angle-sensitive ERG responses from the whole

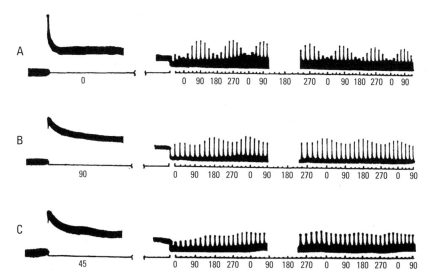

Figure 9.11

Diagram illustrating the effects on the octopus electroretinogram (ERG) of selective adaptation with polarized light. The isolated retina was adapted for about 2 min with bright light passing through a polarizer oriented at 0, 45, or 90 deg to the horizontal plane of the retina (recordings A, B, and C, respectively). The retina was then left in darkness except for regular short test flashes of uniform intensity and duration, between which the polarizer was rotated through steps of 22.5 deg. The left trace with large deflection and slow decay shows the effects of light adaptation on the retina. The traces in the center and at the right are from experiments with the retinas of two different octopuses. (*A*) The largest ERG response following adaptation to light polarized at 0 deg occurs when the polarizer is at 90 or 270 deg. (*B*) Following adaptation at 90 deg, the largest responses are at 0 and 180 deg. (*C*) The effects of adaptation at 45 deg are negligible. (Reprinted with permission from K. Tasaki and Karita, 1966b.)

isolated retina, suggests that the intact system, under normal environmental conditions, responds best to the differences in the polarization characteristics of light entering the eye (discussed further later).

Intracellular recordings from single photoreceptor cells show that each cell has its own characteristic sinusoidal response to changes in the angle of polarization (e-vector), which is obtained without any preadaptation (Sugawara et al., 1971; Tsukahara and Tasaki, 1972). These studies have detected approximately equal numbers of cells with a polarization sensitivity maximum for light polarized in the horizontal or the vertical orientation (with respect to the orientation of the retina in the intact animal). Recordings from the optic nerves have shown that differential activity of cells that is due to the angle of polarization is conveyed to the brain in the form of a spike activity code (figure 9.12) (Saidel et al., 1983).

The fact that octopuses are color blind yet have a retina highly sensitive to the e-vector of light strongly suggests that polarization detection plays an important role in their life. Animals with polarization sensitivity can put it to use in one or more of several ways (see Leggett, 1976). It can be used for navigation in the absence of the sun by using the polarization pattern of scattered UV light in the sky (Wehner, 1989b). It can be used as an underwater, artificial horizon by making use of the predominantly horizontally polarized light at the air/water interface (e.g., Schwind, 1991; Horváth and Varjú, 1997). It can also be used to detect reflective surfaces (Kriska et al., 1998)

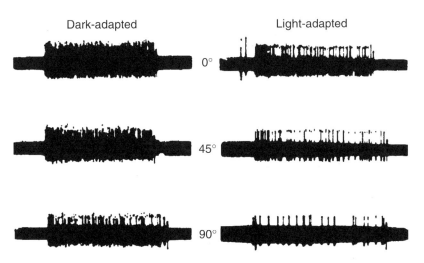

Figure 9.12
Dark- (left) and light- (right) adapted responses (from an optic nerve bundle within a suction electrode) to light stimuli whose plane of polarization was set to the preferred plane (0 deg), orthogonal plane (90 deg), or midway between the two planes (45 deg). The stimulus durations were about 10 s. (Reprinted with permission from Saidel et al., 1983. Copyright 1983 the Nature Publishing Group.)

and to screen out the predominantly horizontally polarized glare reflected from water, which allows clear vision across the air/water interface. It can improve photon capture in dim light (A. W. Snyder et al., 1973) and enhance contrast discrimination (Saidel et al., 1983; Tsukahara, 1989). Finally, it can be used to obtain information on the structure or shape of a remote object (M. F. Land, 1993).

Of these various uses, it seems unnecessary for a benthic creature such as an octopus to detect the air/water interface, although captive cuttlefish can accurately attack prey held well above the water surface (Nesis, 1974), implying that in general, cephalopod eyes see clearly across the water/air interface. Polarization sensitivity might be used for navigation, since orientation to polarization patterns has been reported for loliginid and sepiolid squids (R. Jander et al., 1963). However, bilateral symmetry in patterns of polarized sky light can produce errors of ambiguity because alignment can be in one of two directions, at 180 deg to each other (e.g., Wehner, 1989b). In ants and bees, which are well known to orient to polarization patterns, there are mechanisms to obviate this 180-deg ambiguity (Wehner, 1989b), but no such mechanism has been demonstrated in cephalopods.

In crustaceans, behavioral studies have demonstrated orientation to polarized sky patterns and their use for local navigation. More recently it has been shown that polarized light can be detected as a special sensory quality, termed *polarization vision*, separate from intensity or color (Marshall et al., 1999). Polarization vision is used in communication and in enhancing visual contrast. Similar functions for polarization vision have recently been demonstrated for cephalopods. For example, young squids can use their sensitivity to polarized light to detect transparent objects and to improve the range of their detection (Shashar et al., 1995, 1998; cf. Lythgoe and Hemming, 1967).

Polarization Vision as an Analogue of Color Vision

Learning experiments have demonstrated not only a high degree of visual acuity (comparable to vertebrates) in the octopus (Muntz and Gwyther, 1988a), but also that cephalopods are sensitive to lights of different *e*-vector orientation and to lights filtered with different experimental *e*-vector contrast patterns (Moody and Parriss, 1961; Rowell and Wells, 1961; Moody, 1962; Shashar and Cronin, 1996). The finding that the octopus eye possesses polarization sensitivity based on two separable channels of orthogonal orientation suggests the presence of retinal properties potentially analogous to the color-opponent channels found in dichromatic color vision (see, for example, Hemmi, 1999).

When investigating color vision in animals, it is necessary to demonstrate that they possess photoreceptors with different spectral absorbance characteristics in the same part of the retina; that receptor outputs signal information about color, independent of intensity; and that brain areas are able to map color signals into a color-based representation of the visual world. Similar criteria should apply for demonstrating polarization vision, with "polarization" and "preferred *e*-vector angle" substituted for "color" and "spectral absorbance," respectively. However, as yet we do not know the exact form in which polarization contrast differences are represented in the octopus brain.

Pommes and Primate Color Vision: Finding Ripe Fruit

Objects are recognized, in great part, through their contrast with adjacent objects or the background. For vertebrates, including humans, there are (in simple terms) two ways in which this can be done: via luminance (brightness) contrast and via color contrast (but see Syrkin and Gur, 1997; Switkes and Crognale, 1999).

Color vision is based on the opponency between the information provided by two or more populations of cells with different wavelength sensitivities, and much of the opponency occurs in the early stages of retinal processing (e.g., Ventura et al., 2001). In mammals, color vision is thought to have arisen from a dichromatic system; that is, a system based on the opponency between two cell types, each containing a different visual pigment (G. H. Jacobs, 1993; Hemmi, 1999). In primates, red-green color discrimination probably arose to enable the detection of yellow and orange (i.e., ripe, edible) fruits against a background of green foliage (Regan, et al., 2001). Similarly, yellow-blue discrimination aids in assessing leaf quality (Dominy and Lucas, 2001).

Kippers and Polarization Vision: Finding the Fruits of the Sea

In the octopus's colorless world, a major function of the visual system is to detect fishes, crustaceans, and gastropod mollusks; in other words, the fruits of the sea. M. F. Land (1984) suggested that cephalopods might use polarization opponency to detect the light reflected from teleost fishes, which include both predators and prey. Teleosts have mirrorlike scales that provide brightness- and color-matched camouflage when viewed side-on because they reflect the same intensity and wavelength components found in the ambient light. However, the scales also polarize reflected light (Denton, 1970; Denton and Land, 1971; Shashar et al., 2000), as do the carapaces of crabs (Zeil and Hofman, 2001) and certain regions on the surface of stomatopods (Marshall et al., 1999), rendering them visible when they are otherwise camouflaged. Detecting these isoluminous, isochromatic reflections by differences in polarization may be comparable to detecting the differences in hue that characterize color vision, or it may be merely a method of increasing the contrast in the image.

Octopuses can be trained to discriminate between uniform polarization patterns (Moody and Parriss, 1960) or among mixed patterns in which, for instance, a central disk is vertically polarized and its surround is horizontally polarized, in contrast to a center and surround polarized at the same orientation (figure 9.13). The limit of these discriminations is when orientation differences lie between 10 and 20 deg (Shashar and Cronin, 1996). This finding is important behavioral evidence for recognition of an object based on polarization.

Other behavioral experiments demonstrate that squid hatchlings can detect transparent planktonic prey animals at a 70% greater distance in polarized than in unpolarized light (Shashar et al., 1998), providing further evidence that cephalopods

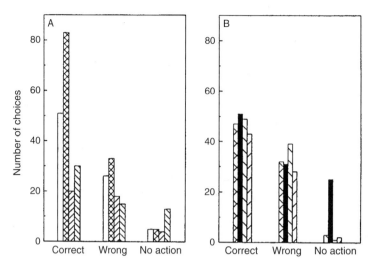

Figure 9.13
Target choices in associative learning experiments with octopuses to assess their ability to select targets containing (*A*) a 90-deg polarization contrast, or (*B*) no contrast, when presented simultaneously with both types of targets. The targets' left-right position, polarization horizontal-vertical orientation, and probes containing the polarization filters were randomized. Each of eight different animals is represented by a different bar pattern. The black bars were from a single *Octopus briareus*; all other individuals were *O. vulgaris*. In both groups of four animals, the octopuses learned to choose the correct target on the basis of the presence or absence of polarization contrast. (Reprinted with permission from Shashar and Cronin, 1996.)

can use their polarization sensitivity to enhance the contrast of objects. Also, an adult cuttlefish preferentially attacks fish when the light reflected from them contains a polarized component but not when the reflected light has been depolarized with a polarization-distorting filter (Shashar et al., 2000).

It is still unclear whether cephalopods can perceive the degree and orientation of the electric vector of light (rather as we see colors) or if polarization simply serves as a contrast enhancer in the intensity domain. The principle of contrast enhancement by polarization vision was first demonstrated by Lythgoe and Hemming (1967). They published two pictures of a row of three plates of different reflectance (black, gray, and white) taken underwater at the same level of illumination—one through a horizontal polarizer and the other through a vertical polarizer. The pictures revealed clearly different contrasts between the objects and the background. At one orientation, the white objects were seen most vividly and black was almost invisible, and vice versa at the other orientation. Clearly, if the information from these two orientations could be combined within the visual system (i.e., a form of polarization opponency), the result would be contrast enhancement that can modify the intensity (gray scale) image to reveal patterns that would be otherwise undetectable (Saidel et al., 1983; Rowe et al., 1995). Useful information can be obtained with only partial analysis and recognition of only polarization contrasts (Tyo et al., 1996). Alternatively, it is possible that polarization information is coded as an independent type of (qualitative) visual input that provides the ability to make discriminations analogous to distinguishing colors (Bernard and Wehner, 1977; Nilsson and Warrant, 1999).

Three Types of Processing within the Octopus Retina

Despite the relative organizational simplicity of the octopus retina, responses recorded in various experiments have revealed a surprising level of complexity, involving mechanisms of adaptation (e.g., Lange and Hartline, 1974; Gleadall et al., 1993) and processing interactions among the photoreceptors.

Processing within the retina can be reasonably assigned to three kinds of activity (Lange et al., 1976; Saidel et al., 1983). The first is opponency like activity, which consists of relatively localized physical interactions (current flow) between adjacent photoreceptor cells. The second is inhibitory interactions over a relatively large area in the plexiform layer, involving the photoreceptor collaterals. The third includes phenomena attributable to activity in efferent nerves arriving from the optic lobe. A similar separation of functions occurs in the vertebrate retina. For example, midget ganglion cells and their associated amacrine cells in the monkey retina are indiscriminate for color, subserving only fine spatial vision but not cone opponency (Calkins and Sterling, 1996).

Opponency

In figure 9.14a, the polarization sensitivity of the receptor potential of the impaled cell is 4.2 (0.26 on the logarithmic scale), but the polarization sensitivity of the axonal output, measured as spike number (figure 9.14b), has improved to 8.5 (0.71 on the logarithmic scale). So, between the arrival of light (indicated by the receptor potential) and transduction of the signal sent to the brain (encoded as an intensity-related train of spikes), something has occurred to improve the cell's polarization sensitivity. This suggests that polarization sensitivity is improved by the interaction between photoreceptor cells, probably as a result of current flow between the two sets of photoreceptors that have their microvilli arranged orthogonally (Tsukahara, 1989).

Shaw (1975) demonstrated that the local electrical properties between photoreceptors are such that the surrounding (nonstimulated) cells will tend to be inhibited electrically. This also explains the classic phenomenon in which preadaptation to light polarized in the preferred plane of polarization of one set of octopus retinula cells subsequently produces a sinusoidal ERG response upon rotation of the polarization angle of a light-flash stimulus of uniform intensity (K. Tasaki and Karita, 1966a,b) (figure 9.11).

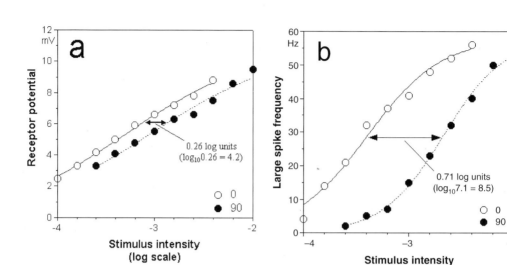

Figure 9.14
Intracellular recordings of responses to intensity series of polarized light. (*a*) Receptor potentials of a single photoreceptor. (*b*) Large spike frequencies of the main axonal output, recorded simultaneously with the data in (*a*). The polarizer was adjusted to evoke either maximum responses (0 deg, open circles) or minimum responses (after rotation through 90 deg, solid circles). Polarization sensitivity is measured as the approximate mean distance between linear sections of the two response curves, as indicated by the double-headed arrows. The continuous lines are derived using a Boltzmann sigmoidal function, calculated by GraphPad Prism, ver. 3 for Windows (GraphPad Software, San Diego, California, www.graphpad.com).

The ERG recorded from the outer region of the octopus retina in response to a light flash is a *negative-going* signal (figure 9.15), consisting of the summed depolarizations of active photoreceptors caused by the influx of (mostly) sodium ions (Nasi et al., 2000). The composition of this current flow includes the sum of opponent (mutual inhibitory) interactions between adjacent photoreceptors, and its spread across the retina is relatively symmetric and local (Norton et al., 1965; cf. Shaw, 1975). A cut in the retina makes little difference to the pattern of spread across the cut region (Norton et al., 1965), emphasizing the physical nature of this current. These effects demonstrate the presence of opponent processing in which cells serving the same part of the visual field respond maximally to different stimuli and the output generated is a function of mutual inhibition between the two cell types.

Lateral Inhibition in the Plexiform Layer
Lateral inhibition is a fundamental process in the retina, a ubiquitous strategy used throughout the animal kingdom to enhance spatial resolution (Yang and Wu, 1991),

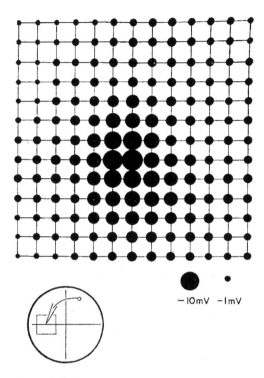

-10mV -1mV

Figure 9.15
Diagram of the relative size of the ERG surface response obtained from the region surrounding an extracellular microelectrode among the outer segments of the isolated octopus
retina. The light stimulus was repositioned systematically across the retina. The circle below
the grid represents the retina and within it, the relative position of the microelectrode
and the area of the stimulus application. (Reprinted with permission from A. C. Norton, Y.
Fukada, K. Motokawa, and K. Tasaki, An investigation of the lateral spread of potentials in
the octopus retina. *Vision Research* 5: 253–267, 1965. Copyright 1965, Elsevier.)

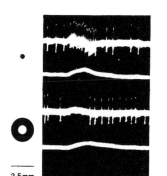

Figure 9.16
Intracellular recording from an isolated octopus retina, illustrating the effects of lateral inhibition. The top and third traces show spike discharges in response to focal and annular (2.5 mm maximum diameter) illumination, respectively; scale bar: 1 mV. The second and fourth traces are direct-current records from the same electrode; scale bar: 30 mV. The bottom trace is a stimulus pulse. (Reprinted with permission from T. Y. Yamamoto et al., 1976.)

edge detection, image sharpening, dynamic range, and regulation of sensitivity (Tsukahara, 1989; X. L. Yang and Wu, 1991; Roska et al., 2000). Lateral inhibition also exists in the less sophisticated eyes of mollusks such as bivalves (T. Y. Yamamoto et al., 1976), emphasizing that it is a fundamental or "primitive" property of molluscan eyes. In the cephalopod retina, there is good evidence that lateral inhibition in the plexiform layer is mediated via the photoreceptor collaterals. Intracellular recordings have demonstrated that octopus photoreceptors receive an inhibitory influence from other nearby photoreceptor cells, since spontaneous activity in the absence of light is abolished during stimulation with an off-center–on-surround annular light stimulus (T. Y. Yamamoto et al., 1976) (figure 9.16).

When a photoreceptor cell is impaled with a microelectrode close to the region from which the collaterals originate (i.e., just beneath the basement membrane, where the ERG is positive-going) and a light stimulus illuminates the recording site, large and small spikes are elicited (figure 9.17) (T. Y. Yamamoto et al., 1976; Tsukahara, 1989). If the microelectrode is retracted or advanced (i.e., at regions more distal or proximal), only large spikes are recorded, suggesting that the large and small spikes are discharges of the main axon and of the fine collaterals, respectively. The large and small spikes have different stimulus-response characteristics (figure 9.18a), although the angle of maximum polarization sensitivity is the same for both. They are therefore assumed to have their own morphologically and electrically independent impulse generator sites (Tsukahara, 1989). Their responses to increases in the diameter of a spot stimulus are dramatically different. The large spikes decrease rapidly in number with

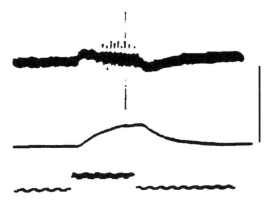

Figure 9.17
Intracellular recording at the level of the collaterals. (*a*) Note the single large spike and several small ones propagated along the axonal and collateral processes, respectively (see text); scale bar: 1 mV. (*b*) direct-current recording; scale bar: 30 mV. (*c*) A 50-ms stimulus pulse. (Reprinted with permission from Tsukahara, 1989.)

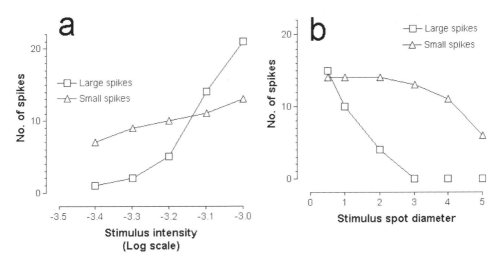

Figure 9.18
(*a*) Intensity-response functions of large (axonal) spikes and small (collateral) spikes from an octopus photoreceptor (each pair of values was counted from intracellular recordings; see figure 9.17). (*b*) The effect of the stimulus spot diameter on large and small spike frequency. Plotted from data in Tsukahara (1989).

increasing stimulus diameter, reaching zero at a spot diameter of 3 mm. The number
of small spikes remains constant for spots of 0.5–2.0 mm, and only begins to decrease
gradually as the spot is enlarged to 3 mm or more (figure 9.18b). The dramatic fall in
the number of large spikes is thought to be the result of an increasing inhibitory effect
as greater numbers of neighboring photoreceptors are stimulated.

If the octopus ERG is recorded beneath the basement lamina, in the cell body
layer and plexiform region, a light-flash stimulus applied to photoreceptors near the
microelectrode elicits a positive-going potential that represents the movement of
current out of the photoreceptors. This indicates that with the high-resistance basement lamina between the outer segments and the inner layer of cell bodies, the (very
long) photoreceptors comprise a dipole (Shaw, 1975). However, if the stimulus is
applied away from the vicinity of the microelectrode, the positive-going potential

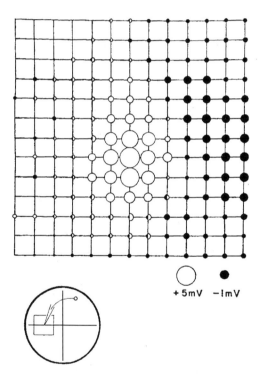

Figure 9.19
Diagram of the relative size of the ERG deep response obtained from an extracellular microelectrode in the region of the photoreceptor cell bodies beneath the basement lamina of
the isolated octopus retina. Conventions as in figure 9.15. (Reprinted with permission from
A. C. Norton, Y. Fukada, K. Motokawa, and K. Tasaki, An investigation of the lateral spread
of potentials in the octopus retina. *Vision Research* 5: 253–267, 1965. Copyright 1965,
Elsevier.)

declines rapidly and then becomes negative-going (figure 9.19). The distribution of this deep negative-going potential is asymmetric, with a bias toward the central part of the retina (K. Tasaki et al., 1963; Norton et al., 1965). This asymmetry disappears if the retina is cut, suggesting that the deep negative-going potential involves some form of lateral processing within the plexiform layer.

The asymmetric spread of the deep negative-going potential toward the center can be attributed to one or more specializations in the central region of the octopus retina. The outer segments are longer (J. Z. Young, 1963), presumably with more microvilli, carrying correspondingly larger numbers of visual pigments and membrane channel molecules, and are therefore able to produce more powerful responses. Next, there is a tendency for the outer segments to contain less screening pigment distally (Young, 1963), exposing more visual pigment to interaction with photons, again suggesting relatively larger current flows. Finally, perhaps the collaterals of more central photoreceptors are more numerous and/or longer centrally than those of peripheral photoreceptors, providing central photoreceptors with a larger area of influence.

The Effects of Efferent Nerves from the Optic Lobe

Experiments in squids and octopuses have demonstrated that dopaminergic efferents from the optic lobe synapse in the plexiform layer of the retina (Lam et al., 1974; Suzuki and Tasaki, 1983). It has also been shown that dopamine arriving via these efferents increases retinal sensitivity to light by causing retraction of screening pigment (Gleadall et al., 1993).

Electrical stimulation (50 Hz for 2.5 s) of an optic nerve bundle causes a 75% reduction in the size of its visual field (figure 9.20), but the significance and implications of this effect on visual performance are unclear.

Polarization-Based Patterns and Behavioral Displays

Although we know little about postretinal processing within the optic lobes and central brain (see Williamson et al., 1994), our knowledge of the electrical activity within the octopus retina suggests clearly that even in unpolarized light, an object will be enhanced at its edge against its background because lateral inhibition via the photoreceptor collaterals will enhance small differences in brightness. More interesting, though, an object reflecting polarized light will be clearly delineated against a background of unpolarized light, even if the light intensity from the object and background is uniform, because of the presence of the two opponent polarization channels.

The use of novel techniques for imaging polarization patterns reveals that squid, octopuses, and cuttlefish can present behavioral displays of polarization patterns on different parts of their bodies, predominantly on the arms and head and around the eyes (Cronin et al., 1995; Shashar et al., 1996; Shashar and Hanlon, 1997; Hanlon et al., 1999b). These patterns can be turned on and off rapidly, possibly through innervation of specialized iridophores (Shashar et al., 2001). For example, in *Sepia*

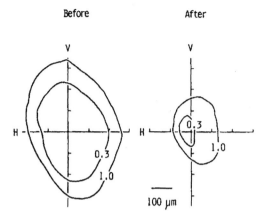

Figure 9.20
Diagram illustrating the effects of optic nerve stimulation on the receptive field of an optic nerve bundle in the octopus retina. The responses were recorded (with a suction electrode) from a cut nerve bundle still attached to the back of the isolated retina. A test flash (50 μm diameter) was moved across the retina at 65-μm intervals and the response was plotted by connecting points of equal sensitivity: 0.3 represents 50% sensitivity and 1.0 represents 10%. H and V represent horizontal and vertical directions on the retina. (Reprinted with permission from H. Suzuki and K. Tasaki, Inhibitory retinal efferents from dopaminergic cells in the optic lobe of the octopus. *Vision Research* 23: 451–457, 1983. Copyright 1983, Elsevier.)

officinalis, polarization stripes appear on the arms within 0.2 s and can be noticed when the animals are normally alert (swimming, or lying alert on the substrate), but they are not displayed when the animals are camouflaged on the substrate, when the female is laying eggs, just before and during attacks on prey, and during aggressive behavior between two males (Shashar et al., 1996).

Polarization patterns can be recorded from cuttlefish only a few weeks old, well before sexual maturity (figure 9.21; plate 18). In the squid *Loligo pealei*, a wide range of polarization patterns have been recorded in the field and in laboratory conditions, during courtship, agonistic displays, feeding, and shoaling (Hanlon et al., 1999b). Although polarization-based signals are less prone to misinterpretation in the intensity and spectrally dynamic marine environment, no specific message has yet been associated with any polarization display and hence their function is still unclear.

The occurrence of body surface polarization patterning has also been demonstrated in mantis shrimp, another group of animals possessing polarization vision (Marshall et al., 1999). Some crab species, too, reflect highly polarized light (Zeil and Hofmann, 2001; N. Shashar, unpublished results), but whether this helps in detecting them, and the extent to which octopuses may use this potential, has yet to be investigated.

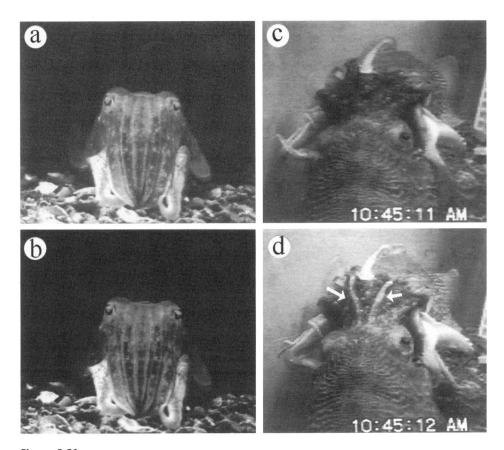

Figure 9.21
Examples of polarization displays in the cuttlefish, *Sepia officinalis*. (*a*) Full color image. (*b*) False color rendering of the same image. Polarization orientation is coded to hue (horizontal polarization presented as red); the percentage of polarization is coded as saturation: full saturation, fully polarized; gray shades, nonpolarized light; and lightness is proportional to the intensity of light reflected from the object. (*c*), (*d*) Example of a male switching on the polarization pattern during mating (images photographed through a filter transmitting horizontally polarized light). (*c*) No polarization pattern visible. (*d*) Polarization pattern displayed 1 s later (indicated by arrows). (Modified after Shashar et al., 1996.) (See plate 18 for color version.)

Life at the Bottom of the Octopus's Garden

Cephalopods are represented in all regions of the world's oceans, including the deepest parts of the sea floor. Many species live at mesopelagic depths (Hanlon and Messenger, 1996) where the only light penetrating from the surface is dim and restricted to a narrow spectrum peaking in the blue or blue-green range (MacFarland and Munz, 1975a,b; Lythgoe, 1976, 1985). However, this down-welling light is still about 200 times brighter than any light reflected from below (Lythgoe, 1985; Widder, 1999), so any organism viewed from underneath appears as a dark silhouette against the surface light, making an attack from below a successful hunting strategy (MacFarland and Munz, 1975b). To defend against this, many mesopelagic animals have evolved photophores (light organs) that emit light downward to camouflage their silhouette. In the firefly squid *Watasenia scintillans*, these include numerous small photophores on the ventral surface of the body and arms, and five large photophores underneath each eye (Sasaki, 1914; Michinomae et al., 1994; Kawahara et al., 1998). These photophores are thought to be highly effective in reducing the probability of the squid being attacked from below. Conversely, however, its eyes have specializations that enhance its ability to attack prey swimming above it.

What Firefly Squids See: The Retina of *Watasenia scintillans*

Watasenia scintillans is a small species of squid belonging to the family Enoploteuthidae. The adults reach only 60 mm in body length and spend most of their time living in semidarkness at a depth of about 400 m. *Watasenia* is unique in possessing three different visual pigment chromophores, which combine with a protein (opsin) to form three different visual pigments. Each photoreceptor cell contains only one of these visual pigments, but two types of photoreceptors receive light from the same part of the visual field. This is compelling evidence that *Watasenia* is capable of distinguishing different wavelengths of light (Michinomae et al., 1994).

The ventral region of *Watasenia*'s retina is highly specialized (Seidou et al., 1990, 1995; Michinomae et al., 1994). There are some unusually long (600 μm) photoreceptors and an arrangement of rhabdoms in well-defined layers, which have been compared to the banked retina of certain deep-sea fishes (Denton and Locket, 1989). The nonspecialized part of *Watasenia*'s retina appears similar in cross-section to any other cephalopod retina, with rhabdoms consisting of microvilli aligned in two orthogonal planes, and a visual pigment with a λ_{max} (wavelength of maximum sensitivity) of 484 nm and retinal (A1) as the chromophore. The outer layer of the ventral retina is similarly organized (figure 9.22), except that 4-hydroxyretinal (A4) is the chromophore, with a λ_{max} that is blue shifted to 470 nm (the α cells of Michinomae et al., 1994). In deeper layers of the ventral retina there are two additional sets of rhabdoms (from β and γ cells) with orthogonal microvilli offset by 45 deg from those of the distal rhabdoms; and the most proximal layer has a fourth, loose type of rhabdom produced by δ cells. The latter contain a visual pigment with dehydroretinal (A2) as its chromophore, with a λ_{max} red shifted to 501 nm (Michinomae et al., 1994). The overlying

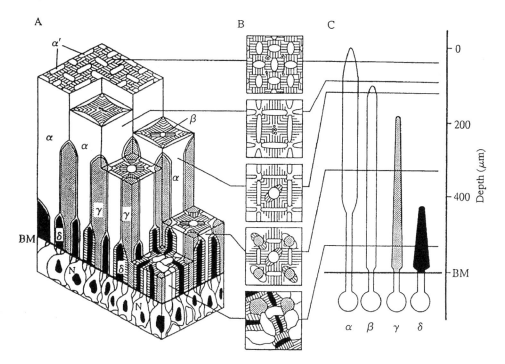

Figure 9.22
Diagram of the ventral region of the retina of the firefly squid, *Watasenia scintillans*, to illustrate the arrangement of the outer segments of the four photoreceptor cell types (α, β, γ, and δ) with depth. (*a*) Block stereogram of the retinal elements. (*b*) Cross-sectional patterns at the levels indicated in (*a*). (*c*) Representation of the relative positions of the outer segments of the four cell types. The scale at the right indicates the depth from the surface of the retina. The longest cells become much narrower distally, producing smaller-sized rhabdoms (α'). The parallel lines indicate the orientation of microvilli. BM, basement lamina; N, nucleus in photoreceptor cell body. (Reprinted with permission from Michinomae et al., 1994.)

rhabdoms containing A4 act as a short-wavelength cutoff filter, shifting the λ_{max} of the A2-containing cells another 50 nm, to 550 nm, which coincides with the peak wavelength of bioluminescence produced by green photophores in the ventral skin (figure 9.23) (Seidou et al., 1995).

It is therefore interesting to note that any color sensitivity in the eyes of blue-water oceanic species has been predicted to be a blue-green opponent system, since the presence of yellow substances in the water is always low, and red light varies the most in quantity with depth in the water column (Lythgoe, 1976). However, the fact of the basic polarization sensitivity of the cephalopod retina raises questions about the role of different wavelength sensitivities in the firefly squid's visual system.

Bending the Rules: Color Vision and Polarization Vision in the Same Part of the Eye
It is expected that in a given rhabdom, intensity will be used to code only one additional (qualitative) parameter—either color or polarization. This is because each component cell can produce only a quantitative neurological signal representing its own photon catch and its efficiency in absorbing and transducing the light. The latter is influenced by the cell's degree of adaptation to a given light intensity, but a photoreceptor's absorption efficiency depends on its spectral sensitivity range and its polarization sensitivity characteristics. In attempting to discern contrast based on one of these qualitative parameters, any mixing of their contribution would produce a confusing signal, such as the false color phenomenon predicted and observed in certain butterflies (Bernard and Wehner, 1977; Rossel, 1989; Wehner and Bernard, 1993; Kelber et al., 2001).

For a thorough analysis of polarization information within a color-blind system, measurement of three independent parameters is required: luminance, percent polarization, and orientation of polarization. However, the extraction of unambiguous information from the interactions between the color and polarization components of a visual system requires additional measurements (Wehner and Bernard, 1993).

Many cases are known in which an organism's eyes assess two qualitative stimulus parameters; however, the analysis of each is usually restricted to a specific region of the eye. For instance, bees possess a form of color vision based on the rhabdomere input from all of the ommatidia except for a mediodorsal strip that is sensitive only to polarization (Rossel, 1989; Wehner, 1989b; Backhaus, 1992a; Chittka et al., 1992). The microvilli of the cells used for color vision are spirally twisted, counteracting any polarization sensitivity.

Mantis shrimps have a very complex system that involves six rows of ommatidia in a midband across the eye. Four of these rows are specialized for color information, while the other two rows (5 and 6) are sensitive only to polarization. The color-sensitive cells contribute equal numbers of microvilli, in each of two orthogonal orientations, to their color-signaling rhabdom, which annuls their ability to respond to polarization. On the other hand, the polarization-signaling rhabdoms are made up of cells that have only one type of visual pigment and no color filters, ensuring that they are wavelength insensitive (Marshall et al., 1991a,b).

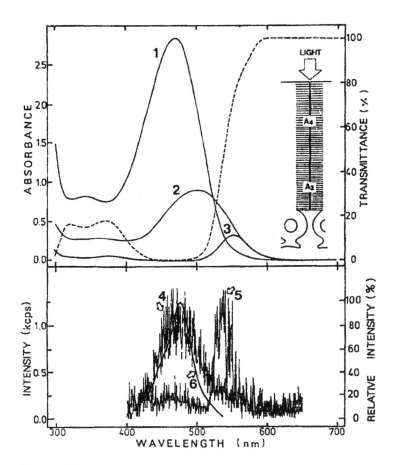

Figure 9.23
Diagram comparing the visual pigment absorption spectra (curves 1–3) for *Watasenia scintillans*, the emission spectra (curves 4 and 5) of its photophores, and (curve 6) the spectrum of light available at 500 m in clear ocean water. Curves 1–3 are the respective absorption spectra of visual pigments: 1, in the distal region (containing the chromophore 4-hydroxyretinal); 2, in the ventral region (containing 3-dehydroretinal); and 3, in the ventral region after modification by the filter effect of the distal region (dashed line, transmittance of distal region). Curves 4 and 5 represent the emission spectra of the ventral photophores exhibiting peaks in blue (curve 4; cf. curves 1 and 6), and green (curve 5; cf. curve 3). (Reprinted from Seidou et al., 1995 by permission of Oxford University Press.)

For most cephalopods, the problem of potential confusion of parameters does not arise because they are color-blind. In *Watasenia*, however, there is no evidence so far that polarization sensitivity is eliminated in any of the photoreceptors, so it is necessary to explain the presence of two different visual pigments in the part of a retina that is obviously polarization sensitive.

Significance of the Polarization and Wavelength Sensitivities of the Ventral Retina
Unfortunately, as yet there has been no successful electrophysiological investigation of the eye of the firefly squid. Michinomae et al. (1994) provided evidence that the two ventral retina visual pigments are never found in the same rhabdom. This suggests strongly that individual rhabdoms cannot provide a wavelength-derived contrast signal. That is, intrarhabdomal color opponency is unlikely in the firefly squid. Having two different visual pigments overlying each other means that the most distal will act as a filter, selectively modifying the light stimuli reaching the proximal rhabdoms (Seidou et al., 1995). There is little doubt, therefore, that the distal and most proximal photoreceptors will show quite different spectral response characteristics. However, if any color opponency occurs, it will be at higher levels of processing (between rhabdoms or during processing in the optic lobes).

The ventral retina shows changes not only in wavelength sensitivity, the β and γ cells have the orientation of their rhabdoms offset by 45 deg with respect to the microvilli of the α-cell rhabdoms (cf. the orientation of the microvilli of figure 9.6b with that in figure 9.6c). This 45-deg offset presumably enhances the sensitivity of their microvilli by enabling optimal absorption of the remaining light with *e*-vectors least likely to be absorbed by the distal layers. It also suggests the possibility of sensitivity to circular polarization (although detailed anatomical and physiological examinations are required to investigate this). If the upper layer has a retarding function, then incoming circular polarization might be converted into partly linear polarization that can be detected by the deeper photoreceptors.

Figure 9.24 summarizes the qualitative parameters used in the ventral retina. Note that for each cell type, the rhabdom has two orthogonal components and is expected to contribute to polarization sensitivity, possibly as contrast enhancement. Shifting the sensitivity of the visual pigments toward longer wavelengths at greater depths in the ventral retina has two consequences. First, it will take advantage of the fact that short-wavelength light is more easily diverted from its path (by being scattered and/or absorbed), so the relative proportion of long-wavelength light available will tend to increase rapidly with depth in the retina. Rayleigh's law predicts that light at 470 nm is about twice as likely to be scattered from its original path as light at 530 nm (Jenkins and White, 1976). Second, offsetting the λ_{max} from the transmission maximum of the environmental light increases sensitivity to contrast, particularly with regard to detecting nonmatching (green) bioluminescence against the background of down-welling (blue) light from the surface (e.g., Lythgoe, 1972; Lythgoe and Partridge, 1989). The stepwise shifting of both qualitative parameters with depth in the ventral retina suggests that a major function is the enhancement of information available in the quantitatively light-deficient mesopelagic environment.

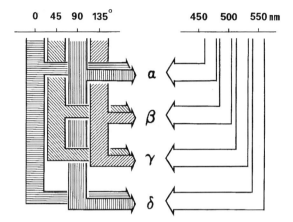

Figure 9.24
Diagram illustrating the qualitative parameters optimal for the absorption of light by different cell types (α, β, γ, and δ) in the firefly squid ventral retina with respect to their occurrence (depth) within the retina. Data from Michinomae et al. (1994) and Seidou et al. (1995). The left side represents the paired (orthogonal) polarization sensitivities of each cell type (0 versus 90 deg or 45 versus 135 deg), and the right side represents their estimated wavelengths of maximum sensitivity. (Adapted from Gleadall, 1994.)

There is little doubt, then, that this retina is exquisitely sensitive. The highly ordered rhabdoms and depth of the (average) cephalopod retina have long been recognized for their photon capture efficiency, yet the firefly squid's ventral retina is more than double the usual depth (J. Z. Young, 1971). It also manifests the earlier-mentioned parameter shifts that further enhance sensitivity. Furthermore, these squids live in water that is about 4°C, which minimizes heat-dependent noise (Aho et al., 1988). These facts suggest strongly that the firefly squid retina compensates for the low intensities of light available for vision in its mesopelagic environment by enhancing both its basic (quantitative) sensitivity and its ability to extract information based on the qualitative parameters of the incident light.

Life in the Twilight Zone: Proposed Functions of the Firefly Squid Ventral Retina
The firefly squid's ventral retina receives the strongest incident light emanating from directly above in a narrow, near-vertical beam (Michinomae et al., 1994). In the squid's deep-sea habitat, this light has a narrow spectrum, with a peak at around 470 nm (curve 6 in figure 9.23) (Lythgoe, 1972; Seidou et al., 1995), so this is the wavelength where receptors sensitive to either color information or polarization patterns function at their best. (Underwater, the percent of polarization varies little with wavelength; Cronin and Shashar, 2001). The outermost layer of photoreceptors may therefore become adapted to the intensity and polarization pattern of the down-welling light, so that any minute changes (e.g., from a counterilluminating organism swimming between the squid and the surface) will be readily detected (see earlier discussion; Gleadall, 1994).

It is interesting that 470 nm is also the peak of the blue bioluminescent light emitted by most of the photophores of this squid's ventral surface, emphasizing their likely role in counterillumination to camouflage the squid's silhouette as seen from below (cf. R. E. Young and Roper, 1976; R. E. Young et al., 1979). The high sensitivity of the outer layer of the ventral retina to this wavelength, and the fact that light guides in the photophores appear to generate a random pattern of polarization, suggest that this outer region may also be capable of detecting the intensity-matched counterillumination of conspecifics. That is, counterillumination closely matching the background surface light intensity and wavelength characteristics may be detected by distinguishing the differences between the polarization pattern of the counterilluminating squid and that of the ambient background light (Kawahara et al., 1998). Detection of bioluminescence may also be aided by the fact that many photophores use layered reflectors, which probably partially polarize emitted light, again enhancing polarization contrast with the background of down-welling light despite matching its intensity (Hanlon and Shashar, 2003).

The 530-nm peak light emission of the green photophores (see curve 5, figure 9.23) on the ventral surface of the mantle, head, and arms is not far from the estimated 550-nm λ_{max} of the deepest (A2-based) δ photoreceptors of the ventral retina (Michinomae et al., 1994; Seidou et al., 1995). The bioluminescent emission from these photophores is characteristically weak (J.-M. Bassot and I. G. Gleadall, unpublished results), but the receptors deep in the ventral retina appear well suited to detecting this light, particularly since a high proportion of the dominant, down-welling blue light will be screened out by the layers of photoreceptors above.

As Seidou et al. (1990) have suggested, these green photophores and their detectors may therefore represent a respective transmitter and receiver operating at a "secret wavelength" for communication among members of this species. Shifting the orientation of optimal polarization sensitivity of these deeper photoreceptors will presumably enhance their sensitivity to light at polarization angles less susceptible to the screening effects of the outer receptor layers.

The specialized ventral region of the retina in *Watasenia* may thus provide the ability to detect (1) organisms swimming above by their low-contrast silhouette and perturbations in the polarization pattern, (2) organisms attempting to camouflage their silhouette by emitting bioluminescence downward, and (3) a "secret code" of downward bioluminescence emitted by conspecifics. All of this is achieved by using stepwise shifts in detection parameters and the screening effects of photoreceptors at different depths within the ventral retina (Gleadall, 1994).

It seems likely that the detection of different hues in this ventral region of the firefly squid retina will be found to serve wavelength-specific behaviors (e.g., Burkhardt, 1983; Goldsmith, 1994), given the dominance in the ventral retina of the basic polarization sensitivity common to many other cephalopods. To fully understand this system, however, it will be necessary to determine how the information from the different photoreceptors layers is processed and represented in the brain. For example, perhaps simultaneous stimulation of several different classes of photoreceptors enables recognition of fellow firefly squids, whereas stimulation of fewer receptor classes signifies prey or predators.

Further research on the visual system of the octopus and firefly squid promises to provide interesting insights into models of retinal function, color and polarization vision, and artificial visual systems.

Conclusions

Cephalopods are among the most exotic and alien life forms imaginable. Their movements, symmetry, relations to space, and body orientation are all completely different from those experienced by humans, as is their ability to coordinate the use of a rather large number of versatile arms. The sensory world of a cephalopod is no less alien, and it is almost amazing that we are able to construct any understanding of their visual experience. However, the fact that they have large eyes, which are surprisingly analogous to those of vertebrates, gives us a wonderful starting point.

From the human's perspective, the cephalopod visual system is simplified somewhat by excluding color information. However, it has acquired a sophisticated polarization-detecting capability. The question of precisely what kind of visual information cephalopods extract from their world is still largely unanswered, and we continue to debate whether polarization is a true, independent component of their visual world or merely a contrast-enhancing device. The answer to this question may be the key that opens the door to the octopus's garden.

The life of cephalopods is intimately entwined with that of fishes and their mutual competition for similar niches. Both groups are highly successful animals, as is evident from their worldwide dominance in both biomass and biodiversity. In their competition with fishes, cephalopods have dramatically enhanced the equipment bequeathed to them by their ancestors. In numerous ways, their enhancements have provided some of the most remarkable examples of convergent evolution known, possibly including a functional equivalent of color vision. It is not surprising that the remarkable beauty and interesting behavior of these wonderful creatures has persuaded a large community of enthusiasts to dedicate long periods of their lives to studying octopuses, cuttlefish, and squid with their fascinating but all-too-short lives.

Acknowledgments

We warmly thank the following persons for their help in our pursuit of understanding the cephalopodan sensory world: Jean-Marie Bassot, Jean Boal, Tom Cronin, Roger Hanlon, Taka Hariyama, Yuji Kito, Ellis Loew, Justin Marshall, John Messenger, Masanao Michinomae, Kohzoh Ohtsu, Bill Saidel, Yasuo Tsukahara, Masamichi Yamamoto, and the late John Z. Young. IGG's research was supported by grants from the Oizumi Applied Information Sciences Research Fund and the Fujiwara Natural History Foundation. NS's research was supported by National Science Foundation grant IBN 9729598 and US-Israel Binational Science Foundation grant 1999040.

III OUT OF SIGHT: CREATING EXTRAVISUAL WORLDS

INTRODUCTION
Moira J. van Staaden

Human experience is so dominated by the visual that we frequently overlook the role of extravisual perceptual worlds, even in our own lives. We are amazed when researchers reveal innate human responses to the pheromones on sweaty T-shirts and astounded that at a cocktail party we can be deeply involved in a discussion on the perils of cloning and yet still hear our name quietly mentioned on the far side of the room. We ought not to be. Such subtle specializations in perception, coupled with higher-level learning and decision processes, are the very foundation of our much-vaunted adaptive abilities. And in this, evolution has ensured that we are not alone.

Light and the light-dark cycle is the most potent selective force ever to have operated on biological organisms. But since most eyes function optimally only in daylight, with a particular light spectrum and direct line of sight, evolution's adaptive tinkering has given rise to alternative modes of acquiring environmental information. Mechanical and chemical modalities are useful in physically complex habitats, utilizing signals that are generally short lived and rapidly modulated, but which have some potential for perception in the absence of a signaler. A chimpanzee hooting in an African rain forest may be clearly audible to his own, as well as rival troops, at substantial distances. But it may be exceedingly difficult to orient to and localize him—which may or may not be a good thing, depending on your motive.

Perception via the mechanical channel is highly developed in just two animal phyla, but dominant ones at that. Arthropods and chordates transduce mechanical signals to neural firings via mechanoreceptors, devices stimulated by some form of kinetic energy. These include many sense organs that monitor internal functions, such as muscle tension or joint position, as well as the senses of touch, balance, and hearing. Operating as reversed signaling devices, mechanoreceptors are constrained by the very same factors that limit signal transmission. They can generate appropriate behavioral responses only if they can correctly identify the source of a stimulus, localize it, and judge its distance. There are essentially two ways of doing this. An animal could use particle velocity receivers that detect the originally disturbed air particles close by, or ears that detect the mechanical disturbance of wave motion originating at some distant point. Systems triggered from close up would need to be very fast and directional indeed, whereas those triggered at greater distance would have more leeway.

In theory, one may describe and evaluate quantitative signal characters by absolute measurements or by measurements relative to either general background intensity or a reference signal. For animals in noisy habitats though, relative evaluations of signal intensity are often more meaningful than absolute ones. Both peripheral and central mechanisms may provide them with this information while preserving the spatial information and sufficient fractionation of the intensity range to estimate distance.

There are few instances in which complete neuronal pathways can be traced from the level of sense organs all the way to that of motor neurons. The startle behavior of insects is a notable exception. While most of an animal's behavioral repertoire is not performed with quite the same urgency as escape, locating a willing and able mate arguably runs a very close second. In this part of the volume we begin to see how neural mechanisms in orthopteroid insects balance the competing selective pressures in inter- and intraspecific interactions, depending on the extent to which the interests of sender and receiver coincide.

10 The Vigilance of the Hunted: Mechanosensory-Visual Integration in Insect Prey

Christopher Comer and Vicky Leung

In order to gain an understanding of the sensory world of another species, it is important to study examples where one can expect to relate the properties of specific nerve cell circuits to an organism's behavior and experience. Insects perform complex analyses on sensory information with circuits made up of relatively few neurons. Thus, they have been important model systems for studying a variety of fundamental issues in cellular neurobiology and animal behavior. This chapter attempts to provide a glimpse of one insect's perceptual world by a consideration of the neuronal circuitry related to a crucial behavior, the detection and evasion of a predatory attack.

The life-and-death struggle between predator and prey provides selective pressures that tend to force nervous system processing toward high levels of efficiency. As Kenneth Roeder explained it, a millisecond or so within the nervous system of an animal can mark the difference between the quick and the dead (Roeder, 1959). Thus, when probing the neuronal substrates of predator detection and evasion, one should expect to encounter sensory processing in its most economical form. This "neural parsimony," as Roeder called it, should be especially profound in insects where there is a numerical limit on the number of neurons that could be involved in any behavioral or perceptual unit.

We focus the discussion on the behavioral challenges faced primarily by two orthopteroidean insects, cockroaches and crickets, and to a smaller extent on mantids and locusts. It was evolutionary thinking that led Roeder to suggest that the relation between predator and prey would be the most revealing place to begin the program of neuroethology (see Roeder, 1963). We believe Roeder's approach is still to be recommended, especially for understanding the uniqueness of an animal's sensory world. In fact, it seems most likely that an analysis of the neural mechanisms underlying predator–prey interactions, situated within the compact central nervous system of an orthopteroidean insect, will yield a glimpse into a perceptual world far from our own.

One of the main conclusions supported by the data reviewed here is the idea that insect model systems are not as simple as many once thought them to be. We now realize that the perception of predatory threat by a cockroach or a cricket involves multiple interacting neural subsystems and is polysensory along a number of different dimensions. Several types of mechanosensation are involved in detecting and evading predators, and vision also plays a role. In fact, vision and mechanical senses are used in overlapping ways to provide an integrated flow of information about moving stimuli within a three-dimensional field surrounding the animal. Thus insects provide valuable "reductions" of the most interesting aspects of sensory perception and neural control as they have been described in animals with much larger nervous systems and much broader behavioral repertoires.

Cerci and the Mechanosensory Spectrum

If one closely examines a cockroach or cricket, it is hard to avoid noticing two short appendages that extend from the rear of their abdomen. These are the cerci, part of a highly conserved mechanosensory system for detecting predatory attack. Cerci are found throughout the orthopteroidean groups (e.g., figure 10.1) and although they are sometimes associated with other behaviors such as courtship, copulation, and orientation with respect to gravity, their most consistent and perhaps original behavioral association is with evasion of terrestrial predators (J. S. Edwards and Reddy, 1986; J. S. Edwards and Palka, 1991; J. S. Edwards, 1997).

Each cercus contains a variety of mechanoreceptors. Prominent among these is a population of long, slender filiform sensory hairs that extend outward from the cuticle surface. Each hair is associated with a primary afferent neuron that has a neurite extending into the cuticular socket where the filiform hair articulates (Nicklaus, 1965). The exact number of hairs and their placement around the cercal circumference varies from species to species. However, two functional attributes seem to be shared by all insect cercal systems. Air movements reaching the cerci from any angle around the animal in the horizontal plane will deflect at least some cercal filiform hairs, and all hairs have certain angles of deflection that will elicit action potentials in their primary afferent neurons. Thus air movements from all directions are detectable with this system, and the angular location of the wind source is encoded by whichever subset of cercal hairs, and associated afferents, is activated.

What an insect will do when a wind stimulus is detected varies across species and behavioral contexts. In active cockroaches such as *Periplaneta americana*, and in crickets such as *Gryllus bimaculatus*, wind movement above a critical level can deflect the filiform hairs sufficiently to release an evasive behavior (e.g., Roeder, 1963; Camhi and Tom, 1978; Gras and Hörner, 1992). When the insect is standing on the substrate, this often takes the form of a body turn that rotates the front (head) end of the insect away from the source of the air movement (figure 10.1A,B). The turn may be followed by running. In crickets the initial response may be a jump rather than a turn, or a turn may be coupled with a jump (Tauber and Camhi, 1995). This system is used to evade a variety of predators, such as toads, lizards, and scorpions, that generate wind currents or air puffs as they strike (Camhi et al., 1978; Sekhar and Reddy, 1988; Comer et al., 1994) (figure 10.1).

This dramatic escape response suggests that these insects have a finely tuned sensory ability to process information about the distance of objects moving toward them. In fact, in now classic studies, Camhi and colleagues showed that *Periplaneta* does not confuse a predator's lunge (which generates a low peak-velocity wind) with ambient wind (which generally has a high peak velocity) (Plummer and Camhi, 1981). Such behavioral selectivity is possible because predator attack movements generate air currents with a substantial acceleration profile to which some filiform cercal hairs and their sensory neurons are specifically tuned (Buño et al., 1981; Shimozawa and Kanou, 1984). As a result, a cockroach or cricket can sense a tiny wind "puff" characteristic

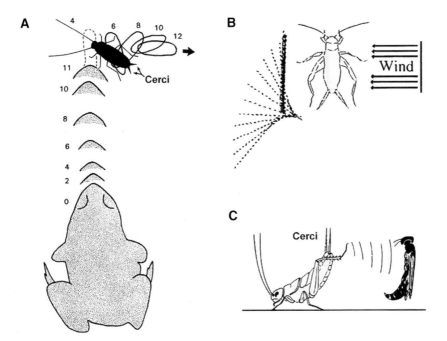

Figure 10.1
Examples of defensive or evasive responses triggered by cercal mechanoreceptors under various circumstances. (*A*) Reconstruction from video records of a marine toad lunging toward a cockroach (*Periplaneta*). The numbers represent individual video frames (1 frame = 16.6 ms). Note that the cockroach begins turning between frames 4 and 6, well before the toad lunges or extends its tongue (dotted outline) from its mouth. (*B*) An example of a turn away from wind by a cricket (*Gryllus*) as reconstructed from high-speed film records. The solid line next to the cricket represents its initial position and the dotted lines show the position of the body axis on subsequent frames (at 4-ms intervals) during the turn away. (*C*) Example of a defensive kicking response during an attack by a wasp (black, on the right). (Drawing *A* from Comer et al., 1994; *B* from Tauber and Camhi, 1995; *C* from Gnatzy and Heusslein, 1986.)

of predatory threat even against the considerable background noise created, for instance, by ambient wind or the animal's own movements.

Studies in crickets have shown that the behavioral repertoire that arises from stimulation of the cercal filiform hairs can be quite broad. For instance, at low wind intensities crickets may make no overt movement. At high intensities they may display limb withdrawal, antennal scanning, kicking, turning, walking, or running (Baba and Shimozawa, 1997). In addition, in crickets, multiple receptor types may contribute to the behavior that is ultimately expressed. For instance, crickets have some filiform cercal hairs that are associated with campaniform sensilla in their sockets. When a wasp lands near a cricket and runs toward it on the substrate, these filiform hairs can detect the approach via air movement and the animal will assume a defense posture (Gnatzy and Kämper, 1990). If the hairs are strongly deflected, however, by being directly touched, the campaniform receptors are activated and the cricket makes a kicking response (Dumpert and Gnatzy, 1977; Gnatzy and Heusslein, 1986) (see figure 10.1C).

Signals from cercal receptors are carried forward from the rear of the abdomen to motor centers in the thorax by a number of interneurons. The best known of these are the uniquely identifiable "giant" interneurons (GIs). These are a set of four to eight bilaterally paired cells that have large-caliber axons ascending through the abdominal portion of the ventral nerve cord to the thoracic ganglia and the brain. A highly similar (and probably homologous) set of such cells (G. A. Jacobs and Murphey, 1987) also with rapidly conducting axons, is found throughout the orthopteroidea (J. S. Edwards and Palka, 1974; Daley et al., 1981; Boyan and Ball, 1986; Boyan et al., 1989) (see figure 10.2). In addition, both cerci and their associated giant interneurons have been described in a primitively wingless thysanuran (the firebrat), and in archaeognathans (bristletails) (J. S. Edwards and Reddy, 1986; J. S. Edwards and Palka, 1991). Hence the ability to sense wind direction is widespread among the basal hexapod groups.

Orthopteroidean GIs are organized in such a way as to preserve the spatial qualities of the sensory information that they encode. For instance, in the terminal abdominal ganglion of the cricket *Acheta*, afferents from filiform hairs form a complex spatiotopic map of wind directions (G. A. Jacobs and Theunissen, 1996). The GIs derive their input from this neural map at the rear of the central nervous system, so that individual GIs display directional selectivity for wind (e.g., Bacon and Murphey, 1984). In turn, the GI system conveys information about wind sensory space to thoracic motor centers via small GI subsets (some with as few as two bilateral pairs) that can represent the location of a wind stimulus by way of an elegant "coarse coding" scheme (J. P. Miller et al., 1991). Cockroach GIs preserve spatial wind sensory information in a manner very similar to that of crickets (e.g., Westin et al., 1977; Daley and Camhi, 1988; Kolton and Camhi, 1995).

Figure 10.3 shows how neural activity within the GI system, and the abdominal nerve cord as a whole, varies as wind stimuli arrive from different directions around a cockroach. This reconstructed functional image draws attention to two important features. First, there are two distinct subsets of GIs on each side of the nerve cord, one

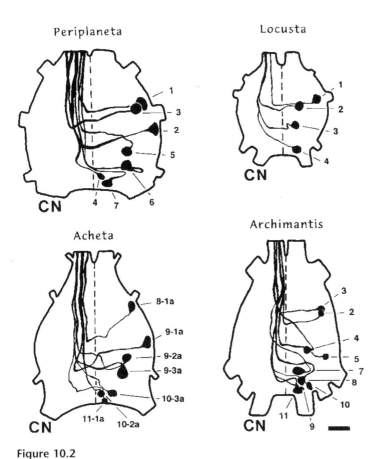

Figure 10.2
Cercal mechanosensory information is transmitted rostrally to thoracic motor circuits and the brain by a conserved system of giant interneurons. Each drawing is of the terminal abdominal ganglion as viewed from above. Rostral is upward on the page. The somata of the giant interneurons (as labeled with dye) that have been identified in each of the species indicated are numbered according to their standard identification scheme. CN, cercal sensory nerve; scale bar = 100 μm. (*Periplaneta* from Daley et al., 1981; *Locusta* adapted from Boyan et al., 1989; *Acheta* adapted from G. A. Jacobs and Murphey, 1987; *Archimantis* adapted from Boyan and Ball, 1986.)

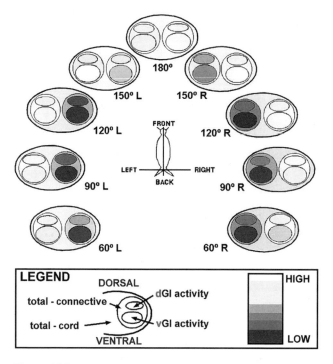

Figure 10.3
A profile of wind-evoked neural activity in interneurons of the cercal wind-sensory system of *Periplaneta*. The legend at bottom is a schematic drawing of a representative section through the ventral nerve cord showing functional groups that could be separated automatically from extracellular multiunit recordings (as described in Smith et al., 1991). Wind stimuli were presented from the indicated angles around the animals in the horizontal plane. Data from five animals were averaged for the figure. The gray level in each neural compartment of the cord schematic, at each angle, indicates the approximate level of wind-evoked neural activity recorded within 50 ms following delivery of a standard wind puff. The scale for relative activity levels is given at the bottom right. White = 100% of the maximal activity recorded from the neural compartment, dark gray = 0% of maximal neural activity. (Adapted from Comer and Dowd, 1993.)

located more dorsally and one more ventrally (dGIs and vGIs, respectively). Second, there are several indicators of wind direction that show up in the population response of wind sensory interneurons. Frontal winds produce larger levels of neural activity overall, and left and right winds produce lateral asymmetries in the amount of neural activity evoked. The latter is especially pronounced in the ventral GI subset.

This GI-based view of wind-sensory space suggests an important role for the vGIs in localizing objects moving around the animal. It also is consistent with a large body of evidence based on lesion, modelling, and stimulation studies that suggests that the vGIs are the primary system underpinning the directional evasive turn that initiates escape behavior (Comer, 1985; Dowd and Comer, 1988; Camhi, 1988; Camhi and Levy, 1989). It is also important to note that the dGIs appear to be functionally distinct from the vGIs in both cockroaches and crickets. The dGI subset also encodes wind direction by its population response, independent of the vGI encoding of wind-sensory space (Mizrahi and Libersat, 1997). The dorsal GIs probably have a role in steering or evading predators while the insect is flying (Ritzmann et al., 1980; Hirota et al., 1993; Libersat, 1992; Ganihar et al., 1994). If so, the dGIs play a role in motor control of flight that parallels the vGI role in directing terrestrial locomotion.

Finally, GI wind-sensory information is integrated with other sensory modalities as it is transformed into motor output, or behavior. It has recently been demonstrated in *Periplaneta* that the same thoracic interneurons (TI_As) that receive vGI input and pass it on to the leg motor neurons also receive a separate converging tactile input from the cuticle, and visual input from the eyes (Ritzmann et al., 1991). Cockroaches will perform escape turns in response to abrupt tactile stimuli (see later discussion), but it is not yet known if the thoracic interneurons represent a specific point of convergence between the wind-activated and touch-activated escape pathways. For example, visual cues alone do not elicit escape responses, but may modulate some aspects of the escape performance (also see later discussion). Hence the polymodality of these interneurons may simply reflect their role in the modulation of wind-evoked escape either by a mechanosensory submodality (touch) or by a different modality altogether (vision).

Antennae and a Broader Mechanosensory Spectrum

It has been known for a while now that cockroaches can also generate escape responses after the cerci are removed or after the ascending GI pathway is completely inactivated (Comer et al., 1988). These animals will turn and run when the cuticle is tapped, and may even escape in response to very intense wind stimuli. However, there does not appear to be a second, noncercal wind sensory system mediating escape behavior. Insects without an intact cercal wind-sensory pathway stop responding to intense winds if the antennae (on their head) are removed (Comer et al., 1988), and do not respond to less intense winds in the range expected to be associated with predatory attacks (Stierle et al., 1994).

These results suggested not only that there is a general somatosensory channel for escape, but also that an important contribution to the channel comes from receptors on the antennae. However, the adequate stimulus for the antennal pathway does not appear to be wind. Cockroaches respond with escape behavior to abrupt tapping of most regions of the body (Ritzmann and Pollack, 1994), and in interactions with real predators the very long, mobile antennae frequently are contacted during strikes (Comer et al., 1994). Some of the predators that seem to be detected by direct contact, especially by the antennae, include spiders, predatory insects such as mantids, and small rodents (Comer et al., 1994) (see figure 10.4A,B). The evasive movements evoked by antennal contact have the same form as those evoked by wind puffs to the cerci.

The success of the cercal system as an escape mechanism is dependent in no small way on its speed. The average time between wind deflection of cercal hairs and the first escape movements directed away from the wind is about 50–60 ms for a stationary cockroach and 50–100 ms for a stationary cricket (Roeder, 1963; Camhi and Tom, 1978; Tauber and Camhi, 1995). However, a system that is not triggered until direct contact occurs must be even faster and directionally specific. Turning responses to abrupt antennal contact are directed away from the side of the stimulated antenna and occur with a latency of only about 25 ms (Comer et al., 1994; Ye and Comer, 1996) (see figure 10.4C).

This antennal touch-evoked evasive behavior depends upon a second system of giant interneurons that rapidly conducts signals from antennal receptors back to thoracic motor centers (Burdohan and Comer, 1990; Stierle et al., 1994). The system is based on two bilateral pairs of large-caliber, descending mechanosensory interneurons (DMIs) related to escape (Burdohan and Comer, 1996) (figure 10.5A). The touch-activated responses of these paired interneurons show a laterality bias. When one antenna is tapped, DMI activity is reliably greater in the connective that is contralateral (versus ipsilateral) to the stimulated antenna (Ye and Comer, 1996). Hence the basic physiology suggests that bilateral integration of touch-evoked DMI neural activity may control escape turning in a manner generally similar to that of wind-evoked GI activity.

Descending mechanosensory interneurons of this general type also are known to exist in crickets, locusts, and mantises. In crickets, several cells with axons descending from the brain and carrying antennal touch information have been described, and some combine visual with mechanosensory input (e.g., Staudacher, 1998; Gebhardt and Honegger, 2001). It is not unusual for descending neurons in orthopteroidean insects to combine visual information from the compound eyes or ocelli with mechanosensory information (e.g., see Bacon, 1980; Mizunami, 1995). Some of the descending mechanosensory interneurons described in crickets and mantises are candidates for homology with cockroach descending mechanosensory interneurons (e.g., Staudacher, 1998; V. Leung, unpublished results). From a comparative perspective, it seems clear that the behavioral significance of the interactions between mechanosensation and vision needs to be investigated. We will return to this point later.

Recordings from the descending mechanosensory interneurons of intact cockroaches during escape responses have demonstrated that the bilateral patterning of activity in the descending mechanosensory interneuron pathway is directly correlated

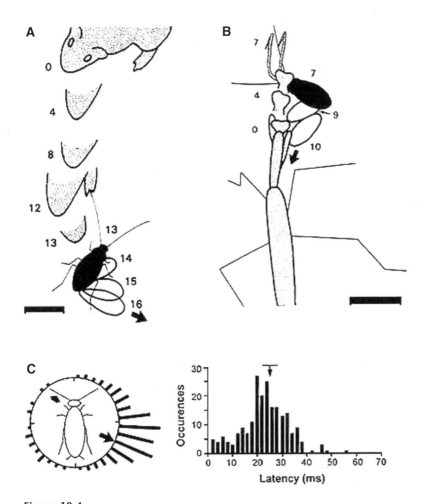

Figure 10.4

Examples from predator–prey interactions and from tests with artificial stimuli to show that some predators are not detected by the cercal system, but rather by antennal mechanoreceptors. (A, B) Reconstructions from video records of a mouse and a mantis (respectively) lunging at cockroaches (predator stippled gray, cockroach black). The frame numbers on the left are for movements of the predator (0 is the start of a lunge). The numbers on the right show the corresponding frames for cockroaches. Note that the cockroaches do not start to move until they are contacted on an antenna by a lunging predator. Scale bar = 1 cm. (C) Circular histogram showing the directionality of escape turns evoked by antennal touch; 215 trials in response to a standard mechanical stimulus are summarized. The short arrow shows the location of the antennal touch; the long arrow shows the mean vector of turns. The linear histogram summarizes the latency of these responses. Cockroaches typically turned away from the side of antennal touch with a latency of about 27 ms (thin arrow). (Drawings A and B from Comer et al., 1994; C from Ye and Comer, 1996.)

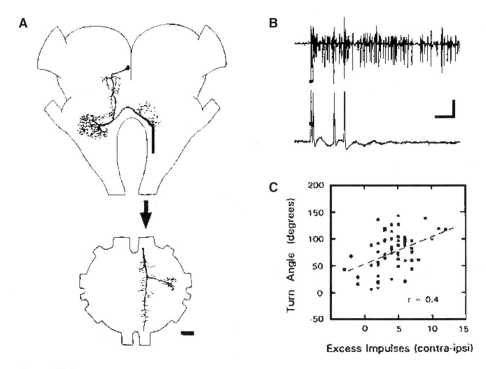

Figure 10.5
Antennal mechanosensory information is transmitted caudally by a second system of giant interneurons and this information is translated into specific angles of escape turns. (*A*) Anatomy of one identified descending mechanosensory neuron, DMIa-1, responsible for touch-evoked escape. A cell is filled with cobalt hexamine and visualized in the brain and metathoracic ganglion (shown in whole mount, viewed from the dorsal surface; other ganglia are omitted). Note that the soma is in the brain side contralateral to the descending axon. Scale bar: 100 μm. (*B*) Simultaneous extracellular (top trace) and intracellular (bottom trace) recording of DMIa-1 responding to a tap on the antenna. The recordings are from the cervical level. Calibration bar: 0.2 mV (extracellular), 10 mV (intracellular), 20 ms. (*C*) Data summary from cockroaches where DMI activity was recorded from chronically implanted electrodes and related on a trial-by-trial basis to escape behavior. The scatter plot gives the relationship between the angle of the turns and the relative numbers of impulses (bilateral differences in spike counts) recorded simultaneously from the cervical connectives on the sides ipsilateral and contralateral to the antenna that was tapped to elicit an escape response. As the number of DMI impulses became relatively greater in the contralateral connective, larger initial angles of contralateral turning were produced. $r = 0.4$, $p < 0.001$. (Drawing *A* from Burdohan and Comer, 1996; *B* and *C* from Ye and Comer, 1996.)

with the direction and specific angle of escape turns (Ye and Comer, 1996) (figure 10.5B,C). This descending interneuron system, which processes direct-touch information, is distinct from the classic GI system that detects predators at a distance using wind cues. The touch-sensory system will detect cues provided by small-bodied predators that do not necessarily generate wind, or that strike from a very close range. In contrast, the wind-sensory system responds to large or abruptly moving predators that strike from father away (Comer et al., 1994). From a perceptual viewpoint, these two interneuron systems tie the escape response of *Periplaneta* to at least two distinguishable mechanosensory subsystems.

Recent work has expanded the potential mechanosensory dimensions that are processed during predator–prey interactions even further. For example, when the antennal flagellum (consisting of about 150 segments) is amputated and a plastic fiber is attached in its place to the basal two segments (the scape and the pedicel) that form the antennal socket, deflection of the "prosthetic" flagellum still activates the descending mechanosensory interneurons and produces a typical escape response (Comer et al., 2003). However, escape behaviors are essentially eliminated by constraining the movement of the two basal segments with wax, for instance, so that tapping the intact flagellum will no longer cause deflections of the basal segments (Comer et al., 2003) (figure 10.6). This indicates that proprioceptors sensitive to the overall displacement of the antennal flagellum actually trigger the escape. In addition, the angle of escape turning can be influenced by the direction an antenna is pointing when it is touched (Comer et al., 1994; Ye et al., 2003). This may indicate a role for the basal proprioceptors in determining escape direction (although an influence from antennomotor reafference has not yet been excluded).

Antennal Receptors

The types of receptors at the antennal base include hair plates and campaniform sensilla at the cuticular surface (e.g., Toh, 1981; Okada and Toh, 2001) and chordotonal organs below the cuticle (e.g., Toh, 1981; Toh and Yokohari, 1985). While there is as yet no definitive information on the basal receptor types related to escape, some observations provide a clue. Scapal hair plate receptors have phasic-tonic discharge characteristics (Okada and Toh, 2001) that would be more appropriate to a role in localizing objects during walking (see Okada and Toh, 2000) than for triggering escape. Furthermore, recordings from descending mechanosensory interneurons in crickets have demonstrated that they receive input from scapal chordotonal organs and perhaps other pedicellar receptors (Gebhardt and Honegger, 2001).

If, then, receptors on the two basal segments are involved in triggering escape, what is the role of the many thousands of receptors on the 150 or so flagellar segments?

The cockroach's antennal flagellum contains tens of thousands of mechanoreceptors, chemoreceptors, and other types of receptors (e.g., Toh, 1977; Schaller, 1978; Hansen-Delkeskamp, 1992). In behavioral studies, cockroaches responded differentially to experimentally controlled antenna contact with conspecifics or natural

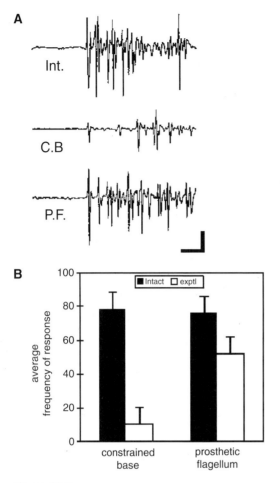

Figure 10.6

The long antennal flagellum does not contain receptors crucial for touch-evoked escape. These receptors are in the scape and pedicel at the antennal base. (*A*) DMIs can be activated in the absence of flagellar receptors. Typical extracellular physiology recordings were obtained from experiments to identify the location of receptors activating key descending interneurons for escape. The upper trace shows representative large-unit (DMI) activity elicited by stimulation of the intact antenna (Int.). The middle trace shows representative activity elicited by stimulation of an antenna with a constrained base (C.B.). The lower trace shows representative activity elicited by stimulation of a prosthetic flagellum (P.F.). All traces are from the connective contralateral to the stimulated antenna. Scale bar: 200 μV; 10 ms. Note that the constraining base nearly eliminates descending neural activity, but this activity remains in the absence of the flagellum. (*B*) Escape behavior can also be triggered in the absence of flagellar receptors, but is almost abolished if displacement of basal segments is prevented. The height of the bars indicates the percentage of escape responses (on average) elicited by touching either the intact antenna (solid) or the experimental antenna (open). The bars on the left show results from animals with one antenna constrained at the base; the bars on the right are from animals with one antennal flagellum replaced with a plastic fiber. Error bars: 1 standard deviation. (Both drawings from Comer et al., 2003.)

predators (such as wolf spiders, genus *Lycosa*; Comer et al., 2003). When cockroaches approach and briefly explore the surface of a spider with their flagellum, they reliably perform escape behaviors in response to subsequent experimentally controlled contact with a spider. However, cockroaches perform escape responses significantly less often in response to experimentally controlled contact from a cockroach after having palpated another cockroach. This relatively sophisticated discrimination requires that the cockroach stroke its antenna across the initial stimulus animal just prior to the subsequent controlled contact (Comer et al., 2003) (see figure 10.7). The nature of the cues obtained initially appears to be related to stimulus texture rather than surface chemicals, although the details have yet to be unraveled. Clearly, the cockroaches are acquiring basic information about stimulus identity during surface exploration via antennal flagellum receptors. However, the integration of sensory input from the basal receptors provides information regarding stimulus location and triggers the motor output for the escape response.

Integrating Antennal Inputs

Experiments have suggested that a very simple algorithm may underlie the interaction of stimulus identity information provided by flagellar receptors with location information provided by basal receptors. Consider first that escape is not elicited at high levels when the antennae are abruptly tapped by a conspecific. However, when the antennae are abruptly tapped by a neutral probe, an escape response is elicited at high levels comparable to the level elicited by a real predator's attack (Comer et al., 2003). These observations do not support a model in which specific cues from a predator increase the likelihood of escape by antennal contact. Rather, they suggest that a default condition exists so that abrupt antennal contact has a high probability of eliciting escape, but the sensory inputs associated with conspecifics tend to lower that probability. This makes sense in that it simplifies the decision process by making it an interaction, at some level, between afferent inputs (Altman and Kien, 1986). This eliminates the requirement to process information about the variety of potential predators that might be detected by antennal contact (Comer et al., 1994). It simply requires that some reliable cue or cues associated with the presence of other cockroaches depress escape behavior.

Vision Complements the Cockroach's Mechanosensory "View" of the World

Cockroaches constantly and spontaneously move their antennae, essentially scanning the world around them for olfactory, mechanosensory, and some other types of sensory information. So any model of antenna-mediated escape behavior must consider both this behavior and the perceptual world that the collected information creates.

It has been known for some time that crickets are able to visually detect the location of moving objects, as evidenced by their antennal movements (Honegger, 1981). Crickets track moving objects by moving the antenna ipsilateral to the visual

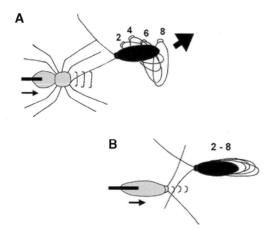

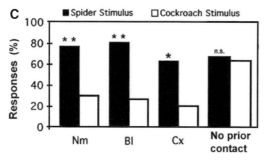

Figure 10.7

Flagellar receptors are involved in distinguishing benign stimuli from threatening stimuli. Shown are reconstructions of typical responses of test animals (black) to spiders (*A*) and cockroaches (*B*) making contact with the antennae. The stimuli were freshly killed specimens mounted on a plastic frame and moved forward (small arrow) by a solenoid-driven armature (black bar). In both cases, movement of the stimulus toward the live cockroach followed brief palpation of the surface of the stimulus. The numbers are video frames where 0 is the frame just prior to the first movement. The large arrow in (*A*) indicates that the cockroach continued with an escape run. In (*B*) the cockroach backed up slightly, but did not turn or run. (*C*) Discrimination of stimulus identity was not abolished by blinding or cercal removal. The histograms give the percent of escape responses observed when a spider stimulus (solid bars) or a cockroach stimulus (open bars) abruptly contacted an antenna. All stimulus presentation occurred after the test animals had palpated the surface of the stimulus for up to 5 s. The data are pooled from twelve cockroaches: six normal (Nm), three blinded (Bl), and three with cerci removed (Cx). Total $n = 217$ trials. *, significant difference between responsiveness to spider and cockroach stimuli at $p < 0.02$; **, difference at $p < 0.01$ (2×2 chi-square test); n.s., no significant difference. Animals that were not allowed to palpate the stimulus before testing (no prior contact) were unable to distinguish between a spider and a cockroach stimulus. (All drawings from Comer et al., 2003.)

stimulus. The antennal tracking movement is spatially accurate, very fast, and sac-cadelike (Honegger, 1981, 1995) (figure 10.8A). This immediately raises the question of to what extent visual information influences antenna placement and perhaps touch-evoked escape responses in their relative, the cockroach.

Observations of free-ranging cockroaches have provided abundant evidence of antennal orienting movements that appear to be under visual guidance. Figure 10.8B shows one example in which coordinated visual tracking of the movements of a nearby conspecific has been documented (Ye et al., 2003). When the cockroach's antennae are in their normal position (60–90 deg from the midline), an object intro-duced into the visual periphery (approximately 120 deg from the midline), at a dis-tance of about one antennal length, reliably elicits ipsilateral antennal movement toward the object. When the cockroach's compound eyes are covered with opaque paint, however, the response is eliminated (Ye et al., 2003) (figure 10.8C). These anten-nal reorientations are also eliminated if the stimulus contrast is reduced to match that of the background against which the stimulus is presented. Surprisingly, then, a cock-roach's visual system plays a role in guiding an antenna to the location of novel objects entering its visual field. These objects can then be palpated by the antennal flagellum.

As we have indicated, when a cockroach palpates an object with its antenna, the probability of an escape response elicited by subsequent antennal contact varies according to whether the second object is perceived as benign (Comer et al., 2003). In this sense, vision plays an indirect role in the stimulus identification that precedes escape behavior. The next logical question is whether visual input is necessary for trig-gering or for normal performance of antenna-mediated escape.

When a cockroach has its vision occluded, there is no effect on its responsiveness to antennal touch, no change in the average latency of touch-evoked escape, and no change in the typical angular size of escape turns (Ye et al., 2003). In contrast to the ineffectiveness of occluding vision on the initiation and performance of escape turning, there is a marked effect on the performance of the subsequent escape "run phase" that follows the initial turn. Animals without visual input run at lower average velocities, and run for much shorter average distances compared with their own pre-lesion behavior (Ye et al., 2003) (figure 10.9).

It is interesting that removal of the cerci also has a marked effect on the run phase. It reduces both run velocity and duration. The lack of visual input has an impact on run performance that is larger than the effect of cercal removal, however, which cannot be explained by a general lowering of motor activity following blinding (N. Mathenia and C. Comer, unpublished results; Ye et al., 2003).

There is very little previous experimental work on the run phase of the cockroach's escape. However, one report has noted that one particular visual cue may be impor-tant in terminating the run phase. When running cockroaches enter an area of decreased illumination, they often terminate running ("the shadow response"; Meyer et al., 1981). A truncated run length for escape following blinding would be consis-tent with a model in which certain types of visual information may be important for continued stimulation of locomotor circuits once running is initiated. Hence, vision

A

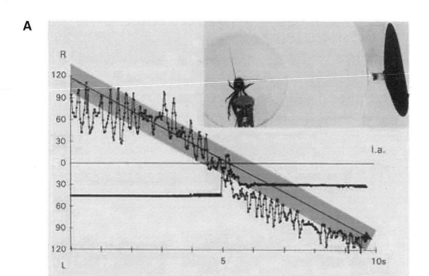

B

C

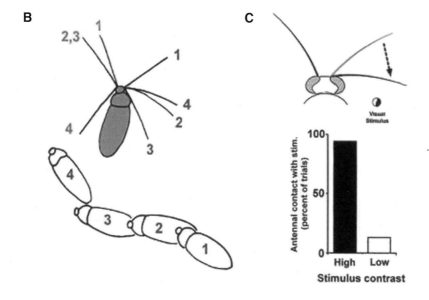

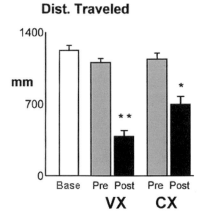

Dist. Traveled

Figure 10.9
While visual stimuli cannot trigger escape behavior, vision can influence the dynamics of the escape run phase in cockroaches. Covering the eyes or removal of the cerci shortened the average length of the run phase of escape. The base consisted of data pooled from twelve animals (n = 631 trials). Pre- and post-test data are from a group of five animals both before and after the eyes were covered (VX; n = 433 total trials) or a group of two animals before and after the cerci were removed (CX; n = 258 total trials). *, significant difference at $p <$ 0.01; **, $p < 0.001$. (From Ye et al., 2003.)

◀ **Figure 10.8**
Moving objects may also be detected visually. (A) Graph of antennal tracking behavior by a cricket *Gryllus campestris* showing angular deviation of the stimulus target (25-deg visual angle, shaded) from the longitudinal axis (l.a.) of the cricket; time in seconds. Angular tracking of the antennae is shown at a resolution of 20 ms. The target moves with an angular speed of 20 deg/s from right (R, upper left) to left (L, lower left). Note that the antennae track trailing or leading edges of the target with rapid saccadelike movements. Inset: One position of the target and antennae during a tracking movement. (B) Apparent visually elicited antennal reorientation in free-ranging cockroaches. As a conspecific approaches from the rear, the right antenna of the focal animal moves toward the conspecific in the right, peripheral visual field, and the left antenna moves to the left peripheral visual field when the conspecific crosses to the left side. The reconstructions are traced from video recordings. (C) Stimuli placed in the periphery reliably evoked ipsilateral antennal movement to contact the stimulus, and these movements depended on visual cues. The schematic illustration of the testing situation shows stimuli placed at about 120 deg in the visual field, a region where antennae are rarely held spontaneously. Positive responses were scored when the ipsilateral antennal flagellum was moved to contact the stimulus within 5 s (arrow). Decreasing the stimulus contrast decreased the responsiveness to visual stimuli. The histograms give the percentage of trials scored positively. The differences between the solid and open bars are highly significant. (Drawing A from Honegger et al., 1995; B and C from Ye et al., 2003.)

is apparently integrated with mechanosensory information to influence the occurrence of escape turning (indirectly) by influencing antennal positioning. Then, during the escape run phase, vision directly influences the distance and duration of the run.

The observation that removal of the cerci causes truncated runs is generally consistent with the observation that cercal input influences flight behavior in orthopteroidean insects (Fraser, 1977; Ritzmann et al., 1980; Boyan and Ball, 1989; Ganihar et al., 1994). It also suggests a role for the dorsal subgroup of the giant interneurons in the run phase of terrestrial escape. This is consistent with the fact that they are activated during locomotion (e.g., Daley and Delcomyn, 1980; Libersat, 1992), and it has been incorporated explicitly into models of the legged escape response (Camhi and Nolen, 1981).

The search for the cells involved in cockroach visual processing pulls the analysis of the cockroach escape behavior out of a mechanistic framework and places it back into a broad evolutionary framework. There are several descending visual interneurons that could signal the fact that a novel visual stimulus has entered an insect's visual field (Leung and Comer, 2001) (figure 10.10). One such interneuron is particularly conspicuous in the cockroach when electrophysiological recordings are made from the ventral nerve cord that is contralateral to the stimulated eye (see figure 10.11A). Simultaneous recordings of this cell's activity and video recordings of antennal movements show that the visual interneuron's activity always precedes antennal movements directed toward a novel visual stimulus (figure 10.10). The interneuron appears to be similar to the descending contralateral movement detector (DCMD) so well known from locusts (e.g., O'Shea et al., 1974; Rind and Simmons, 1992), and apparently present in mantids (chapter 3 in this volume).

In cockroaches, an interneuron with response properties similar to those of the locust DCMD has been reported, based on extracellular recordings (D. H. Edwards, 1982). It has recently been found that an identifiable visual interneuron that reliably discharges prior to antennal orienting movements is the same cell originally described by Edwards (1982). Dye injections and anatomical analysis of this cell support the idea that it may be the cockroach homologue of the locust DCMD (V. Leung, R. M. Robertson, and C. Comer, unpublished results) (figure 10.11B,C). In locusts, the DCMD has been thought for quite some time to play a role in the escape jump (e.g., Burrows and Rowell, 1973; Pearson and O'Shea, 1984). In more recent analyses, it is suggested that the DCMD is involved in visual flight guidance and crash avoidance by detecting looming visual stimuli (Judge and Rind, 1997). The perspective that emerges here is that the DCMD has a pronounced motor control function at the thoracic level in locusts, but may have a significant motor control function at the cephalic level in cockroaches.

Conclusions

The escape behavior of cockroaches should no longer be thought of as a simple, purely wind-evoked behavior. Instead, it should be seen as a complex, variable response

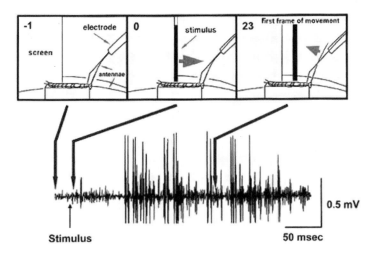

Figure 10.10

Large-amplitude visual activity (primarily from one descending interneuron) precedes directed antennal movements. The drawings of the video frames are numbered (upper left) with respect to the time a stimulus was activated to appear from behind the screen. 0 is the onset of the stimulus (right-facing arrow in the frame). The antenna began moving on frame 23 (left-facing arrow). Simultaneous extracellular recordings were made from the right promesothoracic connective (contralateral to the stimulated visual field). (From V. Leung, unpublished results.)

controlled by a network of interacting sensory guidance systems that support the integrated processing of tactile, wind, and visual information (figure 10.12).

The descending control systems underpinning escape behavior are particularly rich and suggest a wider, more elaborated perceptual world for cockroaches than would be evident if one considered only the processing of wind direction information. Antennomotor control (loop V in figure 10.12) is related to antennal guidance by the cockroach's immobile eyes in ways that bear some formal similarities to the oculomotor control mechanisms in animals with mobile eyes. Antennal orienting movements to approaching objects in the visual field achieve the same ends as do the saccadic movements by which vertebrates foveate novel stimuli that enter their visual field (e.g., P. H. Schiller and Tehovnik, 2001).

The descending mechanosensory interneuron pathway that triggers escape behavior (loop P in figure 10.12) works in concert with a touch-sensory control loop (T) that influences stimulus identification. It also works with the visual control pathway (V) that has some influence, at least indirectly, on stimulus localization and escape directionality. All of these descending systems converge at least at the thoracic level (and perhaps elsewhere) with two kinds of ascending systems, a wind-sensory system (W), and a direct mechanosensory (i.e., campaniform derived) system (M). Hence the control of escape behavior, in its totality, is truly a polymodal phenomenon.

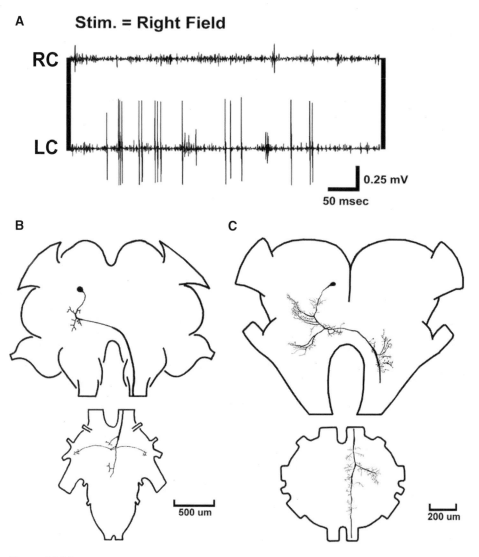

Figure 10.11

The visual interneuron that reliably discharges prior to antennal movements is the cockroach descending contralateral monement detector (DCMD). (*A*) Typical physiological recording of a DCMD in *Periplaneta* taken from the left cervical connective (LC), i.e., contralateral to the visual stimulus. (*B*) Classic anatomical reconstruction of a DCMD filled with cobalt chloride in *Schistocerca vaga*. (*C*) Reconstruction of a DCMD in *Periplaneta americana* filled with cobalt hexamine and silver intensified [the fill in (*B*) is not silver intensified]. The reconstructions show whole mounts of the brain and the metathoracic ganglion as viewed from the dorsal surface. Other ganglia are omitted. (Drawings *A* and *C* from V. Leung, unpublished results; *B* from O'Shea et al., 1974.)

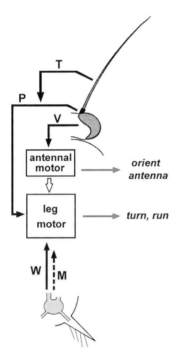

Figure 10.12
Summary of mechanosensory and visual integration underlying the identification and localization of predators by cockroaches and related orthopteroid insects. The right compound eye, antenna, and cercus are shown from above. Pathway W is the giant interneuron pathway where wind stimuli deflect cercal sensory hairs that will trigger an escape response. Pathway M is the mechanosensory pathway from campaniform sensilla (in crickets) that can trigger defensive kicks. Pathway P is the DMI pathway by which stimuli that abruptly displace the antenna trigger an escape turn and run. Pathway T allows information from flagellar receptors to modulate the DMI pathway, for example, to reduce the likelihood of escape toward conspecifics based on cues (perhaps textural) related to stimulus identity. Pathway V allows visual information to be used to orient the antenna toward approaching targets. The white arrow indicates that antennomotor positioning can influence the direction of escape turns. (Adapted from Comer et al., 2003.)

Some researchers have argued that the conserved system of giant interneurons may have been important in setting the stage for wingless insect groups to evolve flight (e.g., J. S. Edwards, 1997). This is an intriguing idea and suggests that wind detection was an early sensory ability that subserved coordinated control of leg motor circuits for predator evasion, but then was co-opted for coordinated control of wing motor circuits. This view could be interpreted as relegating antenna-derived sensation and vision to the status of relative latecomers in an evolutionary sense. However, our review suggests that the close integration of vision with basic somatosensory perception for detecting moving (and perhaps threatening) objects in the immediate sensory field supports a model in which insect escape behavior evolved under multiple sensory influences from very early on. If visual control followed tactile and mechanosensory control in the evolution of insect escape behavior, then vision came to work with circuits that were already used for "viewing" the world through multiple, nonvisual sensory channels.

Acknowledgments

The research described here that was performed in the author's laboratory was supported by several grants from the National Science Foundation, especially grant 9604629. We would like to thank Dr. Yoshichika Baba for a critical reading of the manuscript.

11 A Novel Approach to Hearing: The Acoustic World of Pneumorid Grasshoppers

Moira J. van Staaden, Heiner Römer, and Vanessa C. K. Couldridge

The Pneumorid Grasshopper's Signals

An animal's perceptual representation of the world is a product of sensory systems that have been shaped gradually by natural selection. The evolution of the signal component of the signaler–receiver relationship inherent in the sensory systems that feed the animal's perceptions has been described as an "economical process" that is unlikely to have arisen in isolation but, rather, which has taken shape in terms of the background stimuli against which the signals exist (M. D. Greenfield, 2002). Hence, sense organs function to filter relevant information from a broad background of physical interactions and discard potential input that has not proven useful over the course of evolution. It frequently happens, however, that the real world evolves faster than an animal's cognitive map of it. Hence, sensory-perceptual systems may not be ideally matched to the world in which they operate.

In the case of hearing, most sounds are first detected by specialized receptors in the form of pressure transducers. These cells pick up information from the environment, causing a transduction event that leads to a voltage change across the neuron and a message being transmitted to other parts of the nervous system (i.e., the brain, a central ganglion, or a nerve net). The key selective advantage of hearing throughout evolution is evidenced by its high prevalence in the animal kingdom. Consequently, a remarkable diversity of ears developed as animals converged on different acoustical solutions for collecting and transducing vibrations. Although optimal signaling would occur if there were precise matching of signal and receiver characteristics, recent work suggests that the anticipated co-evolution between signalers and receivers may be much more loosely coupled than generally assumed (Mason and Bailey, 1998; Mason et al., 1999). Because of this less than perfect match, the task of unraveling the evolutionary path of signaling systems, and of understanding the processes responsible for bringing the match about, is significantly more complex than one might initially imagine, and it demands a historical perspective.

As a signaler's repertoire increases, there are concomitant demands on both signalers and recipients, respectively, to choose and produce or detect, decode, and discriminate among the signals. Our research focuses on a taxon that confronts the problem of using auditory cues in a number of behaviors in particularly demanding ways. Specifically, we are interested in how pneumorid, or bladder grasshoppers, detect sounds, decipher meaning in the auditory information that they receive, and how they use information on sound to direct their behaviors.

Bladder grasshoppers (Orthoptera, Pneumoridae) are a small family of seventeen species endemic to the coastal regions of Africa (Dirsh, 1965), with a geographic range spanning forest, savanna, fynbos (fine-leaved bush), and desert habitats. They are cryptic, nocturnal animals with very patchy spatial and temporal distributions. Their most notable features are those relating to acoustic communication; in fact, an absolute reliance on highly exaggerated acoustic signaling was apparent even to Darwin (1871) based solely on his examination of museum specimens. More recent field investigations have demonstrated that pneumorids can detect acoustic signals over a distance of 2 km and these mediate adaptive behavioral responses involved in mate localization, crypsis, and defense (van Staaden and Römer, 1997). These investigations have also shown that pneumorids possess multiple ears of two distinct morphological types (van Staaden and Römer, 1998; van Staaden et al., 2003).

These characteristics are highly improbable in an insect only 5 cm long and completely lacking tympana. This is what makes these creatures so interesting. In this chapter we address the unique auditory world of the bladder grasshoppers and in the tradition of von Uexküll (1934), attempt the salutary task of trying to "think oneself" into the *Umwelt* of another species (Bekoff, 2000).

Auditory Cues that Identify Mates

Mature male bladder grasshoppers are responsible for initiating pair formation by duetting and phonotaxis. They solicit an interaction by repeating a simple, stereotyped, high-intensity call at intervals upward of 4 s, and by flying distances up to 500 m between calls. An acoustic response from a philopatric female elicits more directed male movement and ends in pairing, with no apparent courtship behavior or contribution from other sensory modalities.

In a typical pneumorid, for instance, *Bullacris membracioides*, the male call consists of five short, "noisy" syllables and a sixth long, resonant syllable centered at 1.7 kHz (range 1.58–2.05 kHz; figure 11.1a). The first and second harmonics occur at about 3.4 and 5.1 kHz, attenuated by about 20 and 30 dB, respectively, relative to the carrier frequency and quality factor $Q_{-10\,dB}$ = 4.1–4.6. Signal intensity is high [98 dB sound pressure level (SPL) at 1 m], with the SPL of the introductory syllables attenuated 20 to 25 dB relative to the final note. Typically, receptive females respond with a low-intensity (60 dB SPL at 1 m) and variable series of 1–8 syllables (figure 11.1b). This call has a narrow frequency spectrum (3–11 kHz) with maximum energy between 5 and 7 kHz, a short duration (range 130–175 ms), and a response window within 860 ms of the end of the male's call (range 720–860 ms).

Auditory Cues that Identify Conspecifics

Male mate location calls are species-specific, with a fixed structure of one to six syllables, with the exception of those made by *Pneumora inanis*, in which a fifth syllable may be repeated for several minutes (figure 11.2). The final syllables range in length from 266 to 3800 ms (mean ± S.D. = 988.5 ± 1085) and are always resonant. With the possible exception of *B. membracioides*, the shape of the final syllable has a linear or exponential rise and a relatively sharp decay. Carrier frequencies range from 1.4 to

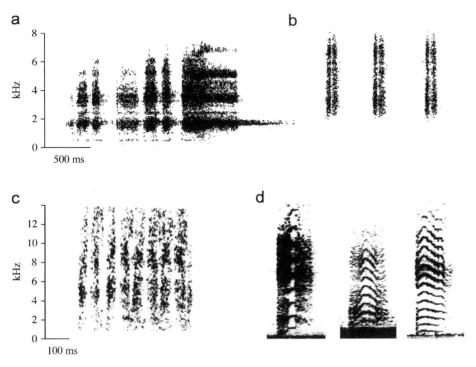

Figure 11.1
Acoustic repertoire of *B. membracioides*: (*a*) Male mating call, (*b*) female response, (*c*) female disturbance call, and (*d*) oral sounds.

3.1 kHz, with potentially sympatric species differing by a minimum of 0.2 kHz and a maximum of 1.1 kHz.

In contrast to the species-specificity of the male signal, evidence suggests that female responses may not be so clearly distinguishable. In the field, males of sympatric *Physemacris variolosus* and *Bullacris discolor* both responded to a model female call given within 1 s of the male signal, simultaneously approaching the acoustic mimic. This is also true for sympatric *Pneumora inanis* and *B. serrata*, suggesting that for males at least, the specific mate recognition system is relatively unsophisticated. This indicates either that the responsibility for species recognition falls disproportionately on females, or that the male response is primarily dependent on temporal rather than frequency characteristics.

A particularly intriguing aspect of the acoustic world of bladder grasshoppers is the production of social "spacing signals," which are not yet well understood. The precise mechanism of sound production is not known, although the form of the calls suggests that some combination of stridulation and airflow is likely (figure 11.1d). Call characteristics are highly variable, and preliminary indications are that these signals

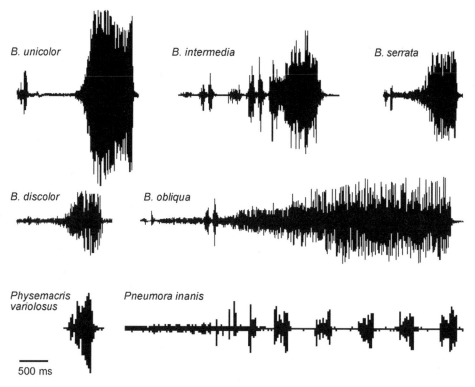

Figure 11.2
Interspecific variation (amplitude versus time displays) in male pair-formation calls of selected pneumorid taxa. With the exception of *P. inanis*, females respond at the end of the complete call as shown. The *P. inanis* call may consist of up to twenty repeated syllables (six shown), each of which generates a female response.

follow motivational-structural rules (Morton, 1975). These acoustic signals are produced by all individuals, but most commonly by nymphs and adult females, and presumably function to space out individuals in order to maintain effective crypsis. Accordingly, they have not been found in forest-living pneumorid species, such as *P. inanis*, which occur at lower densities than those occupying other biomes.

Auditory Cues That Signal Predators
When grasped by a predator, adult female pneumorids produce a sharp stridulation of high intensity that startles the predator, usually causing it to release the potential victim. The physical characteristics of this call are congruent with that of other insect disturbance sounds: a broadband, noisy signal consisting of a variable number of pulses, each about 70 ms in length (figure 11.1c).

The Grasshopper's Auditory System

In general, modern grasshoppers hear via tympanal sensory organs situated on either side of the body in the first abdominal segment. Diagnostic features include a thin membrane backed by a tracheal air space and connected to mechanoreceptors that transform mechanical energy into neural signals. Bladder grasshoppers, however, lack a specialized tympanic membrane but share homologous hearing organs of chordotonal sensilla and an air-filled sac of tracheal origin.

Abdominal Chordotonal Organs

Attached to the pleural cuticle of the first abdominal segment in *B. membracioides* is a large, pear-shaped chordotonal organ (figure 11.3b) composed of about 2000 sensory units. This is comparable to the number of sensory units in the cicada's auditory organ (Fonseca et al., 2000), but is substantially more than the 80–100 units found in the Müller's organ of locusts. The sensilla connect to the cuticle via two bundles of attachment cells that are 15 times longer than those in modern grasshoppers. The smaller bundle contains just thirty sensilla (indicated by the arrows in figure 11.3b, lower right). Small fiber bundles are seen within the organ, but except for the thin attachment, there is no clear anatomical separation, or any unique anatomical features within the organ.

At the ultrastructural level, the sensillum closely resembles the typical insect form. Each sensillum consists of a bipolar sensory-, scolopale-, attachment-, and glial cell. Distally, the sensory cell gives rise to a dendrite, which is surrounded by a Schwann cell. The basal body, situated at the top of the dendrite, is the beginning of the ciliary root that surrounds the basal body with finger-formed processes, and then runs along the dendrite to the soma, where it gives rise to several rootlets. The cilium, which has the typical 9 + 0 structure of an insect sensory cilium, is placed in an extracellular canal maintained by rods within the scolopale cell. The rods are connected to each other, forming a cylinder at the edges, whereas five to seven rods remain separated in the midregion. The cilium protrudes to the scolopale cap, an extracellular structure consisting of fenestrated electron-dense material, at the tip of the scolopale cell. At the proximal end, a long attachment cell surrounds the scolopale cap, to which it is tightly attached by desmosomes. These cells contain densely packed microtubuli and very long nuclei; they are interconnected by desmosomes and are tightly anchored to the epidermis.

Serial Chordotonal Organs

In addition to the chordotonal organ in the first abdominal segment, pneumorid grasshoppers are uniquely endowed with an additional five pairs of pleural chordotonal organs, one each in abdominal segments A2 to A6 (figure 11.3c). These fine strands are closely associated with air sacs emerging from longitudinally oriented trachea, and contain a maximum of eleven sensory cells stretched between the sternal apodeme and an attachment site on the lateral body wall. In *B. membracioides* there

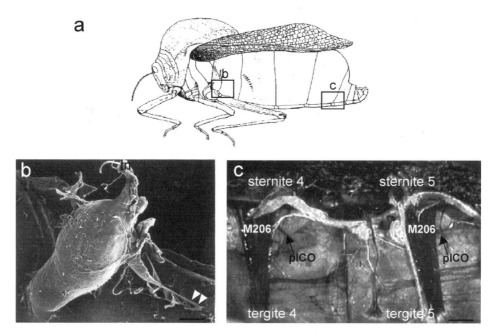

Figure 11.3
Location (*a*) and internal (*b*), (*c*) views of serial hearing organs in a typical pneumorid, *B. membracioides*. (*b*) Scanning electron micrograph of the ear in the first abdominal segment. The arrows (lower right) indicate the small bundle of attachment cells. (*c*) Light microscope view of pleural chordotonal hearing organs 4 and 5 (muscle labeled M206). Scale bars: 200 μm in (*b*) and 5 mm in (*c*).

is a significant decrease in the length of these pleural chordotonal organs from anterior to posterior (range 0.8–2.5 mm). While the functional significance of this trend is not known, it is interesting to note that it mirrors the pattern of neurophysiological sensitivity for this array of ears (van Staaden and Römer, 1998).

Physiological Responses of Chordotonal Organs to Sound

Pneumorid hearing is among the most sensitive known for grasshoppers. At its best frequency of 4 kHz, those in abdominal segment A1 have average thresholds of 20 dB SPL, whereas those in A2–A6 have mean thresholds ranging from 60 to 76 dB SPL at 1.5–2 kHz (figure 11.3). While the latter would generally be considered inordinately high intensities (and low frequencies) for organs to be characterized as functional ears, they are within a biologically meaningful range in the case of *B. membracioides*. The absence of an overt tympanum appears to have no adverse effect on hearing sensitivity, and the intuitively appealing idea of the entire inflated male abdomen acting as a tympanum is patently untrue, since there is no significant sex difference in the auditory thresholds of segments A2–A6 and only minor differences in the absolute sensitivity of A1 at 4 kHz (inflated males 12.8 ± 4.9 dB SPL; alternative males 18 SPL; and females 18 SPL). Some variation in hearing thresholds is introduced by the age and reproductive status of females and morph status in males, with older females and alternative males having lower sensitivity. How the high sensitivity of bladder grasshoppers is achieved is currently not known. However, microscanning laser Doppler vibrometry does show the highest levels of vibrations of the body wall at 4 kHz at the A1 attachment site (D. Robert, M. J. van Staaden, and H. Römer, unpublished results).

Although behavioral playback experiments indicate that the complete temporal structure of the male call is unnecessary to elicit a behavioral response from females, this information is available to the nervous system. When stimulated at the appropriate suprathreshold intensities, spike discharges of the pleural chordotonal organs faithfully represent the temporal song pattern of the male signal.

A striking feature in the neurophysiology of bladder grasshopper hearing is the apparent mismatch between receptors in segment A1 that are best tuned to frequencies of 4 kHz, and the carrier frequency of the male call (1.5–2 kHz; figure 11.4). Such a mismatch is not unique in "primitive" taxa (Mason and Bailey, 1998; Mason et al., 1999), but we may speculate as to its significance in this particular case, where there are multiple signals and ears. Given that tuning of the pleural chordotonal organs in segments A2–A6 matches the species-specific male signal, we can speculate whether these auditory clusters (Yager, 1990) are driven by different selective forces. Perhaps those in A2–A6 evolved to detect intense low-frequency male calls and those in A1 to detect the softer, higher-frequency female calls. Moreover, there could conceivably be a frequency range fractionation beyond that provided by the two types of hearing organ.

Frequency fractionation within the approximately 2000 sensory cells of the hearing organ is an intriguing possibility, particularly in light of recent findings that in cicadas interneurons are sharply tuned to different frequencies, although the recordings of summed action potentials from the afferent nerve show a uniform tuning to low frequencies between 3 and 6 kHz (Fonseca et al., 2000). Although morphological separation of axons into fiber bundles supports this type of functional grouping, there is neither physiological nor behavioral evidence to suggest that pneumorids can finely discriminate different frequencies. In playback experiments, males respond to crude acoustic models across a broad frequency range in an appropriate temporal response window; females respond to any signals of sufficient intensity across the hearing range (M. J. van Staaden, unpublished results). Single-fiber recordings of auditory afferents or interneurons are required to resolve this issue.

The range fractionation observed in the pleural chordotonal organs of pneumorids is a common principle in sensory systems (M. J. Cohen, 1964). Although we do not know why the anterior pleural chordotonal organ is more sensitive than the more posterior ones, the correlation between sensitivity and the length of the pleural chordotonal organs points to a mechanical basis for range fractionation, as reported for the

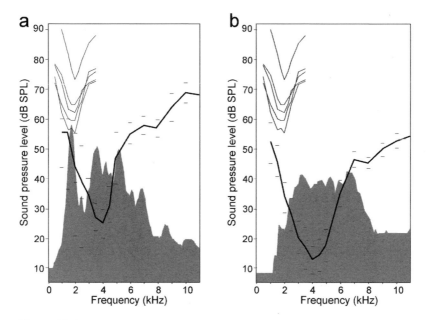

Figure 11.4
Power spectra of pair-formation signals (shaded areas) and neurophysiological tuning curves (A1, heavy line; A2–A6, fine line) for a receiver of the opposite sex. (*a*) Male sender, female receiver; (*b*) female sender, male receiver. The bars indicate the response range (*n* = 10 individuals).

proprioreceptive femoral chordotonal organ in the locust hind leg (Field, 1991; Shelton et al., 1992).

Exteroreceptive Functions of the Chordotonal Organ Receptors

Bilateral ablation of the chordotonal organ in the first abdominal segment has demonstrated conclusively that the pleural organs in pneumorid grasshoppers serve as far-distance exteroreceptors (van Staaden and Römer, 1998). However, given their location in the pleural fold, one might anticipate that pneumorid pleural chordotonal organs have an additional proprioceptive function, such as that of the locust prothoracic cervicosternite chordotonal organ, which combines features of both proprioreceptive mechanoreceptors and hearing organs (Pflüger and Field, 1999). Simultaneous neurophysiological and laser vibrometry measurements detected no correlated activity of the pleural chordotonal organ receptors and ventilatory movement of the tergite in the absence of sound (van Staaden and Römer, 1998). The receptor response was found, however, to be modulated by ventilation during acoustic stimulation, with maximal sensitivity at inspiration when the pleural folds and chordotonal organ strand were stretched.

Although acoustic response is reduced by about 15 dB during expiration, potentially rendering the processing of signals too noisy for reliable detection or discrimination, the reliability and low variance in the acoustic behavior of females responding to calls of different sound pressure levels indicates otherwise (van Staaden and Römer, 1998). Acoustically interacting insects may stop or reduce the amount and/or frequency of ventilation. Pleural chordotonal organs are thus well suited for detecting sounds of potential mates and rivals, although a proprioceptive response may still be possible in other behavioral contexts, such as egg deposition.

Central Nervous System Auditory Projection Patterns

The afferent projections from the tympanal nerve in grasshoppers have been described in detail by several authors (Rehbein, 1976; Riede et al., 1990; K. Jacobs et al., 1999), and more recent efforts have outlined afferent projections from the serially homologous abdominal pleural organs (Hustert, 1978; Prier, 1999; Prier and Boyan, 2000). The projection patterns in *B. membracioides* are not significantly different from those described in other grasshoppers. In the pneumorids, the afferent projection of pleural chordotonal organ afferents from segments A1 to A3, and the more extensive survey by Prier and Boyan (2000) on afferent projections of locust pleural, tympanal, or wing hinge chordotonal organs, have shown that they all arborize in areas of neuropils, such as the ring tract (RT) and the ventral association center (VAC). This projection pattern is a feature of chordotonal organ afferents in all tympanate and several atympanate insects (Boyan, 1993).

The A2–A6 pleural chordotonal organs of females are sufficient to produce a normal response to the male call following ablation of the A1 organ (van Staaden and Römer, 1998). That the few low-frequency receptors in pleural chordotonal organs drive behavior more strongly than the many higher-frequency receptors in segment A1 implies some form of temporal and/or spatial integration at the neuronal level of the auditory pathway—that each low-frequency neuron "speaks more loudly" to the central neural circuits (Pollack and Imaizumi, 1999). In a systematic survey of synaptic inputs of afferents into identified interneurons in the locust, Prier and Boyan (2000) found a convergence of synaptic input into auditory interneurons, and a similar spatial summation may account for the graded acoustic responses observed in the behavior of pneumorid females.

Hearing-Related Behaviors

Female Assessment of Male Separation Distance

As is frequently and understandably the case, stimulus thresholds for behavior are higher than neurophysiological thresholds in *B. membracioides*. For instance, although adult females hear males call at 32 dB SPL, they do not respond until male call intensity reaches 65 dB SPL. This corresponds closely with the neurophysiological threshold of the A2 pleural chordotonal organ, and in playback experiments, the response is elicited much more reliably by pure tones of 2 kHz than 4 kHz. This behavioral tuning strongly suggests that female response is mediated by the chordotonal ears in segments A2–A6. The high SPL of the male call and appropriately tuned pleural receptors means that pleural chordotonal organs can respond at considerable sender-receiver distances. The distance-response functions for pleural chordotonal organs indicate mean activation distances in the field ranging from 80 m for A2 to 10 m for A6 (figure 11.5). Decreasing distance activates receptors more strongly according to both their intensity response function and the attenuation properties of the transmission channel. Consequently, the number of pleural organs activated and the amount of activation within each one provides a calling male with reliable sensory information about a female's distance and constitutes an elementary ranging mechanism.

Male Modulation of Sound Production Levels

In a laboratory situation, males call at a constant intensity of 98–100 dB SPL. However, observations of male calling and phonotactic behavior in the field reveal that this is not always the case, at least not once the males are within the transmission range of a receptive female. As males approach the female, there is a conspicuous downregulation of sound output. This decrease in the active space of the male signal presumably reduces predation risk, and/or competition from conspecifics, particularly from

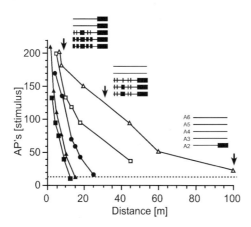

Figure 11.5
Distance-response functions of the discharge of pleural chordotonal organs in segments A2–A6 in response to a male calling song, recorded in a single female (A2, open triangle; A3, open square; A4, solid circle; A5, solid triangle; A6, solid square). The dashed line represents the mean spontaneous activity in all five organs. The arrows and signal ideograms indicate the relative sensory activity of the organs at detection distances (intersection with dashed line) of 100, 30, and 8 m. The male's distance from a female is thus encoded, at least partly, in the output of this hearing organ array.

the alternative male morphs. The decrease in intensity occurs at a distance corresponding to the threshold of the A6 organ, but awaits experimental verification of both the underlying sensory factors and the effect of the corresponding reduction in female response on the efficiency of male phonotactic performance.

Sex Differences in Sound Transmission Range

Social signals, including disturbance calls, are produced predominantly by females in response to predators or to males attempting unwelcome copulation. The mechanism of producing a disturbance sound is a simple stridulation. With the pronotum held at a high angle, the wings are moved rapidly back and forth across the surface of the abdomen, so that teeth-bearing veins on the ventral wing margins contact small pegs in a differentiated region of the tergum. The precise area of contact varies with arousal level. At lower levels it is more lateral and at higher levels it is more dorsal.

Males produce species-specific sexual signals using a power multiplier mechanism in the form of a scraper on the hind leg and a ribbed file located laterally on an inflated abdominal resonator. Species vary in the precise form and number of scraper and file elements, but all tend to be highly symmetrical. In *B. membracioides*, a row of eighteen to twenty-five strong, transverse ridges sitting atop a short, high carina on the proximal side of the hind femur make contact with a file of eight to nine strongly sclerotized ridges on the second abdominal tergite. Impact is spread across the permanently inflated bladder surface, which has a maximal vibration velocity matching the carrier frequency of the male call (1.7 kHz; range 1.6–2.1 kHz) and results in a sound output of 98 dB SPL at 1 m.

In females, by contrast, there is interspecific variation in the mechanism by which sexual signals are produced. In eight of nine observed taxa, responsive females use wing-abdominal stridulation to signal acoustically. The mechanism is similar to that used for disturbance signals, but wing movement is reduced by up to eight repetitions, and contact is made only in the opening phase. Female *Pneumora inanis* are exceptional in using an elytro-leg mechanism, in which the teeth on the edges of the veins of the ventral wing surface contact a rudimentary stridulatory scraper on the proximal surface of the hind leg. *P. inanis* is a forest-dwelling species and presumably represents a derived form for the family.

Factors Affecting Sound Transmission

The consequences of sound transmission over long distances have been fairly well framed by experimental studies (Wiley and Richards, 1978; Wiley, 1991). Physical objects and atmospheric turbulence combine to produce overall attenuation, frequency-dependent attenuation, reverberation, and amplitude fluctuations in acoustic signal transmission (Piercy et al., 1977). In addition to anatomical and neurophysiological adaptations for signal transmission, exploitation of optimal meteorological conditions enhances signal transmission in pneumorids (van Staaden and Römer, 1997).

In a typical pneumorid savanna habitat, temperature decreases with height above the ground surface, creating thermal gradients from midmorning to midafternoon, with moderate turbulent mixing and significant surface wind greater than 7 m/s. A strong temperature inversion occurs shortly after sunset, creating stable conditions with winds less than 2 m/s. Under such conditions, variability in the standard pressure level of a call is lower; both male calls and female responses suffer little or no excess attenuation and attain maximal broadcast areas of 11.3 km^2 and 0.078 km^2, respectively (van Staaden and Römer, 1997).

The significance of this behavior for aspects of signaling other than intensity depends crucially on a more detailed knowledge of the insect's sensory capacity. Few studies of sound transmission have measured the components of degradation in ways that reveal how they might be perceived by a receiver, with signal degradation quantified variously as overall attenuation, frequency-dependent attenuation, reverberation, amplitude fluctuations, or a composite of these (T. J. Brown and Handford, 2000; Naguib and Wiley, 2001).

Although we know that some receivers can attend separately to these different kinds of degradation (Nelson and Stoddard, 1998), we do not know how, or indeed whether, they integrate the different kinds of information. In order to gain insight into how changes in acoustic structure are likely to be perceived and to assess which components of degradation are relevant for pneumorids, we need to measure each of these parameters separately and assess whether their frequency and temporal resolution is adequate to utilize the levels of frequency-dependent attenuation, amplitude fluctuations, and reverberation contained in the natural signals.

Background Noise

Levels of masking noise are known to be relatively high in certain habitats and may result in temporal or spatial segregation, call inhibition, and other behavioral responses (Gogala and Riede, 1995; M. D. Greenfield, 1988; Narins, 1995; Römer et al., 1989).

In the Pneumoridae, competition for airtime derives from both conspecific and heterospecific sources and in general is more severe for pneumorid females, which are unable to change their location. Males, in contrast, could avoid nearby masking sounds by simply flying to another receiver position. Although in the savanna habitat of *B. membracioides* there is no heterospecific sound competition below 2 kHz, the detection of conspecific calls may be seriously compromised by masking noise from a variety of nocturnal cricket species. With song duty cycles of 15–90% and call power spectra from 2 to 6 kHz, these interfere with signal detection since the sensitivity of the pneumorid A1 hearing organ is centered at 4 kHz (van Staaden and Römer, 1997). The background noise level from heterospecifics is extremely irregular in time and space, and determination of its impact will depend substantially on the relative importance and utility of the two forms of hearing organs; i.e., on the extent to which communication depends on the A1 ear.

The Auditory World of the Pneumorid Grasshopper

Differences exist in the sensory perception and, most notably, the transmission distance of the calls of male and female bladder grasshoppers. Hence there are sex differences in the pneumorid's perceptual worlds. Field experiments show that both male and female calls suffer little excess attenuation, or none. However, whereas males achieve a transmission distance of 2 km, the lower broadcast SPL of the female call (60 dB SPL at 1 m) results in a transmission distance of less than 100 m. Given the male hearing threshold of 29.1 dB SPL (van Staaden and Römer, 1997) to the female response, the estimated effective detection distance for the male is only 50 m.

Although the overall form of the male signal is fixed, variation exists in both call length and frequency (according to size) among species. The amplitude of the male call is also variable and is controllable. Whereas males are able to control signal amplitude but not form, the converse is true for females. Playback experiments reveal that variation in the number of syllables per female response depends on the intensity (but not the temporal structure) of the male call. We suggest that the differential tuning and sensitivity of the serial organs mediate this response, providing a ranging mechanism by which the competitive, mobile males locate responsive, flightless females (van Staaden and Römer, 1997).

Laboratory playback experiments indicate significant behavioral tuning to song models of 1.7 kHz, supporting the role of organs A2–A6 in the differential female response. Combined ablation and playback experiments in a naturalistic setting provide more direct evidence for this mechanism and suggest that the neural basis of hearing and sound localization may be asymmetric in bladder grasshopper males and females. Moreover, strong selection on the female response threshold is constrained by her small transmission distance.

The Bias Toward Same-Sex Conspecifics

Sex-specific differences in the transmission distance of signals (40 times greater for males), but not of hearing, result in perceptual worlds biased toward same-sex conspecifics. Whereas inflated males hear even distant male competitors, the female's acoustic world is dominated by the defensive, spacing, and mating calls of her nearby sisters. Moreover, females appear to be more selective in response to the male signals they hear. As noted earlier, females respond only when the male signal intensity exceeds 65 dB SPL, perhaps distinguishing between those within and those beyond their own acoustic transmission range.

The existence of an alternative male morph in at least two pneumorid species poses an exception to this bias (M. J. van Staaden, unpublished results). Alternative males constitute less than 5% of the population and produce no mate location calls, but their ears are similarly tuned to the frequency of the primary male call, with just a minor dropoff in sensitivity (van Staaden et al., 2003). Since both females and alternatives are flightless and restricted to the same food plant, these males live among a predictable abundance of females who are more or less confined in seraglios at the site where the males mature (Hamilton, 1979).

Genetic analyses show that alternative males are significantly more closely related to the females they were caught with than to randomly selected females from the same population (M. J. van Staaden, unpublished results). The evolutionary cost of such seraglios would therefore be some degree of inbreeding. Because alternative males reside in the near vicinity of adult females, they are able to hear both primary males calling at a distance and the calls of receptive females nearby. Alternatives do use a female's response to locate her, but it is unclear as yet whether they capitalize on the distance information contained in her call and their proximity, to reach the female ahead of the primary male (N. Donelson, personal communication).

The Question of Mate Choice

It is not known whether female response to males is a decision-making process, or simply a reflex when a case reaches a high enough amplitude (65 dB). In other words, it is not yet clear whether females are exercising a mating preference by selectively responding to the most desirable signals or if they are responding to every male that is in close proximity. Playback experiments indicate that the complete multisyllabic male call is unnecessary to elicit a female response. Female responses to simple models of the male call with single syllables that exceed a 200-ms duration indicate that there is no internal temporal-acoustic template of the complete male call that must be matched for specific mate recognition to occur. Female age and gravidity status are factors that may be expected to cause variation in the female response threshold.

Evolution through sexual selection may well have forced males to produce an increasingly intense signal. Since the decrease in SPL of the male calling song is rather flat at large distances, a small increase in effective transmission results in a relatively large increase in broadcast range. Certainly, in species with more vagile females, differential attraction to louder male calling songs is quite common (see review by Ryan and Keddy-Hector, 1992), and field studies of mole crickets demonstrated that males calling 2 dB below the loudest male attracted fewer females than the average male (Forrest and Green, 1991).

Selection Pressures and Evolutionary Transitions

Natural selection operates at the level of the phenotype, which, in the case of the nervous system, is behavior. Because of the relationship between calling and reproductive success, singing insects are under selective pressure to optimize the range, while maintaining the specificity, of their calls. The major selection pressure shaping the pneumorid acoustic worldview appears to be the need to maximize call range. Male-male competition is likely to be a principal force driving the evolution of this signaling system, but we know that auditory pathways have a broader communicative function, subserving more than just reproductive behavior. The use of other social signals may impose constraints on receivers. Thus, while the design features of the pneumorid communication system are in accord with all expectations of natural selection to maximize broadcast range (Endler, 1992), the constraints imposed by predation as well as intraspecific competition and communication may be significant.

The Independence of Specialized Tympana and Auditory Organs

Pneumorids clearly demonstrate that conventional tympana are not a necessary condition for a highly sensitive auditory function. If pleural chordotonal organs are the ancestral condition for the detection of airborne sound in Pneumoridae, they would represent a preadaptation for the evolution of a long-distance male call. Completing the evolutionary transition to tympanal hearing would require either a simple increase in the range of detectable frequencies to ultrasound, and/or an increase in the sensitivity.

By linking experimental observations at the anatomical, physiological, and behavioral levels of analysis, studies of bladder grasshoppers provide evidence for the transition in receptor function from proprioception to exteroreception, as well as the selective advantage of evolving complex auditory structures. The number of sensilla in the posterior pleural chordotonal organs is similar in modern grasshoppers (10–15) and pneumorids, and it is not clear whether 2000 sensilla is the ancestral condition or is derived from mutations like those in the rhomboid or abdominal-A genes in *Drosophila*, which affect the number of sensilla in serial homologous organs (Meier et al., 1991). Moreoever, it remains to be investigated in a morphological comparison between insects completely deaf to airborne sound and the pleural chordotonal organs in *B. membracioides*, which parameters of the cuticle and association with the tracheal apparatus exactly turn a proprioreceptive chordotonal organ into a sound-detecting device, albeit with a reduced sensitivity.

The Effects of Directional Selection

Differential Female Responses   Selection cannot act to increase the amplitude of the female call without increasing thoracic muscle mass or resonator space and thereby reducing the resources available for reproduction. However, selection can easily increase information content through repetition and temporal patterning of the call, allowing females to be located more efficiently. There would be a strong selection pressure for females to respond only to sounds that are near enough for the sender to detect the response. A 60-m response distance in females is also the distance at which they might detect an as-yet-unidentified crucial parameter of the male signal.

Male Call Intensity   The relative dearth of information on bladder grasshoppers, despite even Darwin's promotional talents, is largely because they were considered refractory to experimental manipulation. Entering their perceptual world enables us to develop sensitive behavioral assays using ethologically appropriate stimuli, and promises much for unraveling both the proximate and ultimate questions about their sensory abilities. For instance, experiments in directional hearing using an apparent distance paradigm are now possible. In addition to helping us understand the basic neural organization of hearing systems, bladder grasshoppers are shedding light on broader issues regarding the evolution of sensory systems. For instance, the pneumorid's attention to certain specific features of its auditory world can produce reproductive isolation that gives us a starting point for a program to evaluate the mechanisms and genetic architecture of speciation.

Von Uexküll built mechanical devices to try to recreate the perceptual *Weltanschauungen* of his animal subjects. With virtual worlds now a reality, we could certainly do this at a more sophisticated level than was available to von Uexküll. However, whether this is more useful than looking directly at the animals themselves is debatable.

Perceptual systems evolve so as to be "transparent" to much of the variation within natural systems, yet the most deeply embedded evolutionary features of even simple percepts may require rather complex processing. As the pneumorids amply demonstrate, complex asymmetries can arise from very simple ears. Although many neuroanatomical and neurophysiological challenges remain, progress may best be achieved by an intense focus on behavioral studies to define the algorithms most likely to be used by the central nervous system (Gerhardt and Huber, 2002).

Acknowledgments

We thank the students and colleagues who collaborated on experiments in our laboratories and in the field. This material is based upon work supported by the National Science Foundation under grant 0091189 to MvS, and an Austrian Science Foundation (Östereichischen Fonds zur Förderung der Wissenschaftlichen Forschung) grant PO9523-BIO to HR.

References

Aho, A. C., Donner, K., Hyden, C., Larsen, L. O., and Reuter, T. (1988) Low retinal noise in animals with low body-temperature allows high visual sensitivity. *Nature* 334: 348–350.

Ahyong, S. T. and Harling, C. (2000) The phylogeny of the stomatopod Crustacea. *Aust. J. Zool.* 48: 607–642.

Alloway, T. M. (1972) Learning and memory in insects. *Ann. Rev. Entom.* 17: 43–56.

Altman, J. S. and Kien, J. (1986) A model for decision making in the insect nervous system. In M. A. Ali (ed.), *Nervous Systems in Invertebrates*. New York: Plenum, pp. 621–643.

Ameyaw-Akumfi, C. and Hazlett, B. A. (1975) Sex recognition in the crayfish *Procambarus clarkii*. *Science* 190: 1225–1226.

Anderson, C. W. (1993) Modulation of feeding behavior in response to prey type in the frog *Rana pipiens*. *J. Exp. Biol.* 179: 1–11.

Anderson, C. W. and Nishikawa, K. C. (1993) A prey-type dependent hypoglossal feedback system in the frog, *Rana pipiens*. *Brain Behav. Evol.* 42: 189–196.

Anderson, C. W. and Nishikawa, K. C. (1996) The roles of visual and proprioceptive information during motor program choice in frogs. *J. Comp. Physiol. A* 179: 753–762.

Anderson, C. W. and Nishikawa, K. C. (1997a) Sensory modulation and behavioral choice during feeding in the Australian frog, *Cyclorana novaehollandiae*. *J. Comp. Physiol. A* 180: 187–202.

Anderson, C. W. and Nishikawa, K. C. (1997b) The functional anatomy and evolution of hypoglossal afferents in the leopard frog, *Rana pipiens*. *Brain Res.* 771: 285–291.

Antal, M., Matsumoto, N., and Székely, G. (1986) Tectal neurons of the frog: Intracellular recording and labeling with cobalt electrodes. *J. Comp. Neurol.* 246: 238–253.

Arbib, M. A. (1987) Advantages of experimentation in neuroscience. *Behav. Brain Sci.* 10: 368–369.

Arbib, M. A. (1989) Visuomotor coordination: Neural models and perceptual robotics. In J.-P. Ewert and M. A. Arbib (eds.), *Visuomotor Coordination: Amphibians, Comparisons, Models and Robots*. New York: Plenum, pp. 121–171.

Arikawa, K. (1999) Color vision. In E. Eguchi and Y. Tominaga (eds.), *Atlas of Sensory Receptors of Arthropods—Dynamic Morphology in Relation to Function*. Tokyo: Springer-Verlag, pp. 23–32.

Arikawa, K. and Stavenga, D. G. (1997) Random array of colour filters in the eyes of butterflies. *J. Exp. Biol.* 200: 2501–2506.

Arikawa, K. and Kinoshita, M. (2000) Learning by microbrain—From the study of color vision in Papilio. In T. Kato (ed.), *Frontiers of the Mechanisms of Memory and Dementia*. Amsterdam: Elsevier, pp. 3–6.

Arikawa, K. and Uchiyama, H. (1996) Red receptors dominate the proximal tier of the retina in the butterfly *Papilio xuthus*. *J. Comp. Physiol. A* 178: 55–61.

Arikawa, K., Inokuma, K., and Eguchi, E. (1987) Pentachromatic visual system in a butterfly. *Naturwissenschaften* 74: 297–298.

Arikawa, K., Mizuno, S., Scholten, D. G. W., Kinoshita, M., Seki, T., Kitamoto, J., and Stavenga, D. G. (1999a) An ultraviolet absorbing pigment causes a narrow-band violet receptor and a single-peaked green receptor in the eye of the butterfly *Papilio*. *Vision Res.* 39: 1–8.

Arikawa, K., Scholten, D. G. W., Kinoshita, M., and Stavenga, D. G. (1999b) Tuning of photoreceptor spectral sensitivities by red and yellow pigments in the butterfly *Papilio xuthus*. *Zool. Sci.* 16: 17–24.

Aronson, R. B. (1991) Ecology, paleobiology and evolutionary constraint in the octopus. *Bull. Mar. Sci.* 49: 245–255.

Atema, J. (1985) Chemoreceptors in the sea: Adaptations of chemoreceptors and behaviour to aquatic stimulus conditions. *Symp. Soc. Exp. Biol.* 39: 387–423.

Autrum, H. (1950) Die Belichtungspotentiale und das Sehen der Insekten (Untersuchungen an *Calliphora* und *Dixippus*). *Z. Vergl. Physiol.* 32: 176–227.

Autrum, H. and Stöcker, M. (1952) Über optische Verschmelzungsfrequenzen und stroboskopisches Sehen bei Insekten. *Biol. Zentr.* 71: 129–152.

Autrum, H. and von Zwehl, V. (1964) Die spektrale Empfindlichkeit einzelner Sehzellen des Bienenauges. *Z. Vergl. Physiol.* 48: 357–384.

Baba, Y. and Shimozawa, T. (1997) Diversity of motor responses initiated by a wind stimulus in the freely moving cricket, *Gryllus bimaculatus*. *Zool. Sci.* 14: 587–594.

Backhaus, W. (1991) Color opponent coding in the visual system of the honeybee. *Vison Res.* 31: 1381–1397.

Backhaus, W. (1992a) Colour vision in honeybees. *Neurosci. Biobehav. Rev.* 16: 1–12.

Backhaus, W. (1992b) The Bezold-Brücke effect in the color vision system of the honeybee. *Vision Res.* 32: 1425–1431.

Backhaus, W. and Menzel, R. (1987) Color distance derived from a receptor model of color vision in the honeybee. *Biol. Cybern.* 55: 321–331.

Bacon, J. P. (1980) An homologous interneurone in a locust, a cricket and a mantid. *Verh. Dtsch. Zool. Ges.* 73: 300.

Bacon, J. P. and Murphey, R. K. (1984) Receptive fields of cricket (*Acheta domesticus*) interneurones are related to their dendritic structure. *J. Physiol. Lond.* 352: 601–623.

Baddeley, A. (1993) *Your Memory: A User's Guide*. London: Penguin.

Baerends, G. P. (1987) Ethology and physiology: A happy marriage. *Behav. Brain Sci.* 10: 369–370.

Bandai, K., Arikawa, K., and Eguchi, E. (1992) Localization of spectral receptors in the ommatidium of butterfly compound eye determined by polarization sensitivity. *J. Comp. Physiol. A* 171: 289–297.

Banschbach, V. S. (1994) Colour association influences honey bee choice between sucrose concentrations. *J. Comp. Physiol. A* 175: 107–114.

Bardach, J. E. and Villars, T. (1974) The chemical senses of fishes. In P. T. Grant and A. M. Mackie (eds.), *Chemoreception in Marine Organisms*. London: Academic Press, pp. 49–104.

Barlow, H. B. (1953) Summation and inhibition in the frog's retina. *J. Physiol. Lond.* 119: 69–88.

Barlow, H. B. (1982) What causes trichromacy? A theoretical analysis using comb-filtered spectra. *Vison Res.* 22: 635–643.

Barnes, R. D. (1987) *Invertebrate Zoology*, 5th ed. Philadelphia, Pa.: Saunders.

Barth, F. G. (1985) Slit sensilla and the measurement of cuticular strains. In F. G. Barth (ed.), *Neurobiology of Arachnids*. Berlin: Springer-Verlag, pp. 162–188.

Barth, F. G., Wastl, U., Humphrey, J. A. C., and Devarakonda, R. (1993) Dynamics of arthropod filiform hairs. II. Mechanical properties of spider trichobothria (*Cupiennius salei* Keys.). *Phil. Trans. Roy. Soc. Lond. B* 340: 445–461.

Bartley, J. A. (1983) Prey selection and capture by the Chinese mantid (*Tenodera sinensis*, Saussure). Ph.D. dissertation, Univ. of Delaware, Newark, Delaware.

Baumann, F., Mauro, A., Milecchia, R., Nightingale, S., and Young, J. Z. (1970) The extraocular light receptors of the squids *Todarodes* and *Illex*. *Brain Res.* 21: 275–279.

Bekoff, M. (2000) Animal emotions: Exploring passionate natures. *Bioscience* 50: 861–870.

Belisle, C. and Cresswell, J. (1997) The effects of limited memory capacity on foraging behavior. *Theoret. Pop. Biol.* 52: 78–90.

Bennett, A. T. and Cuthill, I. C. (1994) Ultraviolet vision in birds: What is its function? *Vison Res.* 34: 1471–1478.

Berger, F. A. (1985) Morphologie und physiologie einiger visueller interneuronen in den optischen ganglien der gottesanbeterin *Mantis religiosa*. Doctoral dissertation, University of Düsseldorf, Düsseldorf, Germany.

Bernard, G. D. (1979) Red-absorbing visual pigment of butterflies. *Science* 203: 1125–1127.

Bernard, G. D. and Miller, W. H. (1970) What does antenna engineering have to do with insect eyes? *IEEE Stud. J.* 8: 2–8.

Bernard, G. D. and Remington, C. L. (1991) Color vision in Lycaena butterflies: Spectral tuning of receptor arrays in relation to behavioral ecology. *Proc. Natl. Acad. Sci. U.S.A.* 88: 2783–2787.

Bernard, G. D. and Wehner, R. (1977) Functional similarities between polarization vision and color vision. *Vison Res.* 17: 1019–1028.

Bernard, G. D., Douglas, J., and Goldsmith, T. H. (1988) Far-red sensitive visual pigment of a metalmark butterfly. *Invest. Ophthalmol. Suppl.* 29: 350.

Bernhards, H. (1916) Der bau des komplexauges von astacus fluviatilis (*Potamobius astacus* L.). Ein beitrag zur morphologie der decapoden. *Z. Wiss. Zool.* 114: 649–707.

Besharse, J. C. and Iuvone, P. M. (1992) Is dopamine a light-adaptive or a dark-adaptive modulator in retina? *Science* 216: 1250–1252.

Bieger, D. and Neuman, R. S. (1984) Selective accumulation of hydroxytryptamines by frogs' tectal neurons. *Neuroscience* 12: 1167–1177.

Binns, E. E. (1999) The synaptic pharmacology underlying sensory processing in the superior colliculus. *Neurobiology* 59: 129–159.

Bitterman, M. E. (1986) Vertebrate-invertebrate comparisons. In H. J. Jerison and I. Jerison (eds.), *Intelligence and Evolutionary Biology*. NATO Advanced Study Institute on Evolutionary Biology of Intelligence (Popi, Italy), Berlin: Springer-Verlag, pp. 251–276.

Blest, A. D. (1983) Ultrastructure of secondary retinae of primitive and advanced jumping spiders (Araneae, Salticidae). *Zoomorphology* 102: 125–41.

Blest, A. D. (1985a) The fine structure of spider photoreceptors in relation to function. In F. G. Barth (ed.), *Neurobiology of Arachnids*. Berlin: Springer-Verlag, pp. 79–102.

Blest, A. D. (1985b) Retinal mosaics of the principal eyes of jumping spiders (Salticidae) in some neotropical habitats: Optical trade-offs between sizes and habitat illuminances. *J. Comp. Physiol. A* 157: 391–404.

Blest, A. D. (1987a) Comparative aspects of the retinal mosaics of jumping spiders. In A. P. Gupta (ed.), *Arthropod Brain: Its Evolution, Development, Structure and Function*. New York: Wiley, pp. 203–229.

Blest, A. D. (1987b) The retinae of *Euryattus bleekeri*, an aberrant salticid spider from Queensland. *J. Zool. Lond.* 211: 399–408.

Blest, A. D. and Land, M. F. (1977) The physiological optics of *Dinopis subrufus* L. Koch: A fish-lens in a spider. *Proc. Roy. Soc. Lond. B* 196: 197–222.

Blest, A. D. and Price, G. D. (1984) Retinal mosaics of the principal eyes of some jumping spiders (Salticidae: Araneae): Adaptations for high visual acuity. *Protoplasma* 120: 72–84.

Blest, A. D., Hardie, R. C., McIntyre, P., and Williams, D. S. (1981) The spectral sensitivities of identified receptors and the function of retinal tiering in the principal eyes of jumping spiders. *J. Comp. Physiol.* 145: 227–239.

Boal, J. G. and Golden, D. K. (1999) Distance chemoreception in the common cuttlefish, *Sepia officinalis* (Mollusca, Cephalopoda). *J. Exp. Mar. Biol. Ecol.* 235: 307–317.

Bond, A. B. (1983) Visual search and selection of natural stimuli in the pigeon: The attentional threshold hypothesis. *J. Exp. Psychol. Anim. Behav. Process.* 9: 292–306.

Borchers, H.-W. and Ewert, J.-P. (1979) Correlation between behavioral and neuronal activities of toads *Bufo bufo* (L.) in response to moving configurational prey stimuli. *Behav. Processes* 4: 99–106.

Borchers, H.-W., Burghagen, H., and Ewert, J.-P. (1978) Key stimuli of prey for toads (*Bufo bufo* L.): Configuration and movement patterns. *J. Comp. Physiol.* 128: 189–192.

Bowdish, T. I. and Bultman, T. L. (1993) Visual cues used by mantids in learning aversion to aposematically colored prey. *Am. Midl. Nat.* 129: 215–222.

Bowmaker, J. K. (1980) Colour vision in birds and the role of oil droplets. *Trends Neurosci.* 199: 196–199.

Bowmaker, J. K. (1983) Trichromatic colour vision: why only three receptor channels? *Trends Neurosci.* 6: 41–43.

Boyan, G. S. (1993) Another look at insect audition: The tympanic receptors as an evolutionary specialization of the chordotonal system. *J. Insect. Physiol.* 39: 187–200.

Boyan, G. S. and Ball, E. E. (1986) Wind-sensitive interneurones in the terminal ganglion of praying mantids. *J. Comp. Physiol. A* 159: 773–789.

Boyan, G. S. and Ball, E. E. (1989) The wind-sensitive cercal receptor/giant interneurone system of the locust, *Locusta migratoria*. II. Physiology of giant interneurones. *J. Comp. Physiol. A* 165: 511–521.

Boyan, G. S., Williams, J. L. D., and Ball, E. E. (1989) The wind-sensitive cercal receptor/giant interneurone system of the locust, *Locusta migratoria*. I. Anatomy of the system. *J. Comp. Physiol. A* 165: 539–552.

Boyle, P. R. (1977) Receptor units responding to movement in the octopus mantle. *J. Exp. Biol.* 65: 1–9.

Bradley, E. A. and Young, J. Z. (1975) Comparison of visual and tactile learning in Octopus after lesions to one of the two memory systems. *J. Neurosci. Res.* 1: 185–205.

Brandao, M. L., Anseloni, V. Z., Pandossio, J. E., De Araujo, J. E., and Castilho, V. M. (1999) Neurochemical mechnisms of the defensive behavior in the dorsal midbrain. *Neurosci. Biobehav. Rev.* 23: 863–875.

Breithaupt, T., Schmitz, B., and Tautz, J. (1995) Hydrodynamic orientation of crayfish (*Procambaraus clarkii*) to swimming fish prey. *J. Comp. Physiol. A* 177: 481–491.

Bridges, C. D. B. (1972) The rhodopsin-porphyropsin visual system. In H. J. A. Dartnall (ed.), *Handbook of Sensory Physiology*. vol. VII/I, *The Photochemistry of Vision*. Berlin: Springer-Verlag, pp. 417–480.

Brines, M. L. and Gould, J. L. (1982) Skylight polarization patterns and animal orientation. *J. Exp. Biol.* 96: 69–91.

Briscoe, A. D. (2000) Six opsins from the butterfly *Papilio glaucus*: Molecular phylogenetic evidence for paralogous origins of red-sensitive visual pigments in insects. *J. Mol. Evol.* 51: 110–121.

Briscoe, A. D. and Chittka, L. (2001) The evolution of color vision in insects. *Ann. Rev. Entomol.* 46: 471–510.

Briscoe, A. D., Bernard, G. D., Szeto, A. S., Nagy, L. M., and White, R. H. (2003) Not all butterfly eyes are created equal: Rhodopsin absorption spectra, molecular identification and localization of UV-, blue- and green-sensitive rhodopsin encoding mRNA in the retina of *Vanessa cardui*. *J. Comp. Neurol.* 458: 334–349.

Bristowe, W. S. (1958) *The World of Spiders*. London: Collins.

Brodie, E. D. (1977) Hedgehogs use toad venom in their own defense. *Nature* 268: 627–628.

Brooke, R. K., Jr. (1975) A single-lens multiband camera. *Opt. Eng.* 14: 347–350.

Brower, J. V. Z. and Brower, L. P. (1962) Experimental studies of mimicry. 6: the reaction of toads (*Bufo terrestris*) to honey bees (*Apis mellifera*) and their dronefly mimics (*Eristalis vinetorum*). *Am. Naturalist* 96: 297–307.

Browman, H. I. and Hawryshyn, C. W. (2001) Biology of ultraviolet and polarization vision. *J. Exp. Biol.* 204: 2383–2596.

Brown, T. J. and Handford, P. (2000) Sound design for vocalizations: Quality in the woods, consistency in the fields. *The Condor* 102: 81–92.

Brown, W. T. and Marker, W. B. (1977) Unit responses in the frog's caudal thalamus. *Brain Behav. Evol.* 14: 274–297.

Bruce, L. L. and Neary, T. J. (1995) The limbic system of tetrapods: A comparative analysis of cortical and amygdalar populations. *Brain Behav. Evol.* 46: 224–234.

Bryceson, K. P. (1986) Short Communication. The effect of screening pigment migration on spectral sensitivity in a crayfish reflecting superposition eye. *J. Exp. Biol.* 125: 401–404.

Brzoska, J. and Schneider, H. (1978) Modification of prey-catching behavior by learning in the common toad (*Bufo b. bufo* L., Anura, Amphibia): Changes in response to visual objects and effects of auditory stimuli. *Behav. Processes* 3: 125–136.

Buchner, E. (1984) Behavioral analysis of spatial vision in insects. In M. A. Ali (ed.), *Photoreception and Vision in Invertebrates*. New York: Plenum, pp. 561–621.

Budelmann, B. U. (1994) Cephalopod sense organs, nerves and the brain: Adaptations for high performance and life style. *Mar. Freshwater Behav. Physiol.* 25: 13–33.

Budelmann, B. U. (1996) Active marine predators: The sensory world of cephalopods. *Mar. Freshwater Behav. Physiol.* 27: 59–75.

Budelmann, B. U. and Bleckmann, H. (1988) A lateral line analogue in cephalopods: Water waves generate microphonic potentials in the epidermal head lines of *Sepia* and *Lolliguncula*. *J. Comp. Physiol.* A 164: 1–5.

Budelmann, B. U. and Williamson, R. (1994) Directional sensitivity of hair cell afferents in the Octopus statocyst. *J. Exp. Biol.* 187: 245–259.

Budelmann, B. U. and Young, J. Z. (1984) The statocyst-oculomotor system of *Octopus vulgaris*: Extraocular eye muscles, eye muscle nerves, statocyst nerves and oculomotor centre of the central nervous system. *Phil. Trans. Roy. Soc. Lond.* B 306: 159–189.

Budelmann, B. U. and Young, J. Z. (1993) The oculomotor system of decapod cephalopods: Eye muscles, eye muscle nerves and the oculomotor neurons in the central nervous system. *Phil. Trans. Roy. Soc. Lond.* B 340: 93–125.

Budelmann, B. U., Sachse, M., and Staudigl, M. (1987) The angular acceleration receptor system of *Octopus vulgaris*: Morphometry, ultrastructure and neuronal and synaptic organization. *Phil. Trans. Roy. Soc. Lond.* B 315: 305–343.

Budelmann, B. U., Riese, U., and Bleckmann, H. (1991) Structure, function, biological significance of the cuttlefish "lateral lines". In E. Boucaud-Camou (ed.), *La Seiche. The Cuttlefish*. First International Symposium on the Cuttlefish, Sepia. Caen, June 1–3 1989. Caen, France: Institut de Bioclimie et de Biologie Appliquée, Université de Caen, pp. 201–209.

Budelmann, B. U., Schipp, R., and von Boletzky, S. (1997) Cephalopoda. In F. W. Harrison and A. J. Kohn (eds.), *Microscopic Anatomy of Invertebrates*. vol. 6A, *Mollusca II*. New York: Wiley-Liss, pp. 119–414.

Bult, R. and Mastebroek, H. A. K. (1994) Response characteristics of wide-field non-habituating non-directional motion-detecting neurons in the optic lobe of the locust, *Locusta migratoria*. *J. Comp. Physiol.* A 174: 723–729.

Buño, W., Chrispino, L., Monti-Bloch, L., and Mateos, A. (1981) Dynamic analysis of cockroach giant interneuron activity evoked by forced displacement of cercal thread-hair sensilla. *J. Neurobiol.* 12(6): 561–578.

Burdohan, J. A. and Comer, C. M. (1990) An antennal-derived mechanosensory pathway in the cockroach: Descending interneurons as a substrate for evasive behavior. *Brain Res.* 535: 347–352.

Burdohan, J. A. and Comer, C. M. (1996) Cellular organization of an antennal mechanosensory pathway in the cockroach *Periplaneta americana*. *J. Neurosci.* 16: 5830–5843.

Burghagen, H. and Ewert, J.-P. (1982) Question of "head preference" in response to worm-like dummies during prey-capture of toads *Bufo bufo*. *Behav. Processes* 7: 295–306.

Burghagen, H. and Ewert, J.-P. (1983) Influence of the background for discriminating object motion from self-induced motion in toads *Bufo bufo* (L.). *J. Comp. Physiol.* 152: 241–249.

Burkhardt, D. (1983) Wavelength perception and colour vision. *Symp. Soc. Exp. Biol.* 36: 371–397.

Burrows, M. (1996) *The Neurobiology of an Insect Brain*. London: Oxford Univ. Press.

Burrows, M. and Rowell, C. H. F. (1973) Connexions between descending visual interneurons and metathoracic motoneurons in the locust. *J. Comp. Physiol.* 85: 221–234.

Buxbaum-Conradi, H. and Ewert, J.-P. (1995) Pretecto-tectal influences I. What the toad's pretectum tells its tectum: An antidromic stimulation/recording study. *J. Comp. Physiol. A* 176: 169–180.

Buxbaum-Conradi, H. and Ewert, J.-P. (1999) Responses of single neurons in the toad's caudal ventral striatum to moving visual stimuli and test of their efferent projection by extracellular antidromic stimulation/recording techniques. *Brain Behav. Evol.* 54: 338–354.

Cakmak, I., Firatli, C., and Wells, H. (1998) The response of *Apis mellifera syriaca* and *A. m. armeniaca* to nectar differences. *Turk. J. Agri. Forestry* 22: 561–571.

Cakmak, I., Cook, P., Hollis, J., Shah, N., Huntley, D., van Valkenburg, D., and Wells, H. (1999) Africanized honey bee response to differences in reward frequency. *J. Apic. Res.* 38: 125–136.

Caldwell, R. L. and Dingle, H. (1975) Ecology and evolution of agonistic behavior in stomatopods. *Naturwissenschaften* 62: 214–222.

Caldwell, R. L. and Dingle, H. (1976) Stomatopods. *Sci. Am.* 234(1): 80–89.

Calkins, D. J. and Sterling, P. (1996) Absence of spectrally specific lateral inputs to midget ganglion cells in primate retina. *Nature* 381: 613–615.

Camhi, J. M. (1988) Escape behavior in the cockroach: Distributed neural processing. *Experientia* 44(5): 401–408.

Camhi, J. M. and Levy, A. (1989) The code for stimulus direction in a cell assembly in the cockroach. *J. Comp. Physiol.* 165: 83–97.

Camhi, J. M. and Nolen, T. (1981) Properties of the escape system of cockroaches during walking. *J. Comp. Physiol.* 142: 339–346.

Camhi, J. M. and Tom, W. (1978) The escape behavior of the cockroach *Periplaneta americana*. I. Turning response to wind puffs. *J. Comp. Physiol.* 128: 193–201.

Camhi, J. M., Tom, W., and Volman, S. (1978) The escape behavior of the cockroach *Periplaneta americana*. II. Detection of natural predators by air displacement. *J. Comp. Physiol.* 128: 203–212.

Carpenter, R. H. S. (1988) *Movements of the Eyes*. London: Pion.

Cavanagh, P. (1991) What's up in top-down processing? In A. Gorea (ed.), *Representation of Vision—Trend and Tacit Assumptions in Vision Research*. Cambridge: Cambridge Univ. Press, pp. 295–304.

Cervantes-Pérez, F. (1989) Schema theory as a common language to study sensori-motor coordination. In J.-P. Ewert and M. A. Arbib (eds.), *Visuomotor Coordination: Amphibians, Comparisons, Models and Robots*. New York: Plenum, pp. 421–450.

Chapman, A. M. and Debski, E. A. (1995) Neuropeptide Y immunoreactivity of a projection from the lateral thalamic nucleus to the optic tectum of the leopard frog. *Vison Neurosci.* 12: 1–9.

Chapuis, N. (1987) Detour and shortcut abilities in several species of mammals. In P. Ellen and C. Thinus-Blanc (eds.), *Cognitive Processes and Spatial Orientation in Animals and Man.* Dordrecht, Netherlands: Martinus Nijhoff, pp. 97–106.

Cheng, K., Collett, T. S., Pickhard, A., and Wehner, R. (1987) The use of visual landmarks by honeybees: Bees weight landmarks according to their distance from the goal. *J. Comp. Physiol. A* 161: 469–475.

Chevalier, G. and Deniau, J. M. (1990) Disinhibition as a basic process in the expression of striatal functions. *Trends Neurosci.* 13: 277–280.

Chiao, C. C. and Hanlon, R. T. (2001) Cuttlefish camouflage: Visual perception of size, contrast and number of white squares on artificial checkerboard substrata initiates disruptive coloration. *J. Exp. Biol.* 204: 2119–2467.

Chiao, C. C., Cronin, T. W., and Marshall, J. (2000) Eye design and color signaling in a stomatopod crustacean, *Gonodactylus smithii. Brain Behav. Evol.* 56: 107–122.

Chittka, L. (1992) The color hexagon: A chromaticity diagram based on photoreceptor excitations as a generalized representation of colour opponency. *J. Comp. Physiol. A* 170: 533–543.

Chittka, L. (1996) Optimal sets of color receptors and color opponent systems for coding of natural objects in insect vision. *J. Theor. Biol.* 181: 179–196.

Chittka, L. (1998) Sensorimotor learning in bumblebees: Long-term retention and reversal training. *J. Exp. Biol.* 201: 515–524.

Chittka, L. (1999) Bees, white flowers and the color hexagon—a reassessment? No, not yet. *Naturwissenschaften* 86: 595–597.

Chittka, L. (2002) Influence of intermittent rewards in learning to handle flowers in bumblebees. *Entomol. General* 26: 85–91.

Chittka, L. and Briscoe, A. (2001) Why sensory ecology needs to become more evolutionary—insect color vision as a case in point. In F. G. Barth and A. Schmid (eds.), *Ecology of Sensing.* Berlin: Springer-Verlag, pp. 19–37.

Chittka, L. and Geiger, K. (1995) Can honey bees count landmarks? *Anim. Behav.* 49: 159–164.

Chittka, L. and Menzel, R. (1992) The evolutionary adaptation of flower colors and the insect pollinators' color vision systems. *J. Comp. Physiol. A* 171: 171–181.

Chittka, L. and Thomson, J. D. (1997) Sensori-motor learning and its relevance for task specialization in bumble bees. *Behav. Ecol. Sociobiol.* 41: 385–398.

Chittka, L. and Waser, N. M. (1997) Why red flowers are not invisible for bees. *Isr. J. Plant Sci.* 45: 169–183.

Chittka, L., Beier, W., Hertel, H., Steinmann, E., and Menzel, R. (1992) Opponent colour coding is a universal strategy to evaluate the photoreceptor inputs in Hymenoptera. *J. Comp. Physiol. A* 170: 545–563.

Chittka, L., Vorobyev, M., Shmida, A., and Mezel, R. (1993) Bee colour vision—The optimal system for the discrimination of flower colours with three spectral photoreceptor types? In K. Wiese (ed.), *Sensory Systems of Arthropods*. Basel: Switzerland: Birkhaeuser Verlag, pp. 211–218.

Chittka, L., Shmida, A., Troje, N., and Menzel, R. (1994) Ultraviolet as a component of flower reflections and the colour perception of hymenoptera. *Vison Res.* 34: 1489–1508.

Chittka, L., Kunze J., and Geiger, K. (1995) The influences of landmarks on distance estimation of honeybees. *Anim. Behav.* 50: 23–31.

Chittka, L., Thomson, J. D., and Waser, N. M. (1999) Flower constancy, insect psychology and plant evolution. *Naturwissenschaften* 86: 361–377.

Chittka, L., Spaethe, J., Schmidt, A., and Hickelsberger, A. (2001) Adaptation, constraint and chance in the evolution of flower color and pollinator color vision. In L. Chittka and J. D. Thomson (eds.), *Cognitive Ecology of Pollination*. Cambridge: Cambridge Univ. Press, pp. 106–126.

Chou, W. H., Huber, A., Bentrop, J., Schulz, S., Schwab, K., Chadwell, L. V., Paulsen, R., and Britt, S. G. (1999) Patterning of the R7 and R8 photoreceptor cells of *Drosophila*: Evidence for induced and default cell-fate specification. *Development* 126: 607–616.

Clairambault, P. (1976) Development of the prosencephalon. In R. Llinás and W. Precht (eds.), *Frog Neurobiology*. Berlin: Springer-Verlag, pp. 924–945.

Clark, R. J. and Jackson, R. R. (1994a) *Portia labiata*, a cannibalistic jumping spider, discriminates between own and foreign eggsacs. *Int. J. Comp. Psychol.* 7: 38–43.

Clark, R. J. and Jackson, R. R. (1994b) Self-recognition in a jumping spider: *Portia labiata* females discriminate between their own draglines and those of conspecifics. *Ethol. Ecol. Evol.* 6: 371–375.

Clark, R. J. and Jackson, R. R. (1995a) Dragline-mediated sex recognition in two species of jumping spider (Araneae: Salticidae), *Portia labiata* and *Portia fimbriata*. *Ethol. Ecol. Evol.* 7: 73–77.

Clark, R. J. and Jackson, R. R. (1995b) Araneophagic jumping spiders discriminate between the draglines of familiar and unfamiliar conspecifics. *Ethol. Ecol. Evol.* 7: 185–190.

Clark, R. J. and Jackson, R. R. (2000) Web use during predatory encounters between *Portia fimbriata*, an araneophagic jumping spider and its preferred prey, other jumping spiders. *NZ J. Zool.* 27: 129–136.

Clark, R. J., Jackson, R. R., and Harland, D. P. (2001) Speculative hunting by an araneophagic salticid spider. *Behavior* 137: 1601–1612.

Cleal, K. and Prete, F. R. (1996) The predatory strike of free ranging praying mantises, *Sphodromantis lineola* (Burr.). II: Strikes in the horizontal plane. *Brain Behav. Evol.* 48: 191–204.

Clutton-Brock, T. M. and Harvey, P. H. (1980) Primates, brains and ecology. *J. Zool. Lond.* 190: 309–323.

Cobb, C. S., Pope, S. K., and Williamson, R. (1995a) Circadian rhythms to light-dark cycles in the lesser octopus, *Eledone cirrhosa. Mar. Freshwater Behav. Physiol.* 26: 47–57.

Cobb, C. S., Williamson, R., and Pope, S. K. (1995b) The responses of the epistellar photoreceptors to light and their effect on circadian rhythms in the lesser octopus, *Eledone cirrhosa. Mar. Freshwater Behav. Physiol.* 26: 59–69.

Cohen, A. I. (1973) An ultrastructural analysis of the photoreceptors of the squid and their synaptic connections. II. Intraretinal synapses and plexus. *J. Comp. Neurol.* 147: 379–398.

Cohen, M. J. (1964) The peripheral organisation of sensory systems. In R. F. Reiss (ed.), *Neural Theory and Modeling.* Stanford, Calif.: Stanford University Press, pp. 273–292.

Colborn, M., Ahmad-Annuar, A., Fauria K., and Collett, T. S. (1999) Contextual modulation of visuomotor associations in bumble-bees (*Bombus terrestris*). *Proc. Roy. Soc. Lond. B* 266 (1436): 2413–2418.

Collett, T. S. (1977) Stereopsis in toads. *Nature* 267: 349–351.

Collett, T. S. (1982) Do toads plan detours? A study of the detour behaviour of *Bufo viridis. J. Comp. Physiol.* 146: 261–271.

Collett, T. S. (1983) Picking a route: Do toads follow rules or make plans? In J.-P. Ewert, R. R. Capranica, and D. J. Ingle (eds.), *Advances in Vertebrate Neuroethology.* New York: Plenum, pp. 321–330.

Collett, T. S. (1996) Insect navigation en route to the goal—multiple strategies for the use of landmarks. *J. Exp. Biol.* 199: 227–235.

Collett, T. S. and Cartwright, B. A. (1983) Eidetic images in insects: Their role in navigation. *Trends Nevrosci.* 6: 101–105.

Collett, T. S. and Kelber, A. (1988) The retrieval of visuo-spatial memories by honeybees. *J. Comp. Physiol. A* 163: 145–150.

Collett, T. S., Fry, S. N., and Wehner, R. (1993) Sequence learning by honeybees. *J. Comp. Physiol. A* 172: 693–706.

Comer, C. M. (1985) Analyzing cockroach escape behavior with lesions of individual giant interneurons. *Brain Res.* 335: 342–346.

Comer, C. M. (1987) Sensorimotor functions: What is a command, that a code may yield it? A commentary. *Behav. Brain Sci.* 10: 372.

Comer, C. M. and Dowd, J. P. (1993) Multisensory processing for movement: Antennal and cercal mediation of escape turning in the cockroach. In R. D. Beer, R. E. Ritzmann, and T. McKenna (eds.), *Biological Neural Networks in Invertebrate Neuroethology and Robotics.* New York: Academic Press, pp. 89–112.

Comer, C., Schotland, J., and Grobstein, P. (1985) Short and longterm effects of unilateral vestibular lesions on posture and orienting movements in the frog. *Soc. Neurosci. Abstr.* 11: 289.

Comer, C. M., Dowd, J. P., and Stubblefield, G. (1988) Escape responses following elimination of the giant interneuron pathway in the cockroach, *Periplaneta americana. Brain Res.* 445: 370–375.

Comer, C. M., Mara, E., Murphy, K. A., Getman, M., and Mungy, M. C. (1994) Multisensory control of escape in the cockroach *Periplaneta americana* II. Patterns of touch-evoked behavior. *J. Comp. Physiol.* 174: 13–26.

Comer, C. M., Parks, L., Halvorsen, M. B., and Breese-Terteling, A. (2003) The antennal system and cockroach evasive behavior II: Stimulus identification and localization are separable antennal functions. *J. Comp. Physiol. A* 189: 97–103 (in press).

Cooper, R. L., Li, H., Cole, J. E., and Hopper, H. L. (1998) The neuroecology of cave crayfish: Behavioral and anatomical comparisons of vision in blind epigian species raised in a cave and troglobitic species. *Abst. Soc. Neurosci.* 24: 468.10.

Cott, H. B. (1936) The effectiveness of protective adaptations in the hive-bee, illustrated by experiments on the feeding reactions, habit formation and memory of the common toad (*Bufo bufo bufo*). *Proc. Zool. Soc. (Lond.)* 1: 113–133.

Crane, J. (1949) Comparative biology of salticid spiders at Rancho Grande, Venezuela. Part IV. An analysis of display. *Zoolologica, New York* 34: 159–214.

Cronin, T. W. (1985) The visual pigment of a stomatopod crustacean, *Squilla empusa. J. Comp. Physiol.* 156: 679–687.

Cronin, T. W. (1986) Optical design and evolutionary adaptation in crustacean compound eyes. *J. Crust. Biol.* 6: 1–23.

Cronin, T. W. (1994) Polychromatic vision in mantis shrimps. *Sensornie Systemy* 8: 95–106.

Cronin, T. W. and Caldwell, R. L. (2002) Tuning of visual function in three mantis shrimp species that inhabit a range of depths. I: Visual pigments. *J. Comp. Physiol. A* 188: 179–186.

Cronin, T. W. and Goldsmith, T. H. (1981) Fluorescence of crayfish metarhodopsin studied in single rhabdoms. *Biophys. J.* 35: 653–664.

Cronin, T. W. and Marshall, N. J. (1989a) Multiple spectral classes of photoreceptors in the retinas of gonodactyloid stomatopod crustaceans. *J. Comp. Physiol. A* 166: 267–275.

Cronin, T. W. and Marshall, N. J. (1989b) A retina with at least ten spectral types of photoreceptors in a stomatopod crustacean. *Nature* 339: 137–140.

Cronin, T. W. and Marshall, N. J. (2001) Parallel processing and image analysis in the eyes of mantis shrimps. *Biol. Bull.* 200: 177–183.

Cronin, T. W. and Shashar, N. (2001) The linearly polarized light field in clear, tropical marine waters: Spatial and temporal variation of light intensity, degree of polarization and e-vector angle. *J. Exp. Biol.* 204: 2461–2467.

Cronin, T. W., Nair, J. N., Doyle, R. D., and Caldwell, R. L. (1988) Visual tracking of rapidly moving targets by stomatopod crustaceans. *J. Exp. Biol.* 138: 155–179.

Cronin, T. W., Marshall, N. J., and Land, M. F. (1991) Optokinesis in gonodactyloid mantis shrimps (Crustacea; Stomatopoda; Gonodactylidae). *J. Comp. Physiol. A* 168: 233–240.

Cronin, T. W., Yan, H. Y., and Bidle, K. D. (1992) Regional specialization for control of ocular movements in the compound eyes of a stomatopod crustacean. *J. Exp. Biol.* 171: 373–393.

Cronin, T. W., Marshall, N. J., and Caldwell, R. L. (1993) Photoreceptor spectral diversity in the retinas of squilloid and lysiosquilloid stomatopod crustaceans. *J. Comp. Physiol. A* 172: 339–350.

Cronin, T. W., Marshall, N. J., and Caldwell, R. L. (1994a) The intrarhabdomal filters in the retinas of mantis shrimps. *Vison Res.* 34: 279–291.

Cronin, T. W., Marshall, N. J., and Caldwell, R. L. (1994b) The retinas of mantis shrimps from low-light environments (Crustacea; Stomatopoda; Gonodactylidae). *J. Comp. Physiol. A* 174: 607–619.

Cronin, T. W., Marshall, N. J., and Land, M. F. (1994c) Vision in mantis shrimps. *Am. Sci.* 82: 356–365.

Cronin, T. W., Marshall, N. J., Caldwell, R. L., and Shashar, N. (1994d) Specialization of retinal function in the compound eyes of mantis shrimps. *Vison Res.* 34: 2639–2656.

Cronin, T. W., Marshall, N. J., Quinn, C. A., and King, C. A. (1994e) Ultraviolet photoreception in mantis shrimp. *Vison Res.* 34: 1443–1452.

Cronin, T. W., Shashar, N., and Wolff, L. (1995) Imaging technology reveals the polarized light fields that exist in nature. *Biophotonics Int.* 2: 38–41.

Cronin, T. W., Marshall, N. J., and Caldwell, R. L. (1996) Visual pigment diversity in two genera of mantis shrimps implies rapid evolution. *J. Comp. Physiol. A* 179: 371–384.

Cronin, T. W., Marshall, N. J., and Caldwell, R. L. (2000) Spectral tuning and the visual ecology of mantis shrimps. *Phil. Trans. Roy. Soc. B* 355: 1263–1267.

Cronin, T. W., Caldwell, R. L., and Marshall, N. J. (2001) Tunable colour vision in a mantis shrimp. *Nature* 411: 547–548.

Cronin, T. W., Caldwell, R. L., and Erdmann, M. (2002) Tuning of visual function in three mantis shrimp species that inhabit a range of depths. II: Filter pigments. *J. Comp. Physiol. A* 188: 187–197.

Cummins, D. and Goldsmith, T. H. (1981) Cellular identification of the violet receptor in the crayfish eye. *J. Comp. Physiol. A* 142: 199–202.

Curio, E. (1976) *The Ethology of Predation.* Berlin: Springer-Verlag.

Cutting, J. E., Moore, C., and Morrison, R. (1988) Masking the motions of human gait. *Percept. Psychophys.* 44: 339–347.

Dacke, M., Nilsson, D. E., Warrant, E. J., Blest, A. D., Land, M. F., and O'Carroll, D. C. (1999) Built-in polarizers form part of a compass organ in spiders. *Nature* 401: 470–473.

Dafni, A., Bernhardt, P., Shmida, A., Ivri, Y., Greenbaum, S., O'Toole, C., and Losito L. (1990) Red bowl-shaped flowers: Convergence for beetle pollination in the Mediterranean region. *Isr. J. Bot.* 39: 81–92.

Dale, R. H. I. (1988) Spatial memory in pigeons on a four-arm radial maze. *Can. J. Psychol.* 42: 78–83.

Daley, D. L. and Camhi, J. M. (1988) Connectivity pattern of the cercal-to-giant interneuron system of the American cockroach. *J. Neurophysiol.* 60: 1350–1368.

Daley, D. L. and Delcomyn, F. (1980) Modulation of excitability of cockroach giant interneurons during walking I. Simultaneous excitation and inhibition. *J. Comp. Physiol.* 138: 231–239.

Daley, D. L., Vardi, N., Appignani, B., and Camhi, J. M. (1981) Morphology of the giant interneurons and cercal nerve projections of the American cockroach. *J. Comp. Neurol.* 196(1): 41–52.

D'Amato, M. R., Salmon, D. P., and Colombo, M. (1985) Extent and limits of the matching concept in monkeys (*Cebus apella*). *J. Exp. Psychol. Anim. Behav. Proc.* 11: 35–51.

D'Aniello, B., Vallarino M., Pinelli C., Fiorentiono, M., and Rastogi, K. R. (1996) Neuropeptide Y: Localization in the brain and pituitary of the developing frog (*Rana esculenta*). *Cell Tiss. Res.* 285: 253–259.

Darwin, C. (1871) *The Descent of Man and Selection in Relation to Sex*. London: John Murray.

Davis, W. J. (1971) The integrative action of nervous system in crustacean equilibrium reactions. In S. A. Gordon and M. J. Cohen (eds.), *Gravity and Organism*. Chicago: Univ. of Chicago Press, pp. 237–250.

Dawkins, R. (1996) *Climbing Mount Improbable*. New York: W. W. Norton.

de Couet, H. G. and Sigmund, D. (1985) Monoclonal antibodies to crayfish rhodopsin. I. Biochemical characterization and crossreactivity. *Eur. J. Cell Biol.* 38: 106–112.

de Souza, J., Hertel, H., Ventura, D. F., and Menzel, R. (1992) Response properties of stained monopolar cells in the honeybee lamina. *J. Comp. Physiol. A* 170: 267–274.

Dean, J. (1980a) Encounters between bombardier beetles and two species of toads (*Bufo americanus*, *B. marinus*): Speed of prey-capture does not determine success. *J. Comp. Physiol.* 135: 41–50.

Dean, J. (1980b) Effects of thermal and chemical components of bombardier beetle chemical defense: Glossopharyngeal response in two species of toads (*Bufo americanus*, *B. marinus*). *J. Comp. Physiol.* 135: 51–59.

Dean, P. and Redgrave, P. (1991) Approach and avoidance systems in the rat. In M. A. Arbib and J.-P. Ewert (eds.), *Visual Structures and Integrated Functions*. Berlin: Springer-Verlag, pp. 191–204.

Dean, P., Redgrave, P., and Mitchell, I. J. (1988a) Organization of efferent projections from superior colliculus to brainstem in rat: Evidence for functional output channels. *Prog. Brain Res.* 75: 27–36.

Dean, P., Redgrave, P., and Westby, G. W. (1988b) Event or emergency? Two response systems in the mammalian superior colliculus. *Trends Neurosci.* 12: 137–147.

Deeb, S. S. and Motulsky, A. G. (1996) Molecular genetics of human color vision. *Behav. Genet.* 26: 195–207.

Deely, J. (2001) "A sign is what?" *Sign System Studies* 29: 705–744.

Dennett, D. C. (1991) *Consciousness Explained.* London: Penguin.

Dennett, D. C. (1995) Animal consciousness: What matters and why. *Soc. Res.* 62: 691–710.

Dennett, D. C. (1996) *Kinds of minds: Towards an Understanding of Consciousness.* New York: Simon and Schuster.

Denton, E. J. (1970) On the organization of reflecting surfaces in some marine animals. *Phil. Trans. Roy. Soc. Lond. B* 258: 285–313.

Denton, E. J. and Land, M. F. (1971) Mechanism of reflexion in silvery layers of fish and cephalopods. *Proc. Roy. Soc. Lond. B* 178: 43–61.

Denton, E. J. and Locket, N. A. (1989) Possible wavelength discrimination by multi-bank retinae in the deep-sea fishes. *J. Mar. Biol. Assoc. UK* 69: 409–435.

Desimone, R. (1998) Visual attention mediated by biased competition in extrastriate visual cortex. *Phil. Trans. Roy. Soc. Lond. B* 353: 1245–1255.

DeVoe, R. D. (1975) Ultraviolet and green receptors in principal eyes of jumping spiders. *J. Gen. Physiol.* 66: 193–207.

Dicke, U. (1999) Morphology, axonal projection pattern and response types of tectal neurons in plethodontid salamanders. I: Tracer study of projection neurons and their pathways. *J. Comp. Neurol.* 404: 473–488.

Dicke, U. and Roth, G. (1996) Similarities and differences in the cytoarchitecture of the tectum of frogs and salamanders. *Acta. Biol. Hung.* 47: 41–59.

Dicke, U., Roth, G., and Matsushima, T. (1998) Neural substrate for motor control of feeding in amphibians. *Acta Anat.* 163: 127–143.

DiDomenico, R. and Eaton, R. C. (1987) Toward a reformulation of the command concept. *Behav. Brain Sci.* 10: 374–375.

Dirsh, V. M. (1965) Revision of the family Pneumoridae (Orthoptera: Acridoidea). *Bull. Br. Mus. (Nat. Hist.) Entomol.* 15: 325–396.

Disse, D., Ewert, J. C., Hesebeck, O., and Langer, F. (1992) ODANN: Objekt dimensionieren mit ANN. *Abt. Neurobiologie*, University of Kassel.

Dole, J. W., Rose, B. B., and Tachiki, K. H. (1981) Western toads (*Bufo boreas*) learn odor of prey insects. *Herpetologia* 37: 63–68.

Dominy, N. J. and Lucas, P. W. (2001) Ecological importance of trichromatic vision to primates. *Nature* 410: 363–366.

Doty, R. W. (1987) Has the greedy toad lost its soul and if so, what was it? *Behav. Brain Sci.* 10: 375.

Dowd, J. P. and Comer, C. M. (1988) The neural basis of orienting behavior: A computational approach to the escape turn of the cockroach. *Biol. Cybernet.* 60: 37–48.

Drees, O. (1952) Untersuchungen uber die angeborenen Verhaltensweisen bei Springspinnen (Salticidae). *Z. Tierpsychol.* 9: 169–207.

Dukas, R. (1998) Introduction. In R. Dukas (ed.), *Cognitive Ecology: The Evolutionary Ecology of Information Processing and Decision Making.* Chicago: Univ. of Chicago Press.

Dumpert, K. and Gnatzy, W. (1977) Cricket combined mechanoreceptors and kicking response. *J. Comp. Physiol.* 122: 9–25.

Dunham, P. J. (1978) Sex pheromones in crustacea. *Biol. Rev.* 53: 555–583.

Dunham, P. J. (1988) Pheromones and behavior in Crustacea. In H. Laufer and G. H. Downer (eds.), *Endocrinolgy of Selected Invertebrate Types.* New York: Alan R. Liss, pp. 375–392.

Dyer, A. G. (1998) The colour of flowers in spectrally variable illumination and insect pollinator vision. *J. Comp. Physiol. A* 183: 203–212.

Dyer, A. G. (1999) Broad spectral sensitivities in the honeybee's photoreceptors limit colour constancy. *J. Comp. Physiol. A* 185: 445–453.

Dyer, A. G. and Chittka, L. (2004) Biological significance of discriminating between similar colours in spectrally variable illumination: bumblebees as a study case. *J. Comp. Physiol. A,* 190: 105–114.

Eakin, R. M. and Brandenburger, J. L. (1971) Fine structure of the eyes of jumping spiders. *J. Ultrastruct. Res.* 37: 618–663.

Eaton, R. C. (2001) The Mauthner cell and other identified neurons of the brainstem escape network of fish. *Prog. Neurobiol.* 63: 467–485.

Ebbesson, S. O. E. (1980a) *Comparative Neurology of the Telencephalon.* New York: Plenum.

Ebbesson, S. O. E. (1980b) The parcellation theory and its relation to interspecific variability in brain organization, evolutionary and ontogenetic development and neuronal plasticity. *Cell Tiss. Res.* 213: 179–212.

Ebbesson, S. O. E. (1984) Evolution and ontogeny of neural circuits. *Behav. Brain Sci.* 7: 321–366.

Ebbesson, S. O. E. (1987) Prey-catching in toads: An exceptional neuroethological model. *Behav. Brain Sci.* 10: 375–376.

Ebrey, T. G. (1977) New wavelength dependent visual pigment nomograms. *Vision Res.* 17: 147–151.

Edmunds, M. (1972) Defensive behaviour in Ghanaian praying mantids. *Zool. J. Linn. Soc.* 51: 1–32.

Edmunds, M. and Brunner, D. (1999) Ethology of defenses against predators. In F. R. Prete, H. Wells, P. Wells, and L. E. Hurd (eds.), *The Praying Mantids*. Baltimore, Md.: Johns Hopkins Univ. Press, pp. 276–299.

Edrich, W., Neumeyer, C., and von Helversen, O. (1979) "Anti-sun orientation" of bees with regard to a field of ultraviolet light. *J. Comp. Physiol. A* 134: 151–157.

Edwards, D. H. (1982) The cockroach DCMD neurone. II. Dynamics of response habituation and convergence of spectral inputs. *J. Exp. Biol.* 99: 91–107.

Edwards, D. H., Heitler, W. J., and Krasne, F. B. (1999) Fifty years of a command neuron: The neurobiology of escape behavior in the crayfish. *Trends Newrosci.* 22(4): 153–161.

Edwards, J. S. (1997) The evolution of insect flight: Implications for the evolution of the nervous system. *Brain Behav. Evol.* 50: 8–12.

Edwards, J. S. and Palka, J. (1974) The cerci and abdominal giant fibres of the house cricket, *Acheta domesticus*. I. Anatomy and physiology of normal adults. *Proc. Roy. Soc. Lond. B* 185(78): 83–103.

Edwards, J. S. and Palka, J. (1991) Insect neural evolution—a fugue or an opera? *Sem. Neurosci.* 3: 391–398.

Edwards, J. S. and Reddy, R. (1986) Mechanosensory appendages and giant interneurons in the firebrat (*Thermobia domestica*, Thysanura): A prototype system for predator evasion. *J. Comp. Neurol.* 243: 535–546.

Egelhaaf, M. and Borst A. (1990) Bewegungswahrnehmung und visuelle Orientierung bei Fliegen. *Naturwissenschaften* 77: 366–377.

Eggleton, P. (2001) Termites and trees: A review of recent advances in termite phylogenetics. *Insectes Sociaux* 48: 187–193.

Eguchi, E. and Waterman, T. H. (1966) Fine structure patterns in crustacean rhabdoms. In C. G. Bernhard (ed.), *The Functional Organization of the Compound Eye*. Oxford: Pergamon Press, pp. 105–124.

Ehn, R. and Tichy, H. (1994) Hygro- and thermoreceptive tarsal organ in the spider *Cupiennius salei*. *J. Comp. Physiol. A* 174: 345–350.

Eibl-Eibesfeldt, I. (1951) Nahrungserwerb und Beuteschema der Erdkröte (*Bufo bufo* L.). *Behaviour* 4: 1–35.

Eisenberg, J. F. and Wilson, D. E. (1978) Relative brain size and feeding strategies in Chiroptera. *Evolution* 32: 740–751.

Endler, J. A. (1990) On the measurement and classification of colour in studies of animal colour patterns. *Biol. J. Linn. Soc.* 41: 315–352.

Endler, J. A. (1992) Signals, signal conditions and the direction of evolution. *Am. Nat.* 139: S125–S153.

Endler, J. A. (1993) The color of light in forests and its implications. *Ecol. Monogr.* 63: 1–27.

Endler, J. A., Basolo, A., Glowacki, S., and Zerr, J. (2001) Variation in response to artificial selection for light sensitivity in guppies (*Poecilia reticulata*). *Am. Nat.* 158: 36–48.

Epstein, R. (1982) Representation: A concept that fills no gaps. *Behav. Brain Sci.* 5: 377–378.

Ewert, J.-P. (1968) Der Einfluss von Zwischenhirndefekten auf die Visuomotorik im Beutefang- und Fluchtverhalten der Erdkröte (*Bufo bufo* L.). *Z. Vergl. Physiol.* 61: 41–70.

Ewert, J.-P. (1971) Single unit response of the toad (*Bufo americanus*) caudal thalamus to visual objects. *Z. Vergl. Physiol.* 74: 81–102.

Ewert, J.-P. (1974) The neural basis of visually guided behavior. *Sci. Am.* 230: 34–42.

Ewert, J.-P. (1984) Tectal mechanisms that underlie prey-catching and avoidance behaviors in toads. In H. Vanegas (ed.), *Comparative Neurology of the Optic Tectum*. New York: Plenum, pp. 247–416.

Ewert, J.-P. (1987) Neuroethology of releasing mechanisms: Prey catching in toads. *Behav. Brain Sci.* 10: 337–405.

Ewert, J.-P. (1992) Neuroethology of an object features-relating algorithm and its modification by learning. *Rev. Neurosci.* 3: 45–63.

Ewert, J.-P. (1997) Neural correlates of key stimulus and releasing mechanism: A case study and two concepts. *Trends Neurosci.* 20: 332–339.

Ewert, J.-P. (2002) Command neurons and command systems. In M. A. Arbib (ed.), *The Handbook of Brain Theory and Neural Networks*, 2nd ed. Cambridge, Mass.: MIT Press, pp. 233–238.

Ewert, J.-P. and Borchers, W. (1974) Antworten retinaler Ganglienzellen bei freibeweglichen Kröten. *J. Comp. Physiol.* 92: 117–130.

Ewert, J.-P. and Hock, F. J. (1972) Movement sensitive neurones in the toad's retina. *Exp. Brain Res.* 16: 41–59.

Ewert, J.-P. and Traud, R. (1979) Releasing stimuli for antipredator behaviour in the common toad, *Bufo bufo* (L.). *Behaviour* 68: 170–180.

Ewert, J.-P. and von Seelen, W. (1974) Neurobiologie und System-Theorie eines visuellen Muster-Erkennungsmechanismus bei Kröten. *Kybernetik* 14: 167–183.

Ewert, J.-P., Burghagen, H., and Schürg-Pfeiffer, E. (1983) Neuroethological analysis of the innate releasing mechanism for prey-catching behavior in toads. In J.-P. Ewert, R. R. Capranica, and D. J. Ingle (eds.), *Advances in Vertebrate Neuroethology*. New York: Plenum, pp. 413–475.

Ewert, J.-P., Framing, E. M., Schürg-Pfeiffer, E., and Weerasuriya, A. (1990) Responses of medullary neurons to moving visual stimuli in the common toad: I. Characterization of medial reticular neurons by extracellular recording. *J. Comp. Physiol. A* 167: 495–508.

Ewert, J.-P., Dinges, A. W., and Finkenstädt, T. (1994a) Species-universal stimulus responses, modified through conditioning, re-appear after telencephalic lesions in toads. *Naturwissenschaften* 81: 317–320.

Ewert, J.-P., Beneke, T. W., Schürg-Pfeiffer, E., Schwippert, W. W., and Weerasuriya, A. (1994b) Sensorimotor processes that underlie feeding behavior in tetrapods. In V. L. Bels, M. Chardon, and P. Vandevalle (eds.), *Advances in Comparative and Environmental Physiology*. vol. 18, *Biomechanics of Feeding in Vertebrates*. Berlin: Springer-Verlag, pp. 119–161.

Ewert, J.-P. and Borchers, H.-W. (1971) Reaktionscharakteristik von Neuronen aus dem Tectum opticum und Subtectum der Erdkröte *Bufo bufo* (L.). *Z. Vergl. Physiol.* 71: 165–189.

Ewert, J.-P. and Kehl, W. (1978) Configurational prey-selection by individual experience in the toad *Bufo bufo. J. Comp. Physiol.* A 126: 105–114.

Ewert, J.-P., Schürg-Pfeiffer, E., and Schwippert, W. W. (1996) Influence of pretectal lesions on tectal responses to visual stimulation in anurans: Field potential, single neuron and behavior analyses. *Acta Biol. Acad. Sci. Hung.* 47: 223–245.

Ewert, J.-P., Buxbaum-Conradi, H., Dreisvogt, F., Glagow, M., Merkel-Harff, C., Röttgen, A., Schürg-Pfeiffer, E., and Schwippert, W. W. (2001) Neural modulation of visuomotor functions underlying prey-catching behaviour in anurans: Perception, attention, motor performance, learning. *Comp. Biochem. Physiol.* A 128: 417–461.

Exner, S. (1891) *Die Physiologie der Facettirten Augen von Krebsen und Insecten*. Leipzig, Vienna: Deuticke.

Fabre, J.-H. (1912) *Social Life in the Insect World*. (transl. B. Miall) London: T. Fisher Unwin.

Fagan, W. F. and Hurd, L. E. (1994) Hatch density variation of a generalist arthropod predator: Population consequences and community impact. *Ecology* 75: 2022–2032.

Fent, K. (1986) Polarized skylight orientation in the desert ant *Cataglyphis. J. Comp. Physiol.* A 158: 145–150.

Ferguson, G. P., Messenger, J. B., and Budelmann, B. U. (1994) Gravity and light influence the countershading reflexes of the cuttlefish *Sepia officinalis. J. Exp. Biol.* 191: 247–256.

Field, L. H. (1991) Mechanism for range fractionation in chordotonal organs of *Locusta migratoria* (L) and Valanga sp. (Orthoptera: Acrididae). *Int. J. Insect. Morphol. Embryol.* 20: 25–39.

Finkenstädt, T. (1989) Visual associative learning: Searching for behaviorally relevant brain structures in toads. In J.-P. Ewert and M. A. Arbib (eds.), *Visuomotor Coordination: Amphibians, Comparisons, Models and Robots*. New York: Plenum, pp. 799–832.

Finkenstädt, T. and Ewert, J.-P. (1983a) Processing of area dimensions of visual key stimuli by tectal neurons in *Salamandra salamandra. J. Comp. Physiol.* 153: 85–98.

Finkenstädt, T. and Ewert, J.-P. (1983b) Visual pattern discrimination through interactions of neural networks: A combined electrical brain stimulation, brain lesion and extracellular recording study in *Salamandra salamandra. J. Comp. Physiol.* 153: 99–110.

Finkenstädt, T. and Ewert, J.-P. (1985) Glucose utilization in the toad's brain during anesthesia and stimulation of the ascending reticular arousal system: A ^{14}C-2-deoxyglucose study. *Naturwissenschaften* 72: 161–162.

Finkenstädt, T. and Ewert, J.-P. (1988) Stimulus-specific long-term habituation of visually guided orienting behavior toward prey in toads: A ^{14}C-2DG study. *J. Comp. Physiol. A* 163: 1–11.

Finkenstädt, T. and Ewert, J.-P. (1992) Localization of learning-related metabolical changes in brain structures of common toads: A 2-DG-study. In F. Gonzalez-Lima, T. Finkenstädt, and H. Scheich (eds.), *Advances in Metabolic Mapping Techniques for Brain Imaging of Behavioral and Learning Functions*. Dordrecht, Netherlands: Kluwer, pp. 409–445.

Finkenstädt, T., Adler, N. T., Allen, T. O., Ebbesson, S. O. E., and Ewert, J.-P. (1985) Mapping of brain activity in mesencephalic and diencephalic structures of toads during presentation of visual key stimuli: A computer-assisted analysis of 14C-2DG autoradiographs. *J. Comp. Physiol. A* 156: 433–445.

Finkenstädt, T., Adler, N. T., Allen, T. O., and Ewert, J.-P. (1986) Regional distribution of glucose utilization in the telencephalon of toads in response to configurational visual stimuli: A 14C-2DG study. *J. Comp. Physiol. A* 158: 457–467.

Flores, E. E. C. (1983) Visual discrimination testing in the squid *Todarodes pacificus*: Experimental evidence for lack of color vision. *Mem. Nat. Hist. Mus. Victoria* 44: 213–227.

Foelix, R. F. (1996) *Biology of Spiders*. New York: Oxford Univ. Press and Georg Thieme Verlag.

Fonseca, P. J., Münch, D., and Hennig, R. M. (2000) How cicadas interpret acoustic signals. *Nature* 405: 297–298.

Foreman, N. and Stevens, R. (1987) Relationships between the superior colliculus and hippocampus: Neural and behavioral considerations. *Behav. Brain Sci.* 10: 101–151.

Forrest, T. G. and Green, D. M. (1991) Sexual selection and female choice in mole crickets (Scapteriscus: Gryllotalpidae): Modeling the effects of intensity and male spacing. *Bioacoustics* 3: 93–109.

Forster, L. M. (1979) Visual mechanisms of hunting behaviour in *Trite planiceps*, a jumping spider (Araneae: Salticidae). *NZ J. Zool.* 6: 79–93.

Forster, L. M. (1982a) Vision and prey-catching strategies in jumping spiders. *Am. Sci.* 70: 165–175.

Forster, L. M. (1982b) Visual communication in jumping spiders (Salticidae). In P. N. Witt and J. S. Rovner (eds.), *Spider Communication: Mechanisms and Ecological Significance*. Princeton, N.J.: Princeton Univ. Press, pp. 161–212.

Forster, L. M. (1985) Target discrimination in jumping spiders (Araneae: Salticidae) In F. G. Barth (ed.), *Neurobiology of Arachnids*. Berlin: Springer-Verlag, pp. 249–274.

Franceschini, N., Kirschfeld, K., and Minke, B. (1981) Fluorescence of photoreceptor cells observed in vivo. *Science* 213: 1264–1267.

Fraser, P. J. (1977) Cercal ablation modifies tethered flight behaviour of cockroach. *Nature* 268(5620): 523–524.

Frost, B. J. (1982) Mechanisms for discriminating object motion from self-induced motion in the pigeon. In D. J. Ingle, M. A. Goodale, and R. J. W. Mansfield (eds.), *Analysis of Visual Behavior*. Cambridge, Mass: MIT Press, pp. 177–196.

Fujimoto, K., Yanase, T., and Ishizuka, I. (1966) The visual substance of the crayfish, *Procambarus clarkii*. *Mem. Osaka Gakugi Univ.* 15B: 109–114.

Fukushi, T. (1990) Colour discrimination from various shades of grey in the trained blowfly, *Lucilia cuprina*. *J. Insect Physiol.* 36: 69–75.

Fülöp, A. and Menzel, R. (2000) Risk-indifferent foraging behaviour in honeybees. *Anim. Behav.* 60: 657–666.

Gabbiani. F., Krapp, H. G., and Laurent, G. (1999) Computation of object approach by a wide-field, motion-sensitive neuron. *J. Neurosci.* 19: 1122–1141.

Gadagkar, G., Srinivasan, M. V., and Zhang, S. W. (1995) Context-dependent learning in honeybees. *Proc. Austr. Neurosci. Soc.* 6: 226.

Gamlin, P. D. R., Reiner, A., Keyer, K. T., Brecha, N., and Karten, H. J. (1996) Projection of the nucleus pretectalis to a retino-recipient tectal layer in the pigeon (Columba livia). *J. Comp. Neurol.* 368: 424–438.

Ganihar, D., Libersat, F., Wendler, G., and Camhi, J. M. (1994) Wind-evoked escape responses in flying cockroaches. *J. Comp. Physiol.* 175: 49–65.

Gans, C. (1961) A bullfrog and its prey. *Nat. Hist.* 70: 26–37.

Gardenfors, P. (1996) Cued and detached representations in animal cognition. *Behav. Proc.* 35: 263–273.

Gaze, R. M. (1958) The representation of the retina on the optic lobe of the frog. *Quart. J. Exp. Physiol.* 43: 209–314.

Gebhardt, M. and Honegger, H.-W. (2001) Physiological characterization of antennal mechanosensory descending interneurons in an insect (*Gryllus bimaculatus*, *Gryllus campestris*) brain. *J. Exp. Biol.* 204: 2265–2275.

Gegear, R. J. and Laverty, T. M. (2001) The effect of variation among floral traits on the flower constancy of pollinators. In L. Chittka and J. D. Thomson (eds.), *Cognitive Ecology of Pollination*. Cambridge: Cambridge Univ. Press, pp. 1–20.

Gerhardt, H. C. and Huber, F. (2002) *Acoustic Communication in Insects and Anurans: Common Problems and Diverse Solutions*. Chicago: University of Chicago Press.

Gewecke, M. and Hou, T. (1993) Visual brain neurons in *Locusta migratoria*. In K. Weise, F. G. Gribakin, A. V. Popov, and G. Renninger (eds.), *Sensory Systems in Arthropods*. Basel Switzerland: Birkhäuser, pp. 119–144.

Gillespie, P. G. and Walker, R. G. (2001) Molecular basis of mechanosensory transduction. *Nature* 413: 194–202.

Giurfa, M. and Lehrer, M. (2001) Honeybee vision and floral displays: From detection to close-up recognition. In L. Chittka and J. D. Thomson (eds.), *Cognitive Ecology of Pollination*. Cambridge: Cambridge Univ. Press, pp. 61–82.

Giurfa, M., Núñez, J., Chittka, L., and Menzel, R. (1995) Colour preferences of flower-naive honeybees. *J. Comp. Physiol. A* 177: 247–259.

Giurfa, M., Eichmann, B., and Menzel, R. (1996) Symmetry perception in an insect. *Nature* 382: 458–461.

Giurfa, M., Zhang, S. W., Jenett, A., Menzel, R., and Srinivasan, M. V. (2001) The concepts of "sameness" and "difference" in an insect. *Nature* 410: 930–933.

Glantz, R. M. (2001) Polarization analysis in the crayfish visual system. *J. Exp. Biol.* 204: 2383–2390.

Gleadall, I. G. (1994) A model for enhancing the visual information available under low light conditions. *Interdis. Infor. Sci.* 1: 67–75.

Gleadall, I. G., Ohtsu, K., Gleadall, E., and Tsukahara, Y. (1993) Screening-pigment migration in the octopus retina includes control by dopaminergic efferents. *J. Exp. Biol.* 185: 1–16.

Gnatzy, W. and Heusslein, R. (1986) Digger wasp against cricket. *Naturwissenschaften* 73: 212–215.

Gnatzy, W. and Kamper, G. (1990) Digger wasp against crickets. II. An airborne signal produced by a running predator. *J. Comp. Physiol.* 167: 551–556.

Gogala, M. and Riede, K. (1995) Time sharing of song activity by cicadas in Temengor Forest Reserve, Hulu Perak and in Sabah, Malaysia. *Malay. Nat. J.* 49: 48–54.

Goldman, M., Lanson, R., and Rivera, G. (1991) Wavelength categorization by goldfish (*Carassius auratus*). *Int. J. Comp. Psychol.* 4: 195–210.

Goldsmith, T. H. (1978) The effects of screening pigments on the spectral sensitivity of some Crustacea with scotopic (superposition) eyes. *Vision Res.* 18: 475–482.

Goldsmith, T. H. (1990) Optimization, constraint and history in the evolution of eyes. *Quart. Rev. Biol.* 65: 281–322.

Goldsmith, T. H. (1991) *Photoreception and Vision*. New York: Wiley-Liss.

Goldsmith, T. H. (1994) Ultraviolet receptors and color vision: Evolutionary implications and a dissonance of paradigms. *Vision Res.* 34: 1479–1487.

Goldsmith, T. H. and Fernandez, H. R. (1968) Comparative studies of crustacean spectral sensitivity. *Z. Verg. Physiol.* 60: 156–175.

Goldsmith, T. H. and Wehner, R. (1977) Restrictions on rotational and translational diffusion of pigment in the membranes of a rhabdomeric photoreceptor. *J. Gen. Physiol.* 70: 453–490.

Goldstein, E. B. (1989) *Sensation and Perception*. Belmont, Calif.: Wadsworth.

Gombocz, M. (1999) Verhaltensbeobachtungen an der Gottesanbeterin *Empusa fasciata* in ihrer natürlichen Umgebung. Master's thesis, Univ. of Graz, Graz, Austria.

Gonka, M. D., Laurie, T. J., and Prete, F. R. (1999) Responses of movement-sensitive descending visual interneurons to prey-like stimuli in the praying mantis, *Sphodromantis lineola* (Burmeister). *Brain, Behav., Evol.* 54: 243–262.

Gorochov, A. V. (1995) Contribution to the system and evolution of the order Orthoptera. *Zool. Zhur.* 74: 39–45.

Gould, J. L. and Gould, C. G. (1988) *The Sensory World in the Honey Bee.* New York: Scientific American Library, pp. 41–45.

Govardovskii, V. I. (1983) On the role of oil drops in colour vision. *Vision Res.* 23: 1739–1740.

Gras, H. and Horner, M. (1992) Wind-evoked escape running of the cricket *Gryllus bimaculatus*. I. Behavioral analysis. *J. Exp. Biol.* 171: 189–214.

Gray, L. A., O'Reilly, J. C., and Nishikawa, K. C. (1997) Evolution of forelimb movement patterns for prey manipulation in anurans. *J. Exp. Zool.* 277: 417–424.

Graziadei, P. (1962) Receptors in the suckers of the octopus. *Nature (London)* 195: 57–59.

Graziadei, P. (1964) Receptors in the sucker of the cuttlefish. *Nature (London)* 203: 384–386.

Graziadei, P. (1971) The nervous system of the arms. In J. Z. Young (ed.), *The Anatomy of the Nervous System of Octopus vulgaris.* Oxford: Oxford Univ. Press, pp. 45–61.

Graziadei, P. and Gagne, H. T. (1976a) Sensory innervation in the rim of the octopus sucker. *J. Morphol.* 150: 639–680.

Graziadei, P. and Gagne, H. T. (1976b) An unusual receptor in the octopus. *Cell Tiss. Res.* 8: 229–240.

Greenfield, M. D. (1988) Interspecific acoustic interactions among katydids' *neoconocephalus*-inhibition-induced shifts in diel periodicity. *Anim. Behav.* 36: 684–695.

Greenfield, M. D. (2002) *Signalers and Receivers: Mechanisms and Evolution of Arthropod Communication.* Oxford: Oxford Univ. Press.

Gribakin, F. C. (1975) Functional morphology of the compound eye of the bee. In G. A. Horridge (ed.), *The Compound Eye and Vision of Insects.* Oxford: Clarendon Press, pp. 154–176.

Grobstein, P. (1991) Directed movement in the frog: A closer look at a central representation of spatial location. In M. A. Arbib and J.-P. Ewert (eds.), *Visual Structures and Integrated Functions.* Berlin: Springer-Verlag, pp. 125–138.

Grobstein, P., Comer, C. and Kostyk, S. K. (1983) Frog prey capture behavior: Between sensory maps and directed motor output. In J.-P. Ewert, R. R. Capranica, and D. J. Ingle (eds.), *Advances in Vertebrate Neuroethology.* New York: Plenum, pp. 331–347.

Gruberg, E. R. and Ambros, V. R. (1974) A forebrain visual projection in the frog (*Rana pipiens*). *Exp. Brain Res.* 44: 187–197.

Grüsser, O.-J. and Grüsser-Cornehls, U. (1976) Neurophysiology of the anuran visual system. In R. Llinás and W. Precht (eds.), *Frog Neurobiology*. Berlin: Springer-Verlag, pp. 297–385.

Grüsser, O.-J., Grüsser-Cornehls, U., Finkelstein, D., Henn, V., Patutschnik, M., and Butenandt, E. (1967) A quantitative analysis of movement-detecting neurons in the frog retina. *Pflügers Arch.* 293: 100–106.

Guha, K., Jørgensen, C. B., and Larsen, L. O. (1980) Relationship between nutritional state and testes function, together with the observations on patterns of feeding, in the toad. *J. Zool. (Lond.)* 192: 147–155.

Gumbert, A. (2000) Color choices by bumble bees (*Bombus terrestris*): Innate preferences and generalization after learning. *Behav. Ecol. Sociobiol.* 48: 36–43.

Hafner, G. S. and Tokarski, T. R. (1998) Morphogenesis and pattern formation in the retina of the crayfish *Procambarus clarkii. Cell Tiss. Res.* 293: 535–550.

Hamacher, K. and Stieve, H. (1984) Spectral properties of the rhodopsin of the crayfish *Astacus leptodactylus. Photochem. Photobiol.* 39: 379–390.

Hamanaka, T., Kito, Y., Seidou, M., Wakabayashi, K., Michinomae, M., and Amemiya, Y. (1994) X-ray diffraction study of the live squid retina. *J. Mol. Biol.* 238: 139–144.

Hamasaki, D. I. (1968a) The electororetinogram of the intact anesthetized octopus. *Vision Res.* 8: 247–258.

Hamasaki, D. I. (1968b) The ERG-determined spectral sensitivity of the octopus. *Vision Res.* 8: 1013–1021.

Hamdorf, K., Schwemer, J., and Tauber, U. (1968) The visual pigment, the absorption of the photoreceptors and the spectral sensitivity of the retina of *Eledone moschata. Z. Vergl. Physiol.* 60: 375–415.

Hamilton, W. D. (1979) Wingless and fighting males in fig wasps and other insects. In M. S. Blum and N. A. Blum (eds.), *Sexual Selection and Reproductive Competition in Insects.* New York: Academic Press, pp. 167–220.

Hammer, M. and Menzel, R. (1995) Learning and memory in the honeybee. *J. Neurosci.* 15(3): 1617–1630.

Hanlon, R. T. and Messenger, J. B. (1988) Adaptive coloration in young cuttlefish (*Sepia officinalis* L.): The morphology and development of body patterns and their relation to behaviour. *Phil. Trans. Roy. Soc. Lond.* 320: 437–487.

Hanlon, R. T. and Messenger, J. B. (1996) *Cephalopod Behaviour*. Cambridge: Cambridge Univ. Press.

Hanlon, R. T. and Shashar, N. (2003) Aspects of the sensory ecology of cephalopods. In S. P. Collin and J. Marshall (eds.), *Sensory Processing of the Aquatic Environment*. New York: Springer-Verlag.

Hanlon, R. T., Forsythe, J. W., and Joneschild, D. E. (1999a) Crypsis, conspicuousness, mimicry and polyphenism as antipredator defences of foraging octopuses on Indo-Pacific coral reefs, with a method of quantifying crypsis from video tapes. *Biol. J. Linn. Soc.* 66: 1–22.

Hanlon, R. T., Maxwell, M. R., Shashar, N., Loew, E. R., and Boyle, K. L. (1999b) An ethogram of body patterning behavior in the biomedically and commercially valuable squid *Loligo pealei* off Cape Cod, Massachusetts. *Biol. Bull.* 197: 49–62.

Hansen-Delkeskamp, E. (1992) Functional characterization of antennal contact chemoreceptors in the cockroach *Periplaneta americana*. An electrophysiological investigation. *J. Insect Physiol.* 38: 813–822.

Hardie, R. C. (1986) The photoreceptor array of the dipteran retina. *Trends Neurosci.* 9: 419–423.

Hardie, R. C. and Duelli, P. (1978) Properties of single cells in posterior lateral eyes of jumping spiders. *Z. Naturforsch.* 33c: 156–158.

Hardie, R. C., Franceschini, N., Ribi, W., and Kirschfeld, K. (1981) Distribution and properties of sex-specific photoreceptors in the fly *Musca domestica*. *J. Comp. Physiol. A* 145: 139–152.

Hariyama, T. and Tsukahara, Y. (1988) Seasonal variation of spectral sensitivity in crayfish retinula cells. *Comp. Biochem. Physiol.* 91A(3): 529–533.

Hariyama, T., Gleadall, I. G., Liao, L., Gleadall, E., and Tsukahara, Y. (1989) Details of the production of monoclonal antibodies to demonstrate the presence (in winter) of more than one type of opsin in the retinula cells of the crayfish, *Procambarus clarkii* Girard. *Ann. App. Inform. Sci.* 14(2): 101–113.

Harland, D. P. and Jackson, R. R. (2000a) Cues by which *Portia fimbriata*, an araneophagic jumping spider, distinguishes jumping-spider prey from other prey. *J. Exp. Biol.* 203: 3485–3494.

Harland, D. P. and Jackson, R. R. (2000b) "Eight-legged cats" and how they see—a review of recent work on jumping spiders (Araneae: Salticidae). *Cimbebasia* 16: 231–240.

Harland, D. P. and Jackson, R. R. (2001) Prey classification by *Portia fimbriata*, a salticid spider that specializes at preying on other salticids: Species that elicit cryptic stalking. *J. Zool. Lond.* 255: 445–460.

Harland, D. P. and Jackson, R. R. (2002) Influence of cues from the anterior medial eyes of virtual prey on *Portia fimbriata*, an araneophagic jumping spider. *J. Exp. Biol.* 205: 1861–1868.

Harland, D. P., Jackson, R. R., and Macnab, A. (1999) Distances at which jumping spiders (Araneae, Salticidae) distinguish between prey and conspecific rivals. *J. Zool. Lond.* 247: 357–364.

Harling, C. (2000) Re-examination of eye design in the classification of stomatopod crustaceans. *J. Crust. Biol.* 20: 172–185.

Harwood, D. V. and Anderson, C. W. (2000) Evidence for the anatomical origins of hypoglossal afferents in the tongue of the leopard frog, *Rana pipiens. Brain Res.* 862: 288–291.

Hawryshyn, C. W. (1992) Polarization vision in fish. *Am. Sci.* 80: 164–175.

Heide, G., Berger, F., and Mebus, U. (1982) Neurale und neuromuskuläre Korrelate des visuell auslösbaren Kopfstellreflexes bei *Mantis religiosa. Verh. Dtsch. Zool. Ges.* 274.

Heider, E. R. and Olivier, D. C. (1972) The structure of the color space in naming and memory for two languages. *Cog. Psychol.* 3: 337–354.

Heil, K. H. (1936) Beiträge zur Physiologie und Psychologie der Springspinnen. *Z. Vergl. Phsyiol.* 23: 125–149.

Heinrich, B. (1979) *Bumblebee Economics.* Cambridge, Mass.: Harvard Univ. Press.

Heinrich, B., Mudge P. R., and Deringis P. G. (1977) Laboratory analysis of flower constancy in foraging bumblebees: *Bombus ternarius* and *B. terricola. Behav. Ecol. Sociobiol.* 2: 247–265.

Hemmi, J. M. (1999) Dichromatic colour vision in an Australian marsupial, the tammar wallaby. *J. Comp. Physiol. A* 185: 509–515.

Hempel, de Ibarra, N., Giurfa, M., and Vorobyev, M. (2001) Detection of coloured patterns by honeybees through chromatic and achromatic cues. *J. Comp. Physiol. A* 187: 215–224.

Herman, L. M. and Gordon, J. A. (1974) Auditory delayed matching in the bottlenose dolphin. *J. Exp. Anal. Behav.* 21: 19–26.

Herrick, C. J. (1933) The amphibian forebrain. VIII: Cerebral hemispheres and pallial primordia. *J. Comp. Neurol.* 58: 737–759.

Hertel, H. (1980) Chromatic properties of identified interneurons in the optic lobes of the bee. *J. Comp. Physiol.* 137: 215–231.

Hertel, H. and Maronde, U. (1987a) Processing of visual information in the honeybee brain. In R. Menzel and A. Mercer (eds.), *Neurobiology and Behavior of Honeybees*, Berlin: Springer-Verlag, pp. 141–157.

Hertel, H. and Maronde, U. (1987b) The physiology and morphology of centrally projecting visual interneurones in the honeybee brain. *J. Exp. Biol.* 133: 301–315.

Hill, D. E. (1979) Orientation by jumping spiders of the genus *Phidippus* (Araneae: Salticidae) during the pursuit of prey. *Behav. Ecol. Sociobiol.* 5: 301–322.

Hill, P. S. M., Wells, P. H., and Wells, H. (1997) Spontaneous flower constancy and learning in honey bees as a function of colour. *Anim. Behav.* 54: 615–627.

Hill, P. S. M., Hollis, J., and Wells, H. (2001) Foraging decisions in nectarivores: Unexpected interactions between flower constancy and energetic rewards. *Anim. Behav.* 62: 729–737.

Himstedt, W. (1982) Prey selection in salamanders. In D. J. Ingle, M. A. Goodale, and R. J. W. Mansfield (eds.), *Analysis of Visual Behavior.* Cambridge, Mass: MIT Press, pp. 47–66.

Himstedt, W. and Plasa, L. (1979) Home-site orientation by visual cues in salamanders. *Naturwissenschaften* 66: 372–373.

Himstedt, W., Freidank, U., and Singer, E. (1976) Die Veränderung eines Auslösemechanismus im Beutefangverhalten während der Entwicklung von *Salamandra salamandra* (L.). *Z. Tierpsychol.* 41: 235–243.

Himstedt, W., Tempel, R., and Weiler, J. (1978) Responses of salamanders to stationary visual patterns. *J. Comp. Psychol.* 124: 49–52.

Hirota, K., Sonoda, Y., Baba, Y., and Yamaguchi, T. (1993) Distinction in morphology and behavioral role between dorsal and ventral group of cricket giant interneurons. *Zool. Sci.* 10: 705–709.

Holmes, P. W. (1979) Transfer of matching performance in pigeons. *J. Exp. Anal. Behav.* 31: 103–114.

Homann, H. (1928) Beträge zur Physiologie der Spinnenaugen. I. Untersuchungsmethoden, II. Das Sehvermöen der Salticiden. *Z. Vergl. Physiol.* 7: 201–268.

Honegger, H.-W. (1981) A preliminary note on a new optomotor response in crickets: Antennal tracking of moving targets. *J. Comp. Physiol.* 142: 419–421.

Honegger, H.-W., Bartos, M., Gramm, T., and Gebhardt, M. (1995) Peripheral modulation and plasticity of antennal movements in crickets. *Verh. Dtsch. Zool. Ges.* 88.2: 129–137.

Hope, A. J., Partridge, J. C., Dulai, K. S., and Hunt, D. M. (1997) Mechanisms of wavelength tuning in the rod opsins of deep-sea fishes. *Proc. Roy. Soc. Lond. B* 264: 155–163.

Horridge, G. A. (1978) The separation of visual axes in apposition compound eyes. *Phil. Trans. Roy. Soc. Lond. B* 285: 1–59.

Horridge, G. A. (1980) Apposition eyes of large diurnal insects as organs adapted to seeing. *Proc. Roy. Soc. Lond. B* 207: 287–309.

Horridge, G. A. (1996) The honeybee (*Apis mellifera*) detects bilateral symmetry and discriminates its axis. *J. Insect Physiol.* 42(8): 755–764.

Horridge, G. A. (1999) Two-dimensional pattern discrimination by the honeybee. *Physiol. Entomol.* 24: 197–212.

Horridge, G. A. (2000) Seven experiments on pattern vision of the honeybee, with a model. *Vision Res.* 40: 2589–2603.

Horridge, G. A. and Duelli. P. (1979) Anatomy of the regional differences in the eye of the mantis *Ciulfina*. *J. Exp. Biol.* 80: 165–190.

Horridge, G. A. and Zhang, S. W. (1995) Pattern vision in honeybees (*Apis mellifera*): Flower-like patterns with no predominant orientation. *J. Insect Physiol.* 41(8): 681–688.

Horridge, G. A., Zhang, S. W., and O'Carroll, D. (1992a) Insect perception of illusory contours. *Phil. Trans. Roy. Soc. Lond. B* 337: 59–64.

Horridge, G. A., Zhang, S. W., and Lehrer, M. (1992b) Bees can combine range and visual angle to estimate absolute size. *Phil. Trans. Roy. Soc. Lond. B* 337: 49–57.

Horváth, G. and Varjú, D. (1997) Polarization pattern of freshwater habitats recorded by video polarimetry in red, green and blue spectral ranges and its relevance for water detection by aquatic insects. *J. Exp. Biol.* 200: 1155–1163.

Howard, J. (1981) Temporal resolving power of the photoreceptors of *Locusta migratoria*. *J. Comp. Physiol.* 144: 61–66.

Hubel, D. H. and Wiesel T. N. (1962) Receptive fields, binocular interaction and functional architecture in the cat's visual cortex. *J. Physiol.* 160: 106–154.

Huber, F. (1983) Implications of insect neuroethology for studies on vertebrates. In J.-P. Ewert, R. R. Capranica, and D. J. Ingle (eds.), *Advances in Vertebrate Neuroethology*. New York: Plenum, pp. 91–138.

Huber, R. and Delago, A. (1998) Serotonin alters decisions to withdraw in fighting crayfish, *Astacus astacus*: The motivational concept revisited. *J. Comp. Physiol. A* 182: 573–583.

Hurd, L. E. and Eisenberg, R. M. (1984a) Experimental density manipulations of the predator *Tenodera sinensis* (Orthoptera: Mantidae) in an old-field community. I. Mortality, development and dispersal of juvenile mantids. *J. Anim. Ecol.* 53: 269–281.

Hurd, L. E. and Eisenberg, R. M. (1984b) Experimental density manipulations of the predator *Tenodera sinensis* (Orthoptera: Mantidae) in an old-field community. II. The influence of mantids on arthropod community structure. *J. Anim. Ecol.* 53: 955–967.

Hurd, L. E. and Eisenberg, R. M. (1990) Arthropod community responses to manipulation of a bitrophic predator guild. *Ecology* 76: 2107–2114.

Hustert, R. (1978) Segmental and intreganglionic projections from primary fibres of insect mechanoreceptors. *Cell Tiss. Res.* 194: 337–351.

Ibbotson, M. R., Maddess, T., and DuBois, R. (1991) A system of insect neurons sensitive to horizontal and vertical image motion connects the medulla and midbrain. *J. Comp. Physiol. A* 169: 355–367.

Ilse, D. and Vaidya, V. G. (1955) Spontaneous feeding response to colours in *Papilio demoleus* L. *Proc. Ind. Acad. Sci.* 43: 23–31.

Ingle, D. J. (1970) Visuomotor functions of the frog optic tectum. *Brain, Behav. Evol.* 3: 57–71.

Ingle, D. J. (1971) Prey-catching behavior of anurans toward moving and stationary objects. *Vision Res. Suppl.* 3: 447–456.

Ingle, D. J. (1972) Depth vision in monocular frogs. *Psychon. Sci.* 29: 37–38.

Ingle, D. J. (1976a) Spatial vision in anurans. In K. V. Fite (ed.), *The Amphibian Visual System: A Multidisciplinary Approach*. New York: Academic Press, pp. 119–140.

Ingle, D. J. (1976b) Behavioral correlates of central visual function in anurans. In R. Llinás and W. Precht (eds.), *Frog Neurobiology*. Berlin: Springer-Verlag, pp. 435–451.

Ingle, D. J. (1977) Detection of stationary objects by frogs (*Rana pipiens*) after ablation of optic tectum. *J. Comp. Physiol. Psychol.* 91: 1359–1364.

Ingle, D. J. (1979) Effect of pretectum ablation on detection of barriers and apertures by frogs. *Soc. Neurosci. Abstr.* 5: 790.

Ingle, D. J. (1982) Organization of visuomotor behaviors in vertebrates. In D. J. Ingle, M. A. Goodale, and R. J. W. Mansfield (eds.), *Analysis of Visual Behavior*. Cambridge, Mass.: MIT Press, pp. 67–109.

Ingle, D. J. and Cook, J. (1977) The effect of viewing distance upon size preference of frogs for prey. *Vision Res.* 17: 1009–1013.

Ingle, D. J. and McKinley, D. (1978) Effects of stimulus configuration on elicited prey catching by the marine toad (*Bufo marinus*). *Anim. Behav.* 26: 885–891.

Irwin, R. E. and Brody, A. K. (1999) Nectar-robbing bumble bees reduce the fitness of *Ipomopsis aggregata* (Polemoniaceae). *Ecology* 80: 1703–1712.

Ishii S., Kubokawa, K., Kikuchi, M., and Nishio, H. (1995) Orientation of the toad, *Bufo japanicus*, toward the breeding pond. *Zool. Sci.* 12: 475–484.

Ivanoff, A. and Waterman, T. H. (1958) Factors, mainly depth and wavelength, affecting the degree of underwater light polarization. *J. Mar. Res.* 16: 283–307.

Jackson, R. R. (1988) The biology of *Jacksonoides queenslandica*, a jumping spider (Araneae: Salticidae) from Queensland: Intraspecific interactions, web-invasion, predators, and prey. *NZ J. Zool.* 15: 1–37.

Jackson, R. R. (1992) Predator-prey interactions between web-invading jumping spiders and *Argiope appensa* (Araneae, Araneidae), a tropical orb-weaving spider. *J. Zool. Lond.* 228: 509–520.

Jackson, R. R. (1995) Cues for web invasion and aggressive mimicry signalling in *Portia* (Araneae, Salticidae). *J. Zool. Lond.* 236: 131–149.

Jackson, R. R. and Blest, A. D. (1982a) The biology of *Portia fimbriata*, a web-building jumping spider (Araneae, Salticidae) from Queensland: Utilization of webs and predatory versatility. *J. Zool. Lond.* 196: 255–293.

Jackson, R. R. and Blest, A. D. (1982b) The distances at which a primitive jumping spider, *Portia fimbriata*, makes visual discriminations. *J. Exp. Biol.* 97: 441–445.

Jackson, R. R. and Hallas, S. E. A. (1986a) Comparative biology of *Portia africana*, *P. albimana*, *P. fimbriata*, *P. labiata* and *P. schultzi*, araneophagic web-building jumping spiders (Araneae: Salticidae): Utilization of silk, predatory versatility and intraspecific interactions. *NZ J. Zool.* 13: 423–489.

Jackson, R. R. and Hallas, S. E. A. (1986b) Capture efficiencies of web-building jumping spiders (Araneae, Salticidae): Is the jack-of-all-trades the master of none? *J. Zool. Lond.* 209: 1–7.

Jackson, R. R. and Pollard, S. D. (1996) Predatory behavior of jumping spiders. *Ann. Rev. Entomol.* 41: 287–308.

Jackson, R. R. and Wilcox, R. S. (1993a) Spider flexibly chooses aggressive mimicry signals for different prey by trial and error. *Behavior* 127: 21–36.

Jackson, R. R. and Wilcox, R. S. (1993b) Observations in nature of detouring behaviour by *Portia fimbriata*, a web-invading aggressive-mimic jumping spider from Queensland. *J. Zool. Lond.* 230: 135–139.

Jackson, R. R. and Wilcox, R. S. (1998) Spider-eating spiders. *Am. Sci.* 86: 350–357.

Jackson, R. R., Rowe, R. J., and Wilcox, R. S. (1993) Anti-predator defences of *Argiope appensa* (Araneae, Araneidae), a tropical orb-weaving spider. *J. Zool. Lond.* 229: 121–132.

Jackson, R. R., Li, D., Fijn, N., and Barrion, A. (1998) Predatory-prey interactions between aggressive-mimic jumping spiders (Salticidae) and araeneophagic spitting spiders (Scytodidae) from the Philippines. *J. Insect. Behav.* 11: 319–342.

Jackson, R. R., Carter, C. M., and Tarsitano, M. S. (2001) Trial-and-error solving of a confinement problem by a jumping spider, *Portia fimbriata*. *Behavior* 138: 1215–1234.

Jackson, R. R., Clark, R. J., and Harland, D. P. (2002) Behavioural and cognitive influences of kairomones from *Jacksonoides queenslandicus* (Araneae, Salticidae) on *Portia fimbriata*, an araneophagic salticid spider that specializes at preying on other salticids. *Behavior* 139: 749–775.

Jacobs, G. A. and Murphey, R. K. (1987) Segmental origins of the cricket giant interneuron system. *J. Comp. Neurol.* 265: 145–157.

Jacobs, G. A. and Theunissen, F. E. (1996) Functional organization of a neural map in the cricket cercal sensory system. *J. Neurosci.* 16: 769–784.

Jacobs, G. H. (1993) The distribution and nature of colour vision among the mammals. *Biol. Rev. Camb. Phil. Soc.* 68: 413–471.

Jacobs, K., Otte, B., and Lakes-Harlan, R. (1999) Tympanal receptor cells of *Schistocera gregaria*: Correlation of soma positions and dendrite attachment sites, central projections and physiologies. *J. Exp. Zool.* 283: 270–285.

James, A. C. and Osorio, D. (1996) Characterisation of columnar neurons and visual signal processing in the medulla of the locust optic lobe by system identification techniques. *J. Comp. Physiol. A* 178: 183–199.

Jander, R., Daumer, K., and Waterman, T. H. (1963) Polarized light orientation by two Hawaiian decapod cephalopods. *Z. Vergl. Physiol.* 46: 383–394.

Jander, U. and Jander, R. (2002) Allometry and resolution of bee eyes (Apoidea). *Arth. Struct. Dev.* 30: 179–193.

Jenkins, F. A. and White, H. E. (1976) *Fundamentals of Optics*. Tokyo: McGraw-Hill Kogakusha.

Jerison, H. J. (1973) *Evolution of the Brain and Intelligence*. New York: Academic Press.

Jerison, H. J. (1985) On the evolution of mind. In D. A. Oackley (ed.), *Brain and Mind, Psychology in Progress*. London, New York: Methuen, pp. 1–31.

Johnson, M. D. (1976) Concerning the feeding habits of the praying mantis *Tenodera aridifolia sinensis*, Saussure. *J. Kansas Ent. Soc.* 49: 164.

Judd, S. P. D. and Collett, T. S. (1998) Multiple stored views and landmark guidance in ants. *Nature* 392 (6677): 710–714.

Judge, S. J. and Rind, F. C. (1997) The locust DCMD, a movement-detecting neurone tightly tuned to collision trajectories. *J. Exp. Biol.* 200: 2209–2216.

Julesz, B. (1971) *The Foundations of Cyclopean Perception*. Chicago: Univ. of Chicago Press.

Kaiser, W. (1974) The spectral sensitivity of the honeybee optomotor walking response. *J. Comp. Physiol.* 90: 405–408.

Kaiser, W. and Seidl, R. (1977) The participation of all three colour receptors in the phototactic behaviour of fixed walking honeybees. *J. Comp. Physiol.* 122: 27–44.

Kamil, A. C. (1998) On the proper definition of cognitive ethology. In I. M. Pepperberg, A. Kamil, and R. Balda (eds.), *Animal Cognition in Nature*. New York: Academic Press, pp. 1–28.

Kandori, I. and Ohsaki, N. (1996) The learning abilities of the white cabbage butterfly, *Pieris rapae*, foraging for flowers. *Res. Popul. Ecol.* 38: 111–117.

Kaps, F. and Schmid, A. (1996) Mechanisms and possible behavioural relevance of retinal movements in the ctenid spider *Cupiennius salei*. *J. Exp. Biol.* 199: 2451–2458.

Kästner, A. (1950) Reaktionen der Hüpfspinnen (Salticidae) auf unbewegte farblose und farbige Gesichtsreize. *Zool. Beitr.* 1: 13–50.

Katte, O. and Hoffmann, K.-P. (1980) Direction specific neurons in the pretectum of the frog (*Rana esculenta*). *J. Comp. Physiol.* 140: 53–57.

Kawahara, M., Gleadall, I. G., and Tsukahara, Y. (1998) A note on the fibre-optic light-guides in the eye photophores of *Watasenia scintillans*. *S. Afr. J. Mar. Sci.* 20: 123–127.

Kay, P. and McDaniel, C. K. (1978) The linguistic significance of the meanings of basic color terms. *Language* 54: 610–646.

Kelber, A. (1997) Innate preferences for flower features in the hawkmoth *Macroglossum stellatarum*. *J. Exp. Biol.* 200: 827–836.

Kelber, A. (1999a) Ovipositing butterflies use a red receptor to see green. *J. Exp. Biol.* 202: 2619–2630.

Kelber, A. (1999b) Why "false" colours are seen by butterflies. *Nature* 402: 251.

Kelber, A. and Henique, U. (1999) Trichromatic colour vision in the hummingbird hawkmoth, *Macroglossum stellatarum* L. *J. Comp. Physiol. A* 184: 535–541.

Kelber, A. and Pfaff, M. (1999) True colour vision in the orchard butterfly, *Papilio aegeus*. *Naturwissenschaften* 86: 221–224.

Kelber, A., Thunell, C., and Arikawa, K. (2001) Polarisation-dependent colour vision in *Papilio* butterflies. *J. Exp. Biol.* 204: 2469–2480.

Kennedy, D. and Bruno, M. S. (1961) The spectral sensitivity of crayfish and lobster vision. *J. Gen. Physiol.* 44: 1089–1102.

Kennedy, J. S. (1945) Observations on the mass migration of desert locust hoppers. *Trans. Roy. Entomol. Soc. Lond.* 95: 247–262.

Keskinen, E., Takaku, Y., Meyer-Rochow, V. B., and Hariyama, T. (2002) Postembryonic eye growth in the seashore Isopod *Ligia exotica* (Crustacea, Isopoda) *Biol. Bull.* 202: 223–231.

Kevan, P. G., Chittka, L., and Dyer, A. G. (2001) Limits to the salience of ultraviolet: Lessons from colour vision in bees and birds. *J. Exp. Biol.* 204: 2571–2580.

Kicliter, E. (1973) Flux, wavelength and movement discrimination in the frogs: Forebrain and midbrain contributions. *Brain. Behav. Evol.* 8: 340–365.

Kicliter, E. and Goytia, E. J. (1995) A comparison of spectral response functions of positive and negative phototaxis in two anuran amphibians, *Rana pipiens* and *Leptodactylus pentadactylus*. *Neurosci. Lett.* 185: 144–146.

Kien, J. and Menzel, R. (1977a) Chromatic properties of interneurons in the optic lobes of the bee. I.Broad band neurons. *J. Comp. Physiol.* 113: 17–34.

Kien, J. and Menzel, R. (1977b) Chromatic properties of interneurons in the optic lobes of the bee. II. Narrow band and colour opponent neurons. *J. Comp. Physiol. A* 113: 35–53.

King-Leung, K. and Goldsmith, T. H. (1977) Photosensitivity of retinular cells in white-eyed crayfish (*Procambarus clarkii*). *J. Comp. Physiol. A* 122: 273–288.

Kinoshita, M. and Arikawa, K. (2000) Colour constancy of the swallowtail butterfly, *Papilio xuthus*. *J. Exp. Biol.* 203: 3521–3530.

Kinoshita M., Sato, M., and Arikawa, K. (1997) Spectral receptors of nymphalid butterflies. *Naturwissenschaften* 84: 199–201.

Kinoshita, M., Shimada, N., and Arikawa, K. (1999) Colour vision of the foraging swallowtail butterfly *Papilio xuthus*. *J. Exp. Biol.* 202: 95–102.

Kirschfeld, K. (1976) The resolution of lens and compound eyes. In F. Zettler and R. Weiler (eds.), *Neural Principles in Vision*. Berlin: Springer-Verlag, pp. 354–370.

Kitamoto, J., Sakamoto, K., Ozaki, K., Mishina, Y., and Arikawa, K. (1998) Two visual pigments in a single photoreceptor cell: Identification and histological localization of three mRNAs encoding visual pigment opsins in the retina of the butterfly *Papilio xuthus*. *J. Exp. Biol.* 201: 1255–1261.

Kitamoto, J., Ozaki, K., and Arikawa, K. (2000) Ultraviolet and violet receptors express identical mRNA encoding an ultraviolet-absorbing opsin: Identification and histological localization of two mRNAs encoding short-wavelength-absorbing opsins in the retina of the butterfly *Papilio xuthus*. *J. Exp. Biol.* 203: 2887–2894.

Knowles, A. and Dartnall, H. J. A. (1977) Habitat and visual pigments. In H. Davson (ed.), *The Eye*. vol. 2B, *The Photobiology of Vision*. New York: Academic Press, pp. 581–641.

Kolb, G. (1986) Retinal ultrastructure in the dorsal rim and large dorsal area of the eye of *Aglais urticae* (Lepidoptera). *Zoomorphology* 106: 244–246.

Kolb, G. and Scherer, C. (1982) Experiments on wavelength specific behavior of *Pieris brassicae* L. during drumming and egg-laying. *J. Comp. Physiol. A* 149: 325–332.

Kolton, L. and Camhi, J. M. (1995) Cartesian representation of stimulus direction: Parallel processing by two sets of giant interneurons in the cockroach. *J. Comp. Physiol.* 176: 691–702.

Kondrashev, S. L. (1987) Neuroethology and color vision in amphibians. *Behav. Brain Sci.* 10: 385.

Kong, K. L., Fung, Y. M., and Wasserman, G. S. (1980) Filter-mediated color vision with one visual pigment. *Science* 207: 783–786.

Kozicz, T. and Lázár, G. (1994) The origin of tectal NPY immunopositive fibers in the frog. *Brain Res.* 635: 345–348.

Kozicz, T. and Lázár, G. (2001) Colocalization of GABA, enkephalin and neuropeptide Y in the tectum of the green frog *Rana esculenta*. *Peptides* 22: 1071–1077.

Kral, K. (1987) Organization of the first optic neuropile (or lamina) in different insect species. In A. P. Gupta (ed.), The *Arthropod Brain: Its Evolution, Development, Structure and Functions*. New York: Wiley, pp. 181–201.

Kral, K. (1998a) Side-to-side movements to obtain motion depth cues: A short review of research on the praying mantis. *Behav. Proc.* 43: 71–77.

Kral, K. (1998b) Spatial vision in the course of an insect's life. *Brain Behav. Evol.* 52: 1–6.

Kral, K. (1999) Binocular vision and distance estimation. In F. R. Prete, H. Wells, P. Wells, and L. E. Hurd (eds.), *The Praying Mantids*. Baltimore, Md.: Johns Hopkins Univ. Press, pp. 114–140.

Kral, K. and Devetak, D. (1999) The visual orientation strategies of *Mantis religiosa* and *Empusa fasciata* reflect differences in the structure of their visual surroundings. *J. Insect Behav.* 12: 737–752.

Kral, K. and Poteser, M. (1997) Motion parallax as a source of distance information in locusts and mantids. *J. Insect Behav.* 10: 145–163.

Krebs, W. and Lietz, R. (1982) Apical region of the crayfish retinula. *Cell Tiss. Res.* 222: 409–415.

Kretz, R. (1979) A behavioural analysis of colour vision in the ant *Cataglyphis bicolor* (Formicidae, Hymenoptera). *J. Comp. Physiol. A* 131: 217–233.

Kriska, G., Horvath, G., and Andrikovics, S. (1998) Why do mayflies lay their eggs en masse on dry asphalt roads? Water-imitating polarized light reflected from asphalt attracts Ephemeroptera. *J. Exp. Biol.* 201: 2273–2286.

Kristensen, N. P. (1991) Phylogeny of extant hexapods. In I. D. Naumann, P. B. Carne, J. F. Lawrence, E. S. Nielsen, J. P. Spradbery, R. W. Taylor, M. J. Whitten, and M. J. Littlejohn (eds.), *The Insects of Australia: A Textbook for Students and Research Workers.* Melbourne: CSIRO, Melbourne University Press, pp. 125–140.

Krout, K. E., Loewy, A. D., Westby, G. W. M., and Redgrave, P. (2001) Superior colliculus projections to midline and intralaminar thalamic nuclei of the rat. *J. Comp. Neurol.* 431: 198–216.

Kühn, A. (1924) Versuche über das Unterscheidungsvermögen der Bienen und Fische für Spektrallichter. *Nachr. D. Ges. Wiss.* 1: 66–71.

Kunze, J. and Gumbert, A. (2001) The combined effect of color and odor on flower choice behavior of bumble bees in flower mimicry systems. *Behav. Ecol.* 12: 447–456.

Kunze, P. and Boschek, C. B. (1968) Elektronmikroskopische Untersuchung zur Form der achten Retinulazelle bei Ocypode. *Z. Naturforsch.* 23: 568–569.

Kupfermann, I. and Weiss, K. R. (1978) The command neuron concept. *Behav. Brain Sci.* 1: 3–39.

Kurasawa, M., Wakakuwa, M., Kitamoto, J., Giurfa, M., and Arikawa, K. (2002) Spectral heterogeneity of the ommatidia in the retina of worker honeybees: A molecular phylogenetic study demonstrating three types of ommatidia. *Proc. XIV Int. Meeting IUSSI,* Sapporo, Japan. Sapporo, Japan: Hokkaido University, p. 72.

Labhart, T. and Nilsson, D. E. (1995) The dorsal eye of the dragonfly Sympetrum: Specializations for prey detection against the sky. *J. Comp. Physiol. A* 176: 437–453.

Lam, D. M. K., Wiesel, T. N., and Kaneko, A. (1974) Neurotransmitter synthesis in cephalopod retina. *Brain Res.* 82: 365–368.

Laming, P. R. and Cairns, C. (1998) Effects of food, glucose and water ingestion on feeding activity in the toad (*Bufo bufo*). *Behav. Neurosci.* 112: 1266–1272.

Land, E. H. (1977) The retinex theory of color vision. *Sci. Am.* 237: 108–128.

Land, M. F. (1969a) Structure of the retinae of the eyes of jumping spiders (Salticidae: Dendryphantinae) in relation to visual optics. *J. Exp. Biol.* 51: 443–470.

Land, M. F. (1969b) Movements of the retinae of jumping spiders (Salticidae: Dendryphantinae) in response to visual stimuli. *J. Exp. Biol.* 51: 471–493.

Land, M. F. (1971) Orientation by jumping spiders in the absence of visual feedback. *J. Exp. Biol.* 54: 119–139.

Land, M. F. (1972) Stepping movements made by jumping spiders during turns mediated by the lateral eyes. *J. Exp. Biol.* 57: 15–40.

Land, M. F. (1974) A comparison of the visual behaviour of a predatory arthropod with that of a mammal. In C. A. G. Wiersma (ed.), *Invertebrate Neurons and Behavior*. Cambridge, Mass: MIT Press, pp. 411–418.

Land, M. F. (1981) Optics and vision in invertebrates. In H. Autrum (ed.), *Handbook of Sensory Physiology*. vol. VII/6B, *Comparative Physiology and Evolution of Vision in Invertebrates*. Berlin: Springer-Verlag, pp. 471–592.

Land, M. F. (1984) Molluscs. In M. Ali (ed.), *Photoreception and Vision in Invertebrates*. NATO Advanced Science Series A, vol. 74, New York: Plenum, pp. 699–725.

Land, M. F. (1985a) The morphology and optics of spider eyes. In F. G. Barth (ed.), *Neurobiology of Arachnids*. Berlin: Springer-Verlag, pp. 53–78.

Land, M. F. (1985b) Fields of view of the eyes of primitive jumping spiders. *J. Exp. Biol.* 119: 381–384.

Land, M. F. (1993) Old twist in a new tale. *Nature* 363: 581–852.

Land, M. F. (1995) The functions of eye movements in animals remote from man. In J. M. Findlay (ed.), *Eye Movement Research*. Amsterdam: Elsevier, pp. 63–76.

Land, M. F. (1997) Visual acuity in insects. *Annu. Rev. Entomol.* 42: 147–177.

Land, M. F. and Furneaux, S. (1997) The knowledge base of the oculomotor system. *Phil. Trans. Roy. Soc. Lond. B* 352: 1231–1239.

Land, M. F. and Nilsson D. E. (2002) *Animal Eyes*. Oxford: Oxford Univ. Press.

Land, M. F., Marshall, N. J., Brownless, D., and Cronin, T. W. (1990) The eye-movements of the mantis shrimp *Odontodactylus scyllarus* (Crustacea: stomatopods). *J. Comp. Physiol. A* 167: 155–166.

Lange, G. D. and Hartline, P. H. (1974) Retinal responses in squid and octopus. *J. Comp. Physiol.* 93: 19–36.

Lange, G. D., Hartline, P. H., and Hurley, A. C. (1976) The question of lateral interactions in the retinas of cephalopods. In F. Zettler and R. Weiler (eds.), *Neural Principles in Vision*. Berlin: Springer-Verlag, pp. 89–93.

Langley, C. M., Riley, D. A., Bond, A. B. and Goel, N. (1996) Visual search for natural grains in pigeons (*Columba livia*): Search images and selective attention. *J. Exp. Psychol. Anim. Behav. Proc.* 22: 139–151.

Lashley, K. S. (1949) Persistent problems in the evolution of mind. Quart. Rev. Biol. 24: 28–42.

Laughlin, S. B. (1981) Neural principles in the peripheral visual systems of invertebrates. In H. Autrum (ed.), *Handbook of Sensory Physiology*. vol. VII/6B, *Comparative Physiology and Evolution of Vision in Invertebrates*. Berlin: Springer-Verlag, pp. 133–280.

Laughlin, S. B. (1989) Coding efficiency and design in visual processing. In D. G. Stavenga and R. C. Hardie (eds.), *Facets of Vision*. Berlin: Springer-Verlag, pp. 213–234.

Laughlin, S. B., Howard, J., and Blakeslee, B. (1987) Synaptic limitations to contrast coding in the retina of the blowfly *Calliphora. Proc. Roy. Soc. Lond. B* 231: 437–467.

Lázár, G. (1971) The projection of the retinal quadrants on the optic centers in the frog: A terminal degeneration study. *Acta Morph. Acad. Sci. Hung.* 19: 325–334.

Lázár, G. (1973) Role of accessory optic system in the optokinetic nystagmus of the frog. *Brain Behav. Evol.* 5: 443–460.

Lázár, G. (1979) Organization of the frog visual system. In K. Lissák (ed.), *Recent Developments of Neurobiology in Hungary*, vol. 8. Budapest: Akadémiai Kiadò, pp. 9–50.

Lázár, G. (1984) Structure and connections of the frog optic tectum. In H. Vanegas (ed.), *Comparative Neurology of the Optic Tectum*. New York: Plenum, pp. 185–210.

Lázár, G. (1989) Cellular architecture and connectivity of the frog's optic tectum and pretectum. In J.-P. Ewert and M. A. Arbib (eds.), *Visuomotor Coordination: Amphibians, Comparisons, Models and Robots*. New York: Plenum, pp. 175–199.

Lázár, G. (2001) Peptides in frog brain areas processing visual information. *Microscop. Res. Techn.* 54: 201–219.

Lázár, G. and Kozicz, T. (1990) Morphology of neurons and axon terminals associated with descending and ascending pathways of the lateral forebrain bundle in *Rana esculenta. Cell Tiss. Res.* 260: 535–548.

Lázár, G., Tóth, P., Csank, G., and Kicliter, E. (1983b) Morphology and location of tectal projection neurons in frogs: A study with HRP and cobalt-filling. *J. Comp. Neurol.* 215: 108–120.

Lázár, G., Maderdrut, J. L., Trasti, S. L., Liposits, Z., Tóth, P., Kozicz, T., and Merchenthaler I. (1993) Distribution of proneuropeptide Y-derived peptides in the brain of *Rana esculenta* and *Xenopus laevis. J. Comp. Neurol.* 327: 551–571.

Lefebvre, L., Whittle, P., Lascaris, E., and Finkelstein, A. (1997) Feeding innovations and forebrain size in birds. *Anim. Behav.* 53: 549–560.

Leggett, L. M. W. (1976) Polarised light-sensitive neurons in a swimming crab. *Nature (London)* 262: 709–711.

Lehrer, M. (1998) Looking all around: Honeybees use different cues in different eye regions. *J. Exp. Biol.* 201: 3275–3292.

Lehrer, M., Horridge, G. A., Zhang, Z. W., and Gadagkar, R. (1995) Shape vision in bees: Innate preference for flower-like patterns. *Phil. Trans. Roy. Soc. Lond. B* 347: 123–137.

Leitinger, G. (1994) Frühe postembryonale Entwicklung des Komplexauges und der Lamina ganglionaris der Gottesanbeterin nach Photodegeneration der akuten Zone mit Sulforhodamin. Masters thesis, Univ. of Graz, Graz, Austria.

Leitinger, G. (1997) Serotonin-immunoreactive neurones in the visual system of larval and adult praying mantis (*Tenodera sinensis*). Ph.D. thesis, Univ. of Graz, Graz, Austria.

Leitinger, G., Pabst, M. A., and Kral, K. (1999) Serotonin-immunoreactive neurones in the visual system of the praying mantis: An immunohistochemical, confocal laser scanning and electron microscopic study. *Brain Res.* 823: 11–23.

Lettvin, J. Y., Maturana, H. R., McCulloch, W. S., and Pitts, W. H. (1959) What the frog's eye tells the frog's brain. *Proc. Inst. Radio. Engin.* 47: 1940–1951.

Leung, V. and Comer, C. M. (2001) Identification and characterization of a visual interneuron in the cockroach, *Periplaneta americana*, equivalent to DCMD. *Soc. Neurosci. Abstr.* vol. 27, Program No. 308.2.

Levine, J. S. (1980) Vision underwater. *Oceanus* 23: 19–26.

Li, D. and Jackson, R. R. (1996) Prey preferences of *Portia fimbriata*, an araneophagic, web-building jumping spider (Araneae: Salticidae) from Queensland. *J. Insect Behav.* 9: 613–642.

Li, D., Jackson, R. R., and Barrion, A. (1997) Prey preferences of *Portia labiata*, *P. africana* and *P. schultzi*, araneophagic jumping spiders (Araneae: Salticidae) from the Philippines, Sri Lanka, Kenya and Uganda. *NZ J. Zool.* 24: 333–349.

Li, D., Jackson, R. R., and Barrion, A. (1999) Parental and predatory behaviour of *Scytodes* sp., an araneophagic spitting spider (Araneae: Scytodidae) from the Philippines. *J. Zool. Lond.* 247: 293–310.

Li, Z., Fite, K. V., Montgomery, N. M., and Wang, S. R. (1996) Single-unit resoponses to whole-field visual stimulation in the pretectum of *Rana pipiens*. *Neurosci. Lett.* 218: 193–197.

Libersat, F. (1992) Modulation of flight by giant interneurons of the cockroach. *J. Comp. Physiol.* 170: 379–392.

Lima, P. A., Coehlo, M. L., Andrade, J. P., and Brown, E. R. (1995) Do squid school like fish? In A. Guerra, E. Rolán, and F. Rocha (eds.), *Abstracts of the 12th International Malacological Congress*, Vigo, Spain: Instituto de Investigaciones Marinas, pp. 70.

Lindauer, M. (1955) Schwarmbienen auf Wohnungssuche. *Z. Vergl. Physiol.* 37: 263–324.

Lindauer, M. (1959) Angeborene und erlernte Komponenten in der Son-nenorientierung der Bienen. *Z. Vergl. Physiol.* 42: 43–62.

Lindemann, B. (2001) Receptors and transduction in taste. *Nature* 413: 219–225.

Lindemann, S. O. G. and Roth, G. (1999) A fear acquisition system in amphibians. *Neural Plast.* 1: 65.

Lindsay, P. H. and Norman, D. A. (1977) *Human Information Processing: An Introduction to Psychology*. New York: Academic Press.

Liske, E. (1999) The hierarchical organization of mantid behavior. In F. R. Prete, H. Wells, P. Wells, and L. E. Hurd (eds.), *The Praying Mantids*. Baltimore, Md.: Johns Hopkins Univ. Press, pp. 224–250.

Little, E. E. (1975) Chemical communication in maternal behaviour of crayfish. *Nature* 255: 400–1.

Loi, P. K., Saunders, R. G., Young, D. C., and Tublitz, N. J. (1996) Peptidergic regulation of chromatophore function in the European cuttlefish *Sepia officinalis*. *J. Exp. Biol.* 199: 1177–1187.

Lubbock, J. (1889) Die Sinne und das Geistige Leben der Tiere. *Wissenschaftl. Bibliothek Band* 57.

Lucero, M. T. and Gilly, W. T. (1995) Physiology of squid olfaction. In N. J. Abbott, R. Williamson, and L. Maddock (eds.), *Cephalopod Neurobiology. Neuroscience Studies in Squid, Octopus and Cuttlefish*. Oxford: Oxford Univ. Press.

Lucero, M. T., Farrington, H., and Gilly, W. F. (1994) Quantification of L-dopa and dopamine in squid ink: Implications for chemoreception. *Biol. Bull.* 187: 55–63.

Lucero, M. T., Horrigan, F. T., and Gilly, W. F. (1992) Electrical responses to chemical stimulation of squid olfactory receptor cells. *J. Exp. Biol.* 162: 231–249.

Luksch, H. and Roth, G. (1996) Pretecto-tectal interactions: Effects of lesioning and stimulating the pretectum on field potentials in the optic tectum of salamanders in vitro. *Neurosci. Lett.* 217: 137–140.

Luksch, H., Kahl, H., Wiggers, W., and Roth, G. (1998) Connectivity of the salamander pretectum: An in-vitro (whole-brain) intracellular tracing study. *Cell Tiss. Res.* 292: 47–56.

Lunau, K. (1990) Colour saturation triggers innate reactions to flower signals: Flower dummy experiments with bumblebees. *J. Comp. Physiol. A* 166: 827–834.

Lunau, K., Wacht, S., and Chittka, L. (1996) Colour choices of naive bumble bees and their implications for colour perception. *J. Comp. Physiol. A* 178: 477–489.

Luthardt, G. and Roth, G. (1979) The role of stimulus movement patterns in the prey-catching behavior of *Salamandra salamandra*. *Copeia* 1979: 442–447.

Lythgoe, J. N. (1972) The adaptation of visual pigments to the photic environment. In H. J. A. Dartnall (ed.), *Handbook of Sensory Physiology*. VII/1, *Photochemistry of Vision*. Berlin: Springer-Verlag, pp. 566–603.

Lythgoe, J. N. (1976) Underwater vision. *Proc. Roy. Soc. Med.* 69: 67–68.

Lythgoe, J. N. (1979) *The Ecology of Vision*. Oxford: Clarendon Press.

Lythgoe, J. N. (1985) Aspects of photoreception in aquatic environments. *Symp. Soc. Exp. Biol.* 39: 373–386.

Lythgoe, J. N. and Hemming, C. C. (1967) Polarized light and underwater vision. *Nature* 213: 893–894.

Lythgoe, J. N. and Partridge, J. C. (1989) Visual pigments and the acquisition of visual information. *J. Exp. Biol.* 146: 1–20.

Mace, G. M., Harvey, P. H., and Clutton-Brock, T. M. (1981) Brain size and ecology in small mammals. *J. Zool. Lond.* 193: 333–354.

MacFarland, W. N. and Munz, F. W. (1975a) Part II: The photic environment of clear tropical seas during the day. *Vision Res.* 15: 1063–1070.

MacFarland, W. N. and Munz, F. W. (1975b) Part III: The evolution of photopic visual pigments in fishes. *Vision Res.* 15: 1071–1080.

Maddess, T., Dubois, R. A., and Ibbotson, M. R. (1991) Response properties and adaptation of neurones sensitive to image motion in the butterfly *Papilio aegeus. J. Exp. Biol.* 161: 171–199.

Magni, F., Papi, F., Savely, H. E., and Tongiorgi, P. (1964) Research on the structure and physiology of the eyes of a lycosid spider. II. The role of different pairs of eyes in astronomical orientation. *Archs. Ital. Biol.* 102: 123–136.

Magni, F., Papi, F., Savely, H. E., and Tongiorgi, P. (1965) Research on the structure and physiology of the eyes of a lycosid spider. III. Electroretinographic responses to polarised light. *Archs. Ital. Biol.* 103: 146–158.

Maldonado, H. (1970) The deimatic reaction in the praying mantis *Stagmatoptera biocellata. Z. Vergl. Physiol.* 68: 60–71.

Maloney, L. T. (1986) Evaluation of linear models of surface spectral reflectance with small numbers of parameters. *J. Opt. Soc. Am. A* 3: 1673–1683.

Maloney, L. T. and Wandell, B. A. (1986) Color constancy: A method for recovering surface spectral reflectance. *J. Opt. Soc. Am. A* 3: 29–33.

Manning, R. L. (1995) Stomatopod crustacea of Vietnam: The legacy of Raoul Serene. *Crustacean Research Special Number 4.* Carcinol. Soc. Japan, Tokyo.

Manning, R. L., Schiff, H., and Abbott, H. (1984) Eye structure and the classification of the stomatopod Crustacea. *Zool. Scripta.* 13: 41–44.

Marín, O., González, A., and Smeets, W. J. A. J. (1997a) Basal ganglia organization in amphibians: Efferent connections of the striatum and the nucleus accumbens. *J. Comp. Neurol.* 380: 23–50.

Marín, O., González, A., and Smeets, W. J. A. J. (1997b) Anatomical substrate of amphibian basal ganglia involvement in visuomotor behaviour. *Eur. J. Neurosci.* 9: 2100–2109.

Marín, O., Smeets, W. J. A. J., and González, A. (1997c) Basal ganglia organization in amphibians: Development of striatal and nucleus accumbens connections with emphasis on the catecholaminergic inputs. *J. Comp. Neurol.* 383: 349–369.

Marín, O., Smeets, W. J. A. J., and González, A. (1997d) Basal ganglia organization in amphibians: Catecholaminergic innervation of the striatum and the nucleus accumbens. *J. Comp. Neurol.* 378: 50–69.

Marín, O., González, A., and Smeets, W. J. A. J. (1998a) Basal ganglia organization in amphibians: Chemoarchitecture. *J. Comp. Neurol.* 392: 285–312.

Marín, O., Smeets, W. J. A. J., and González A. (1998b) Evolution of the basal ganglia in tetrapods: A new perspective based on recent studies in amphibians. *Trends Neurosci.* 21: 487–494.

Marín, O., Smeets, W. J. A. J., Munoz, M., Sanchez-Camacho, C., Pena, J. J., Lopez, J. M., and González, A. (1999) Cholinergic and catecholaminergic neurons relay striatal information to the optic tectum in amphibians. *Eur. J. Morphol.* 37: 155–159.

Marshall, N. J. (1988) A unique colour and polarisation vision system in mantis shrimps. *Nature* 333: 557–560.

Marshall, N. J. and Land, M. F. (1993a) Some optical features of the eyes of stomatopods. I. Eye shape, optical axis and resolution. *J. Comp. Physiol. A* 173: 565–582.

Marshall, N. J. and Land, M. F. (1993b) Some optical features of the eyes of stomatopods. II. Ommatidial design, sensitivity and habitat. *J. Comp. Physiol. A* 173: 583–594.

Marshall, N. J. and Messenger, J. B. (1996) Colour-blind camouflage. *Nature (London)* 382: 408–409.

Marshall, N. J. and Oberwinkler, J. (1999) The colourful world of the mantis shrimp. *Nature (London)* 401: 873–874.

Marshall, N. J., Land, M. F., King, C. A., and Cronin, T. W. (1991a) The compound eyes of mantis shrimps (Crustacea, Hoplocarida, Stomatopoda). I. Compound eye structure: The detection of polarized light. *Phil. Trans. Roy. Soc. Lond. B* 334: 33–56.

Marshall, N. J., Land, M. F., King, C. A., and Cronin, T. W. (1991b) The compound eye of mantis shrimps (Crustacea, Hoplocarida, Stomatopoda). II. Colour pigments in the eyes of stomatopod crustaceans: Polychromatic vision by serial and lateral filtering. *Phil. Trans. Roy. Soc. Lond. B* 334: 57–84.

Marshall, N. J., Land, M. F., and Cronin, T. W. (1994) The six-eyed stomatopod. *Endeavour* 18: 17–26.

Marshall, N. J., Jones, J. P., and Cronin, T. W. (1996) Behavioural evidence for color vision in stomatopod crustaceans. *J. Comp. Physiol. A* 179: 473–481.

Marshall, N. J., Cronin, T. W., and Shashar, N. (1999) Behavioural evidence for polarization vision in stomatopods reveals a potential channel for communication. *Curr. Biol.* 9: 755–758.

Masino, T. and Grobstein, P. (1989a) The organization of descending tectofugal pathways underlying orienting in the frog, *Rana pipiens*. I. Lateralization, parcellation and an intermediate spatial representation. *Exp. Brain Res.* 75: 227–244.

Masino, T. and Grobstein, P. (1989b) The organization of descending tectofugal pathways underlying orienting in the frog, *Rana pipiens*. II. Evidence for the involvement of a tecto-tegmento-spinal pathway. *Exp. Brain Res.* 75: 245–264.

Masino, T. and Grobstein, P. (1990) Tectal connectivity in the frog *Rana pipiens*: Tectotegmental projections and a general analysis of topographic organization. *J. Comp. Neurol.* 291: 103–127.

Mason, A. C. and Bailey, W. J. (1998) Ultrasound hearing and male-male competition in Australian katydids (Tettigoniidae, Zaprochilinae) with sexually dimorphic ears. *Physiol. Entomol.* 23: 139–149.

Mason, A. C., Morris G. K., and Hoy, R. R. (1999) Peripheral frequency mis-match in the primitive ensiferan *Cyphoderris monstrosa* (Orthoptera: Hagilidae). *J. Comp. Physiol. A* 184: 543–551.

Masters, W. M., Markl, H., and Moffat, A. J. M. (1986) Transmission of vibration in a spider's web. In W. A. Shear (ed.), *Spiders: Webs, Behavior and Evolution*. Stanford, Calif: Stanford Univ. Press, pp. 49–69.

Mathger, L. M. and Denton, E. J. (2001) Reflective properties of iridophores and fluorescent "eyespots" in the loliginid squid *Alloteuthis subulata* and *Loligo vulgaris*. *J. Exp. Biol.* 204: 2103–2118.

Matic, T. (1983) Electrical inhibition in the retina of the butterfly *Papilio*. I. Four spectral types of photoreceptors. *J. Comp. Physiol. A* 152: 169–182.

Matsui, S., Seidou, M., Uchiyama, I., Sekiya, N., Hiraki, K., Yoshihara, K., and Kito, Y. (1988) 4-hydroxyretinal, a new visual pigment chromophore found in the bioluminescent squid, *Watacenia scintillans*. *Biochem. Biophys. Acta*. 966: 370–374.

Matsumoto, N. (1989) Morphological and physiological studies of tectal and pretectal neurons in the frog. In J.-P. Ewert and M. A. Arbib (eds.), *Visuomotor Coordination: Amphibians, Comparisons, Models and Robots*. New York: Plenum, pp. 201–222.

Matsumoto, N., Schwippert, W. W., and Ewert, J.-P. (1986) Intracellular activity of morphologically identified neurons of the grass frog's optic tectum in response to moving configurational visual stimuli. *J. Comp. Physiol. A* 159: 721–739.

Matsumoto, N., Schwippert, W. W., Beneke, T. W., and Ewert, J.-P. (1991) Forebrain-mediated control of visually guided prey-catching in toads: Investigation of striato-pretectal connections with intracellular recording/labeling methods. *Behav. Proc.* 25: 27–40.

Matsushima, T., Satou, M., and Ueda, K. (1989) Medullary reticular neurons in the Japanese toad: Morphology and excitatory inputs from the optic tectum. *J. Comp. Physiol. A* 166: 7–22.

Mazokhin-Porshnyakov, G. A. (1966) Recognition of coloured objects by insects. In C. G. Bernhard (ed.), *The Functional Organization of the Compound Eye*. Oxford: Pergamon Press, pp. 163–170.

McFarland, D. and Bosser, T. (1993) *Intelligent Behavior in Animals and Robots*. Cambridge, Mass: MIT Press.

McIlwain, J. T. (1996) *An Introduction to the Biology of Vision*. Cambridge: Cambridge University Press.

Medina, L. and Reiner, A. (1995) Neurotransmitter organization and connectivity of the basal ganglia in vertebrates: Implications for the evolution of basal ganglia. *Brain, Behav. Evol.* 46: 235–258.

Medina, L., Jiao, Y., and Reiner, A. (1999) The functional anatomy of the basal ganglia in birds. *Eur. J. Morphol.* 37: 160–165.

Meier, T., Chabaud, F., and Reichert, H. (1991) Homologous patterns in the embryonic development of the peripheral nervous system in the grasshopper *Schistocera gregaria* and the fly *Drosophila melanogaster*. *Development* 112: 241–253.

Meinecke, C. C. and Langer, H. (1984) Localization of visual pigments within rhabdoms of the compound eye of *Spodoptera exempta* (Insecta, Noctuidae). *Cell Tiss. Res.* 238: 359–368.

Meinertzhagen, I. A. (1991) Evolution of the cellular organization of the arthropod compound eye and optic lobe. In J. R. Cronly-Dillon and R. L. Gregory (eds.), *Evolution of the Eye and Visual System: Vision and Visual Dysfunction*. New York: Macmillan, pp. 341–363.

Mengual, E., de las Heras, S., Erro, E., Lanciego, J. L., and Bimenez-Amaya, J. M. (1999) Thalamic interaction between the input and the output system of the basal ganglia. *J. Chem. Neuroanat.* 16: 187–200.

Menzel, R. (1979) Spectral sensitivity and colour vision in invertebrates. In H. Autrum (ed.), *Handbook of Sensory Physiology*. vol. VII/6A, *Invertebrate Photoreceptors*. Berlin: Springer-Verlag, pp. 503–580.

Menzel, R. (1985) Learning in honey bees in an ecological and behavioral context. In B. Hölldobler and M. Lindauer (eds.), *Experimental Behavioral Ecology*. Stuttgart: Gustav Fischer Verlag, pp. 55–74.

Menzel, R. (1990) Learning, memory and "cognition" in honey bees. In R. P. Kesner and D. S. Olton (eds.), *Neurobiology of Comparative Cognition*. Hillsdale, N.J.: IEA Publishers, pp. 237–292.

Menzel, R. (2001) Behavioral and neural mechanisms of learning and memory as determinants of flower constancy. In L. Chittka and J. D. Thomson (eds.), *Cognitive Ecology of Pollination*. Cambridge: Cambridge Univ. Press, pp. 21–40.

Menzel, R. and Backhaus, W. (1989) Color vision in honey bees: Phenomena and physiological mechanisms. In D. Stavenga and R. Hardie (eds.), *Facets of Vision*. Berlin: Springer-Verlag, pp. 281–297.

Menzel, R. and Backhaus, W. (1991) Colour vision in insects. In P. Gouras (ed.), *The Perception of Colour*. London: Macmillan, pp. 262–293.

Menzel, R. and Bitterman, M. E. (1983) Learning by honeybees in an unnatural situation. In F. Huber and H. Markl (eds.), *Neurobiology and Behavioral Physiology*. Berlin: Springer-Verlag, pp. 206–215.

Menzel, R. and Blakers, M. (1976) Colour receptors in the bee eye—Morphology and spectral sensitivity. *J. Comp. Physiol.* 108: 11–33.

Menzel, R. and Greggers, U. (1985) Natural phototaxis and its relationship to colour vision in honeybees. *J. Comp. Physiol.* 157: 311–321.

Menzel, R. and Lieke, E. (1983) Antagonistic color effects in spatial vision of honeybees. *J. Comp. Physiol. A* 151: 441–448.

Menzel, R. and Muller, U. (1996) Learning and memory in honeybees: From behavior to neural substrates. *Ann. Rev. Neurosci.* 19: 379–404.

Menzel, R., Bicker, G., Carew, T. J., Fischbach, K. F., Gould, J. L., Heinrich, B., Heisenberg, M. A., Lindauer, M., Markl, H. S., Quinn, W. G., Sahley, C. L., and Wagner, A. R. (1984) Biology of invertebrate learning. In P. Marler and H. S. Terrace (eds.), *The Biology of Learning: Report of the Dahlem Workshop on the Biology of Learning*. Berlin: Springer-Verlag, pp. 249–270.

Merchenthaler, I., Lázár, G., and Maderdrut, J. L. (1989) Distribution of proenkephalin-derived peptides in the brain of *Rana esculenta*. *J. Comp. Neurol.* 281: 23–39.

Meredith, M. A. and Stein, B. E. (1986) Visual, auditory and somato-sensory convergence on cells in superior colliculus results in multisensory integration. *J. Neurophysiol.* 75: 1843–1857.

Merkel-Harff, C. and Ewert, J.-P. (1991) Learning-related modulation of toad's responses to prey by neural loops involving the forebrain. In M. A. Arbib and J.-P. Ewert (eds.), *Visual Structures and Integrated Functions*. Berlin: Springer-Verlag, pp. 417–426.

Messenger, J. B. (1971) The optic tract lobes. In J. Z. Young (ed.), *The Anatomy of the Nervous System of Octopus vulgaris*. Oxford: Oxford Univ. Press, pp. 481–506.

Messenger, J. B. (1974) Reflective elements in cephalopod skin and their importance for camouflage. *J. Zool. Lond.* 174: 387–395.

Messenger, J. B. (1977) Evidence that Octopus is colour blind. *J. Exp. Biol.* 70: 49–55.

Messenger, J. B. (1979a) The nervous system of *Loligo* IV. The peduncle and olfactory lobes. *Phil. Trans. Roy. Soc. Lond. B* 285: 275–309.

Messenger, J. B. (1979b) The eyes and skin of Octopus: Compensating for sensory deficiencies. *Endeavour* 3: 92–98.

Messenger, J. B. (1981) Comparative physiology of vision in molluscs. In H. Autrum (ed.), *Handbook of Sensory Physiology*. vol. VII/6C, *Comparative Physiology and Evolution of Vision in Invertebrates*. Berlin: Springer-Verlag, pp. 93–200.

Messenger, J. B. (1991) Photoreception and vision in molluscs. In J. R. Cronly-Dillon and R. L. Gregory (eds.), *Evolution of the Eye and Visual System*. London: Macmillan, pp. 364–397.

Messenger, J. B. (2001) Cephalopod chromatophores: Neurobiology and natural history. *Biol. Rev. Camb. Phil. Soc.* 76: 473–528.

Messenger, J. B., Wilson, A. P., and Hedge, A. (1973) Some evidence for colour blindness in Octopus. *J. Exp. Biol.* 59: 77–94.

Meyer, D. J., Margiotta, J. F., and Walcott, B. (1981) The shadow response of the cockroach *Periplaneta americana*. *J. Neurobiol.* 12(1): 93–96.

Meyer-Rochow, V. B. and Eguchi, E. (1984) The effects of temperature and light on particles associated with crayfish visual membrane: A freeze-fracture analysis and electrophysiological study. *J. Neurocytol.* 13: 935–959.

Michinomae, M., Masuda, H., Seidou, M., and Kito, Y. (1994) Structural basis for wavelength discrimination in the banked retina of the firefly squid, *Watasenia scintillans*. *J. Exp. Biol.* 193: 1–12.

Miller, J. P., Jacobs, G. A., and Theunissen, F. E. (1991) Representation of sensory information in the cricket cercal sensory system I. Response properties of the primary interneurons. *J. Neurophysiol.* 66: 1680–1689.

Miller, W. H. (1979) Ocular optical filtering. In H. Autrum (ed.), *Handbook of Sensory Physiology.* Vol. VII/6C, *Comparative Physiology and Evolution of Vision in Invertebrates.* Berlin: Springer-Verlag, pp. 69–143.

Mitaku, T. (1951) The distribution of two species of crayfish imported from America in Japan (in Japanese). *Zool. Sci.* 68: 124.

Mittelstaedt, H. (1962) Control systems of orientation in insects. *Ann. Rev. Ent.* 7: 177–198.

Mize, R. (1983) Patterns of convergence and divergence of retinal and cortical synaptic terminals in the cat superior colliculus. *Exp. Brain Res.* 269: 211–221.

Mizrahi, A. and Libersat, F. (1997) Independent coding of wind direction in cockroach giant interneurons. *J. Neurophysiol.* 78(5): 2655–2661.

Mizunami, M. (1995) Morphology of higher-order ocellar interneurons in the cockroach brain. *J. Comp. Neurol.* 362: 293–304.

Montgomery, N. M. and Fite, K. V. (1991) Organization of ascending projections from the optic tectum and mesencephalic pretectal gray in *Rana pipiens. Vision Neurosci.* 7: 459–478.

Montgomery, N. M., Fite, K. V., Taylor, M., and Bengston, L. (1982) Neural correlates of optokinetic nystagmus in the mesencephalon of *Rana pipiens*: Functional analysis. *Brain, Behav. Evol.* 21: 137–150.

Montgomery, N. M., Fite, K. V., and Li, Z. (1991) Anatomical evidence for an intergeniculate leaflet in *Rana pipiens. Neurosci. Lett.* 133: 105–108.

Moody, M. F. (1962) Evidence for the intraocular discrimination of vertically and horizontally polarized light by Octopus. *J. Exp. Biol.* 39: 21–30.

Moody, M. F. and Parriss, J. R. (1960) Discrimination of polarized light by Octopus. *Nature* 186: 839–840.

Moody, M. F. and Parriss, J. R. (1961) The discrimination of polarized light by Octopus: A behavioral and morphological study. *Z. Vergl. Physiol.* 44: 268–291.

Moran, M. D. and Hurd, L. E. (1994) Environmentally determined male-biased sex ratio in a praying mantid. *Am. Midl. Nat.* 132: 205–208.

Morton, E. S. (1975) Ecological sources of selection on avian sounds. *Am. Nat.* 109: 17–34.

Muntz, W. R. A. (1962a) Microelectrode recordings from the diencephalon of the frog (*Rana pipiens*) and a blue-sensitive system. *J. Neurophysiol.* 25: 699–711.

Muntz, W. R. A. (1962b) Effectiveness of different colours of light in releasing the positive phototactic behavior of frogs and a possible function of the retinal projection to the diencephalon. *J. Neurophysiol.* 25: 712–720.

Muntz, W. R. A. (1977a) Pupillary response of cephalopods. *Symp. Zool. Soc. Lond.* 38: 277–285.

Muntz, W. R. A. (1977b) The visual world of amphibia. In H. Autrum, R. Jung, W. R. Loewenstein, D. M. McKay, and H. L. Teuber (eds.), *Handbook of Sensory Physiology.* vol. VII/5, *The Visual System in Vertebrates.* Berlin: Springer-Verlag, pp. 275–307.

Muntz, W. R. A. and Gwyther, J. (1988) Visual acuity in *Octopus pallidus* and *Octopus australis. J. Exp. Biol.* 134: 119–129.

Muntz, W. R. A. and Johnson, M. S. (1978) Rhodopsins of oceanic decapods. *Vision Res.* 18: 601–602.

Nagel, T. (1974) What is it like to be a bat? *Phil. Rev.* 83(4): 435–450.

Naguib, M. and Wiley, R. H. (2001) Estimating the distance to a source of sound: Mechanisms and adaptations for long-range communication. *Anim. Behav.* 62: 825–837.

Nakamura, T. and Yamashita, S. (2000) Learning and discrimination of colored papers in jumping spiders (Araneae, Salticidae). *J. Comp. Physiol. A* 186: 897–901.

Narins, P. M. (1995) Frog communication. *Sci. Am.* 273: 78–83.

Nasi, E., Pilar Gomez, M., and Payne, R. (2000) Phototransduction mechanisms in microvillar and ciliary photoreceptors of invertebrates. In D. G. Stavenga, W. J. DeGrip, and E. N. Pugh (eds.), *Handbook of Biological Physics.* vol. 3, *Molecular Mechanisms in Visual Transduction.* Amsterdam: Elsevier, pp. 389–448.

Neary, T. J. (1990) The pallium of anuran amphibians. In E. G. Jones and A. Peters (eds.), *Comparative Structure and Evolution of Cerebral Cortex, Part I: Cerebral Cortex,* vol. 8A, New York: Plenum, pp. 107–138.

Neary, T. J. and Northcutt, R. G. (1983) Nuclear organization of the bullfrog diencephalon. *J. Comp. Neurol.* 213: 262–278.

Nel, A. and Roy, R. (1996) Revision of the fossil "mantid" and "ephemerid" species described by Piton from the Paleocene of Menat (France) (Mantodea: Chaeteessidae, Mantidae; Ensifera: Tettigonioidea) *Eur. J. Entomol.* 93: 223–234.

Nelson, B. S. and Stoddard, P. K. (1998) Accuracy of auditory distance and azimuth perception by a passerine bird in natural habitat. *Anim. Behav.* 56: 467–477.

Nesis, K. N. (1974) Cuttlefishes catch prey in the air. *Priroda* 1974(5): 107–109 (in Russian).

Neumeyer, C. (1981) Chromatic adaptation in honeybee: Successive color contrast and color constancy. *J. Comp. Physiol. A* 144: 543–553.

Neumeyer, C. (1991) Evolution of colour vision. In J. R. Cronly-Dillon and R. L. Gregory (eds.), *Vision and Visual Dysfunction: Evolution of the Eye and Visual System,* vol. 2. London: Macmillan, pp. 284–305.

Neumeyer, C. (1998) Color vision in lower vertebrates. In W. G. K. Backhaus, R. Kliegl, and J. S. Werner (eds.), *Color Vision: Perspectives from Different Disciplines.* Berlin, New York: Walter de Gruyter, pp. 149–162.

Neumeyer, C. and Kitschmann, M. (1998) Color categories in goldfish and humans. *Invest. Ophthal. Vision Sci.* 39: 155.

Neville, A. C. and Luke, B. M. (1971) Form optical activity in crustacean cuticle. *J. Insect Physiol.* 17: 519–526.

Nicklaus, R. (1965) Die Erregung einzellner Fadenhaare von *Periplaneta americana* in abhängigkeit von der Grösse und Richtung der Auslenkung. *Z. Vergl. Physiol.* 50: 331–362.

Nickle, D. A. (1981) Predation on a mouse by the Chinese mantid *Tenodera aridifolia sinensis*, Saussure (Dictyoptera: Mantoidea). *Proc. Ent. Soc. Wash.* 83: 802–803.

Nilsson, D.-E. (1983) Evolutionary links between apposition and superposition optics in crustacean eyes. *Nature (London)* 302: 818–821.

Nilsson, D.-E. (1989) Optics and evolution of the compound eye. In D. G. Stavenga and R. C. Hardie (eds.), *Facets of Vision*. Berlin: Springer-Verlag, pp. 30–73.

Nilsson, D.-E. and Warrant, E. J. (1999) Visual discrimination: Seeing the third quality of light. *Curr. Biol.* 9: R535–R357.

Nilsson, D.-E., Labhart, T., and Meyer, E. (1987) Photoreceptor design and optical properties affecting polarization sensitivity in ants and crickets. *J. Comp. Physiol. A* 161: 645–658.

Nilsson, D.-E., Land, M. F., and Howard, J. (1988) Optics of the butterfly eye. *J. Comp. Physiol. A* 162: 341–366.

Nishikawa, K. C. (1999) Neuromuscular control of prey capture in frogs. *Phil. Trans. Roy. Soc. Lond. B. Sci.* 354: 941–954.

Nishikawa, K. C. and Gans, C. (1992) The role of hypoglossal sensory feedback during feeding in the marine toad, *Bufo marinus. J. Exp. Zool.* 264: 245–252.

Nishikawa, K. C., Roth, G., and Dicke, U. (1991) Motor neurons and motor columns of the anterior spinal cord of salamanders: Posthatching development and phylogenetic distribution. *Brain, Behav. Evol.* 37: 368–382.

Nishikawa, K. C., Anderson, C. W., Deban, S. M., and O'Reilly, J. C. (1992) The evolution of neural circuits controlling feeding behavior in frogs. *Brain, Behav. Evol.* 40: 125–140.

Norman, M. D. (2000) *Cephalopods, a World Guide*. Hackenheim, Germany: ConchBooks.

Norman, M. D., Finn, J., and Tregenza, T. (2001) Dynamic mimicry in an Indo-Malayan octopus. *Proc. Roy. Soc. Lond. B* 268: 1755–1758.

Northcutt, R. G. and Ronan, M. (1992) Afferent and efferent connections of the bullfrog medial pallium. *Brain, Behav. Evol.* 40: 1–16.

Norton, A. C., Fukada, Y., Motokawa, K., and Tasaki, K. (1965) An investigation of the lateral spread of potentials in the octopus retina. *Vision Res.* 5: 253–267.

Nosaki, H. (1969) Electrophysiological study of color encoding in the compound eye of crayfish, *Procambarus clarkia. Z. vergl. Physiol.* 64: 318–323.

Obara, Y. and Majerus, M. E. N. (2000) Initial mate recognition in the British cabbage but-terfly, *Pierisrapae rapae. Zool. Sci.* 17: 725–730.

Okada, J. and Toh, Y. (2000) The role of antennal hair plates in object-guided tactile ori-entation of the cockroach (*Periplaneta americana*). *J. Comp. Physiol. A* 186: 849–857.

Okada, J. and Toh, Y. (2001) Peripheral representation of antennal orientation by the scapal hair plate of the cockroach *Periplaneta americana. J. Exp. Biol.* 204: 4301–4309.

Okano, T., Fukada, Y., and Yoshizawa, T. (1995) Molecular basis for tetrachromatic color vision. *Comp. Biochem. Physiol. B* 112: 405–414.

Olivo, R. F. and Larsen, M. E. (1978) Brief exposure to light intensities screening pigment migration in retinula cells of the crayfish, *Procambarus. J. Comp. Physiol.* 125: 91–96.

O'Shea, M. and Rowell, C. H. F. (1976) The neuronal basis of a sensory analyzer, the acridid movement detector system. II. Response decrement, convergence and the nature of the excitatory afferents to the fan-like dendrites of the LGMD. *J. Exp. Biol.* 65: 289–308.

O'Shea, M., Rowell, C. H. F., and Williams, J. L. D. (1974) The anatomy of a locust visual interneurone: The descending contralateral movement detector. *J. Exp. Biol.* 60: 1–12.

Osorio, D. (1986) Directionally selective cells in the locust medulla. *J. Comp. Physiol. A* 159: 841–847.

Osorio, D., Averof, M., and Bacon, J. P. (1995) Arthropod evolution: Great brains, beauti-ful bodies. *Ecol. Evol.* 10: 449–454.

Osorio, D., Marshall, N. J., and Cronin, T. W. (1997) Stomatopod photoreceptor spectral tuning as an adaptation for colour constancy in water. *Vision Res.* 37: 3299–3309.

Otis, T. and Gilly, W. F. (1990) Jet-propelled escape in the squid *Loligo opalescens*: Concerted control by giant and non-giant motor axon pathways. *Proc. Nat. Acad. Sci. U.S.A* 87: 2911–2915.

O'Tousa, J. E., Baehr, W., Martin, R. L., Hirsch, J., Pak, W. L., and Applebury, M. L. (1985) The *Drosophila* ninaE gene encodes an opsin. *Cell* 40: 839–850.

Ott, M., Schaeffel, F., and Kirmse, W. (1998) Binocular vision and accommodation in prey-catching chameleons. *J. Comp. Physiol. A* 182: 319–330.

Packard, A. (1969a) Operational convergence between cephalopods and fish: An exercise in functional anatomy. *Arch. Zool. Ital.* 51: 523–542.

Packard, A. (1969b) Visual acuity and eye growth in *Octopus vulgaris* (Lamarck). *Monitore. Zool. Ital.* 3: 19–32.

Packard, A. (1972) Cephalopods and fish: The limits of convergence. *Biol. Rev.* 47: 241–307.

Packard, A. (1995) Organization of cephalopod chromatophore systems: A neuromuscular image-generator. In N. J. Abbott, R. Williamson, and L. Maddock (eds.), *Cephalopod Neuro-biology. Neuroscience Studies in Squid, Octopus and Cuttlefish*. Oxford: Oxford Univ. Press, pp. 331–367.

Packard, A. and Hochberg, F. G. (1977) Skin patterning in Octopus and other genera. *Sym. Zool. Soc. Lond.* 38: 191–231.

Packard, A. and Sanders, G. D. (1969) What the octopus shows to the world. *Endeavour* 28: 992–999.

Palka, J. (1967) An inhibitory process influencing visual responses in a fiber of the ventral nerve cord of locusts. *J. Insect Physiol.* 41: 235–248.

Papini, M. R., Muzio, R. N., and Segura, E. T. (1995) Instrumental learning in toads (*Bufo arenarum*): Reinforcer magnitude and the medial pallium. *Brain, Behav. Evol.* 46: 61–71.

Partridge, J. C. (1989) The visual ecology of avian cone oil droplets. *J. Comp. Physiol. A* 165: 415–426.

Patton, P. and Grobstein, P. (1998a) The effects of telencephalic lesions on the visually mediated prey orienting behavior in the leopard frog (*Rana pipiens*). I. The effects of complete removal of one telencephalic lobe, with a comparison to the effect of unilateral tectal lobe lesions. *Brain, Behav. Evol.* 51: 123–143.

Patton, P. and Grobstein, P. (1998b) The effects of telencephalic lesions on the visually mediated prey-orienting behavior in the leopard frog (*Rana pipiens*). II. The effects of limited lesions to the telencephalon. *Brain, Behav. Evol.* 51: 144–161.

Pearson, K. G. and O'Shea, M. (1984) Escape behavior of the locust. The jump and its initiation by visual stimuli. In R. C. Eaton (ed.), *Neural Mechanisms of Startle Behavior*. New York: Plenum, pp. 163–178.

Peaslee, A. G. and Wilson, G. (1989) Spectral sensitivity in jumping spiders (Araneae, Salticidae). *J. Comp. Physiol. A* 164: 359–363.

Peckham, G. W. and Peckham, E. G. (1887) Some observations on the mental powers of spiders. *J. Morphol.* 1: 383–419.

Peitsch, D., Fietz, A., Hertel, H., de Souza, J., Ventura, D. F., and Menzel, R. (1992) The spectral input systems of hymenopteran insects and their receptor-based colour vision. *J. Comp. Physiol. A* 170: 23–40.

Perez, S. M., Taylor, O. R., and Jander, R. (1997) A sun compass in monarch butterflies. *Nature* 387: 29.

Pettigrew, J. D. and Collin, S. P. (1995) Terrestrial optics in an aquatic eye: The sandlance, *Limnichthytes fasciatus* Creediidae, Teleostei. *J. Comp. Physiol. A* 177: 397–408.

Pflüger, H. J. and Field, L. H. (1999) A locust chordotonal organ coding for proprioceptive and acoustic stimuli. *J. Comp. Physiol.* 184: 169–183.

Pick, C. G. and Yanai, J. (1983) Eight arm maze for mice. *Int. J. Neurosci.* 21: 63–66.

Piercy, J. E., Embleton, T. F. W., and Sutherland, L. C. (1977) Review of noise propagation in the atmosphere. *J. Acoust. Soc. Am.* 61: 1402–1418.

Plummer, M. R. and Camhi, J. M. (1981) Discrimination of sensory signals from noise in the escape system of the cockroach: The role of wind acceleration. *J. Comp. Physiol.* 142: 347–357.

Pollack, G. S. and Imaizumi, K. (1999) Neural analysis of sound frequency in insects. *BioEssays* 21: 295–303.

Pollard, S. D., Macnab, A. M., and Jackson, R. R. (1987) Communication with chemicals: Pheromones and spiders. In W. Nentwig (ed.), *Ecophysiology of Spiders*. Heidelberg: Springer-Verlag, pp. 133–141.

Porter, K. R. (1972) *Herpetology*. Philadelphia, Pa.: Saunders.

Poteser, M. and Kral, K. (1995) Visual distance discrimination in praying mantis larvae: An index of the use of motion parallax. *J. Exp. Biol.* 198: 2127–2137.

Poteser, M., Pabst, M. A., and Kral, K. (1998) Proprioceptive contribution to distance estimation by motion parallax in a praying mantid. *J. Exp. Biol.* 201: 1483–1491.

Prazdny, K. (1985) Detection of binocular disparities. *Biol. Cybern.* 52: 93–99.

Prete, F. R. (1992a) Discrimination of visual stimuli representing prey versus non-prey by the praying mantis *Sphodromantis lineola* (Burr.). *Brain, Behav. Evol.* 39: 285–288.

Prete, F. R. (1992b) The effects of background pattern and contrast on prey discrimination by the praying mantis *Sphodromantis lineola* (Burr.). *Brain, Behav. Evol.* 40: 311–320.

Prete, F. R. (1993) Stimulus direction and retinal image location affect appetitive responses to computer-generated stimuli by the praying mantis *Sphodromantis lineola* (Burr.). *Vis. Neurosci.* 10: 997–1005.

Prete, F. R. (1999) Prey Recognition. In F. R. Prete, H. Wells, P. Wells, and L. E. Hurd (eds.), *The Praying Mantids*. Baltimore, Md.: Johns Hopkins Univ. Press, pp. 141–179.

Prete, F. R. and Cleal, K. (1996) The predatory strike of free ranging praying mantises, *Sphodromantis lineola* (Burr.) I: Strikes in the midsagittal plane. *Brain, Behav. Evol.* 48: 173–190.

Prete, F. R. and Mahaffey, R. J. (1993) Appetitive responses to computer-generated visual stimuli by the praying mantis *Sphodromantis lineola* (Burm.). *Vis. Neurosci.* 10: 669–679.

Prete, F. R. and Mclean, T. (1996) Responses to moving small-field stimuli by the praying mantis, *Sphodromantis lineola* (Burmeister). *Brain, Behav. Evol.* 47: 42–54.

Prete, F. R. and Wolf, M. M. (1992) Religious supplicant, seductive cannibal, or reflex machine? In search of the praying mantis. *J. Hist. Biol.* 25: 91–136.

Prete, F. R., Klimek, C. A., and Grossman, S. P. (1990) The predatory strike of the praying mantis, *Tenodera aridifolia sinensis* (Sauss.). *J. Insect. Physiol.* 36: 561–565.

Prete, F. R., Lum, H., and Grossman, S. P. (1992) Non-predatory ingestive behaviors of the praying mantids *Tenodera aridifolia sinensis* (Sauss.) and *Sphodromantis lineola* (Burm.). *Brain, Behav. Evol.* 39: 124–132.

Prete, F. R., Placek, P. J., Wilson, M. A., Mahaffey, J., and Nemcek, R. R. (1993) Stimulus speed and order of presentation effect the visually released predatory behaviors of the praying mantis *Sphodromantis lineola* (Burm.). *Brain, Behav. Evol.* 42: 281–294.

Prete, F. R., Hurd, L. E., Branstrator, D., and Johnson, A. (2002) Responses to computer-generated visual stimuli by the male praying mantis, *Sphodromantis lineola* (Burmeister). *Anim. Behav.* 63: 503–510.

Prete, F. R., Wells, H., Wells, P., and Hurd, L. E. (eds.) (1999) *The Praying Mantids*. Baltimore: Johns Hopkins University Press.

Preuss, T. and Budelmann, B. U. (1995a) A dorsal light reflex in a squid. *J. Exp. Biol.* 198: 1157–1159.

Preuss, T. and Budelmann, B. U. (1995b) Proprioceptive hair cells on the neck of the squid *Lolliguncula brevis*: A sense organ in cephalopods for the control of head-to-body position. *Phil. Trans. Roy. Soc. Lond. B* 349: 153–178.

Prier, K. R. (1999) The axonal projections and central connections of a set of serially repeating sensory organs in the locust, *Schistocerca gregaria*. Doctoral dissertation, University of Basel, Switzerland.

Prier, K. R. and Boyan, G. S. (2000) Synaptic input from serial chordotonal organs onto segmentally homologous interneurons in the grasshopper *Schistocerca gregaria*. *J. Insect Physiol.* 46: 298–312.

Pumphrey, R. J. (1961) Concerning vision. In J. A. Ramsay and V. B. Wigglesworth (eds.), *The Cell and the Organism. Essays Presented to Sir James Gray*. Cambridge: Cambridge Univ. Press, pp. 193–208.

Qiu, X. and Arikawa, K. (2003) The photoreceptor localization confirms the spectral heterogeneity of ommatidia in the male small white butterfly, *Pieris rapae crucivora*. *J. Comp. Physiol. A* 189: 81–88.

Qiu, X., Vanhoutte, K. A. J., Stavenga, D. G., and Arikawa, K. (2002) Ommatidial heterogeneity in the compound eye of the male small white butterfly, *Pieris rapae crucivora*. *Cell Tiss. Res.* 307: 371–379.

Raguso, R. A. (2001) Floral scent, olfaction and scent-driven foraging behavior. In L. Chittka and J. D. Thomson (eds.), *Cognitive Ecology of Pollination*. Cambridge: Cambridge Univ. Press, pp. 83–105.

Rashotte, M. E. (1987) Behavior in relation to objects in space: Some historical perspectives. In P. Ellen and C. Thinus-Blanc (eds.), *Cognitive Processes and Spatial Orientation in Animals and Man*. Dordrecht, Netherlands: Martinus Nijhoff, pp. 97–106.

Ratliff, F. (1976) On the psychophysiological bases of universal color terms. *Proc. Am. Phil. Soc.* 120: 311–330.

Regan, B. C., Julliot, C., Simmen, B. Viénot, F., Charles-Dominique, P., and Mollon, J. D. (2001) Fruits, foliage and the evolution of primate colour vision. *Phil. Trans. Roy. Soc. Lond. B* 356: 229–283.

Regolin, L., Vallortigara, G., and Zanforlin, M. (1994) Perceptual and motivational aspects of detour behaviour in young chicks. *Anim. Behav.* 47: 123–131.

Regolin, L., Vallortigara, G., and Zanforlin, M. (1995a) Object and spatial representations in detour problems by chicks. *Anim. Behav.* 49: 195–199.

Regolin, L., Vallortigara, G., and Zanforlin, M. (1995b) Detour behaviour in the domestic chick: Searching for a disappearing prey or a disappearing social partner. *Anim. Behav.* 50: 203–211.

Rehbein, H. G. (1976) Auditory neurons in the ventral cord of the locust; orphological and functional properties. *J. Comp. Physiol. A* 110: 233–250.

Reiner, A. (1987) The distribution of proenkephalin-derived peptides in the central nervous system of turtles. *J. Comp. Neurol.* 259: 65–91.

Reiner, A., Brauth, S. E., and Karten, H. J. (1980) Basal ganglionic pathways to the tectum: Studies in reptiles. *J. Comp. Neurol.* 193: 565–589.

Reiner, A., Karten, H. J., and Brecha, N. C. (1982a) Enkephalin-mediated basal ganglia influences over the optic tectum: Immunohistochemistry of the tectum and the lateral spiriform nucleus in pigeon. *J. Comp. Neurol.* 208: 37–53.

Reiner, A., Brecha, N. C., and Karten, H. J. (1982b) Basal ganglia pathways to the tectum: The afferent and efferent connections of the lateral spiriform nucleus of pigeon. *J. Comp. Neurol.* 208: 16–36.

Reiner, A., Brauth, S. E., and Karten, H. J. (1984) Evolution of the amniote basal ganglia. *Trends Neurosci.* 7: 320–325.

Reiner, A., Medina, L., and Veenman, C. L. (1998) Structural and functional evolution of the basal ganglia in vertebrates. *Brain Res. Rev.* 28: 235–285.

Rensch, B. (1956) Increase in learning capability with increase of brain-size. *Am. Nat.* 90: 81–95.

Reuther, T. and Virtanen, K. (1972) Border and colour coding in the retina of the frog. *Nature* 239: 260–263.

Ribi, W. A. (1978a) Colour receptors in the eye of the digger wasp, *Sphex cognatus* Smith: Evaluation by selective adaptation. *Cell Tiss. Res.* 195: 471–483.

Ribi, W. A. (1978b) A unique hymenopteran compound eye. The retina fine structure of the digger wasp *Sphex cognatus* Smith (Hymenoptera, Sphecidae). *Zool. Jb. Anat. Bd.* 100: 299–342.

Richman, D. B. and Jackson, R. R. (1992) A review of the ethology of jumping spiders (Araneae, Salticidae). *Bull. Br. Arachnol. Soc.* 9: 33–37.

Ridpath, M. G. (1977) Predation on frogs and small birds by *Hierodula werneri* (G.T) (Mantidae) in tropical Australia. *J. Aust. Ent. Soc.* 16: 153–154.

Riede, K., Kämper, G., and Höfler, I. (1990) Tympana, auditory thresholds and projection areas of tympanal nerves in singing and silent grasshoppers (Insecta, Acridoidea). *Z. Morphol.* 109: 223–230.

Rind, F. C. (1987) Non-directional movement-sensitive neurons of the locust optic lobe. *J. Comp. Physiol. A* 161: 477–494.

Rind, F. C. (1990a) A directionally selective motion-detecting neuron in the brain of a locust: Physiological and morphological characterization. *J. Exp. Biol.* 149: 1–19.

Rind, F. C. (1990b) Identification of directionally selective motion-detecting neurons in the locust lobula and their synaptic connections with an identified descending neuron. *J. Exp. Biol.* 149: 21–43.

Rind, F. C. and Simmons, P. J. (1992) Orthopteran DCMD neuron: A reevaluation of responses to moving objects. I. Selective responses to approaching objects. *J. Neurophysiol.* 68: 1654–1666.

Rind, F. C. and Simmons, P. J. (1997) Signaling of object approach by the DCMD neuron of the locust. *J. Neurophysiol.* 77: 1029–1033.

Ritzmann, R. E. and Pollack, A. J. (1994) Responses of thoracic interneurons to tactile stimulation in the cockroach, *Periplaneta americana. J. Neurobiol.* 25: 1113–1128.

Ritzmann, R. E., Tobias, M. L., and Fourtner, C. R. (1980) Flight activity initiated via giant interneurons of the cockroach: Evidence for bifunctional trigger interneurons. *Science* 210: 443–445.

Ritzmann, R. E., Pollack, A. J., Hudson, S. E., and Hyvonen, A. (1991) Convergence of multimodal sensory signals at thoracic interneurons of the escape system of the cockroach, *Periplaneta americana. Brain Res.* 563: 175–183.

Roberts, W. A. (1972) Short-term memory in the pigeon: Effects of repetition and spacing. *J. Exp. Psychol. Anim. Behav. Proc.* 6: 217–237.

Roche King, J. and Comer, C. M. (1996) Visually elicited turning behavior in *Rana pipiens*: Comparative organization and neural control of escape and prey capture. *J. Comp. Physiol. A* 178: 293–305.

Roeder, K. D. (1959) A physiological approach to the relation between prey and predator. *Smithson. Misc. Coll.* 137: 287–306.

Roeder, K. D. (1963) *Nerve Cells and Insect Behavior*. Reprinted 1998. Cambridge, Mass.: Harvard Univ. Press.

Roffe, T. (1975) Spectral perception in Octopus: A behavioral study. *Vision Res.* 15: 353–356.

Roitblat, H. L. (1982) The meaning of representation in animal memory. *Behav. Brain Sci.* 5: 353–372.

Roitblat, H. L. (1987) *Introduction to Comparative Cognition*. New York: W.H. Freeman.

Römer, H., Bailey, W. J., and Dadour, I. (1989) Insect hearing in the field. III. Masking by noise. *J. Comp. Physiol. A* 164: 609–620.

Ronacher, B. (1992) Pattern recognition in honeybees: Multidimensional scaling reveals a city-block metric. *Vison Res.* 32: 1837–1843.

Roper, C. F. E. and Hochberg, F. G. (1988) Behavior and systematics of cephalopods from Lizard Island, Australia based on color and body patterns. *Malacologia* 29: 153–193.

Roska, B., Nemeth, E., Orzo, L., and Werblin, F. S. (2000) Three levels of lateral inhibition: A space-time study of the retina of the tiger salamander. *J. Neurosci.* 20: 1941–1951.

Rossel, S. (1979) Regional differences in photoreceptor performance in the eye of the praying mantis. *J. Comp. Physiol.* 131: 95–112.

Rossel, S. (1989) Polarization sensitivity in compound eyes. In D. G. Stavenga and R. C. Hardie (eds.), *Facets of Vision*. Berlin: Springer-Verlag, pp. 298–316.

Rossel, S. and Wehner, R. (1984) Celestial orientation in bees: The use of spectral cues. *J. Comp. Physiol.* 155: 605–613.

Roth, G. (ed.) (1987) *Visual Behavior in Salamanders*. Berlin, New York: Springer-Verlag.

Roth, G. and Grunwald, W. (2000) Morphology, axonal projection pattern and responses to optic nerve stimulation of thalamic neurons in the salamander *Plethodon jordani*. *J. Comp. Neurol.* 428: 543–557.

Roth, G. and Jordan, M. (1982) Response characteristics and stratification of tectal neurons in the toad *Bufo bufo* (L.). *Exp. Brain Res.* 45: 393–398.

Roth, G. and Westhoff, G. (1999) Cytoarchitecture and connectivity of the amphibian medial pallium. *Eur. J. Morphol.* 37: 166–171.

Roth, G., Naujoks-Manteuffel, C., and Grunwald, W. (1990) Cytoarchitecture of the tectum mesencephali in salamanders: A Golgi and HRP study. *J. Comp. Neurol.* 291: 27–42.

Roth, G., Dicke, U., and Grunwald, W. (1999) Morphology, axonal projection pattern and response types of tectal neurons in plethodontid salamanders. II: Intracellular recording and labeling experiments. *J. Comp. Neurol.* 404: 489–504.

Rowe, M. P., Pugh, E. N., Jr., Tyo, J. S., and Engheta, N. (1995) Polarization difference imaging: A biologically inspired technique for observation through scattering media. *Opt. Lett.* 20: 608–610.

Rowell, C. H. F. and O'Shea, M. (1976a) The neuronal basis of a sensory analyzer, the acridid movement detector system. I. Effects of simple incremental and decremental stimuli in light and dark adapted animals. *J. Exp. Biol.* 65: 273–288.

Rowell, C. H. F. and O'Shea, M. (1976b) The neuronal basis of a sensory analyzer, the acridid movement detector system. III. Control of response amplitude by tonic lateral inhibition. *J. Exp. Biol.* 65: 273–288.

Rowell, C. H. F. and Wells, M. J. (1961) Retinal orientation and the discrimination of polarized light by octopuses. *J. Exp. Biol.* 38: 827–831.

Rowell, C. H. F., O'Shea, M., and Williams, J. L. D. (1977) The neuronal basis of a sensory analyzer, the acridid movement detector system. IV. The preference for small field stimuli. *J. Exp. Biol.* 68: 157–185.

Ryan, E. P. (1966) Pheromone: Evidence in a decapod crustacean. *Science* 151(708): 340–341.

Ryan, M. J. and Keddy-Hector, A. (1992) Directional patterns of female mate choice and the role of sensory biases. *Am. Nat.* 139: S4–S35.

Sabra, R. and Glantz, R. M. (1985) Polarization sensitivity of crayfish photoreceptors is correlated with their termination sites in the lamina ganglionaris. *J. Comp. Physiol. A* 156: 315–318.

Saibil, H. and Hewat, E. (1987) Ordered transmembrane and extracellular structure in squid photoreceptor microvilli. *J. Cell. Biol.* 105: 19–28.

Saidel, W. M., Lettvin, J. Y., and MacNichol, E. F. J. (1983) Processing of polarized light by squid photoreceptors. *Nature* 304: 534–536.

Salcedo, E., Huber, A., Henrich, S., Chadwell, L. V., Chou, W. H., Paulsen, R., and Britt, S. G. (1999) Blue- and green-absorbing visual pigments of *Drosophila*: Ectopic expression and physiological characterization of the R8 photoreceptor cell-specific Rh5 and Rh6 rhodopsins. *J. Neurosci.* 19: 10716–10726.

Sandeman, D. C. (1985) Crayfish antennae as tactile organs: Their mobility and the responses of their proprioceptors to displacement. *J. Comp. Physiol. A* 157: 363–373.

Sandeman, D. C., Erber, J., and Kien, J. (1975) Optokinetic eye movements in the crab *Carcinus maenas*. I. Eye torque. *J. Comp. Physiol.* 101: 243–258.

Sasaki, M. (1914) Observations on hotaru-ika *Watasenia scintillans*. *J. Coll. Agric., Tohoku Imperial Univ., Sapporo* 6: 75–107.

Satou, M. and Ewert, J.-P. (1985) The antidromic activation of tectal neurons by electrical stimuli applied to the caudal medulla oblongata in the toad *Bufo bufo* L. *J. Comp. Physiol. A* 157: 739–748.

Satou, M., Matsushima, T., Takeuchi, H., and Ueda, K. (1985) Tongue-muscle-controlling motoneurons in the Japanese toad: Topography, morphology and neuronal pathways from the "snapping-evoking area" in the optic tectum. *J. Comp. Physiol. A* 157: 717–737.

Sauer, W. H., Roberts, M. J., Lipinski, M. R., Smale, M. J., Hanlon, R. T., Webber, D. M., and O'Dor, R. K. (1997) Choreography of the squid's nuptial dance. *Biol. Bull.* 192: 203–207.

Saunders, B. A. C. and van Brakel, J. (1997) Are there nontrivial constraints on colour categorization? *Behav. Brain. Sci.* 20: 167–228.

Savory, T. H. (1928) *The Biology of Spiders*. London: Sidgwick and Jackson.

Scalia, F. (1976) The optic pathway of the frog: Nuclear organization and connections. In R. Llinás and W. Precht (eds.), *Frog Neurobiology*. Berlin: Springer-Verlag, pp. 386–406.

Schaller, D. (1978) Antennal sensory system of *Periplaneta americana* L.: Distribution and frequency of morphologic types of sensilla and their sex-specific changes during postembryonic development. *Cell. Tiss. Res.* 191(1): 121–139.

Scherer, C. and Kolb, G. (1987a) Behavioural experiments on the visual processing of colour stimuli in *Pieris brassicae* L. (Lepidoptera). *J. Comp. Physiol. A* 160: 645–656.

Scherer, C. and Kolb, G. (1987b) The influence of colour stimuli on visually controlled behaviour in *Aglais urticae* L., *Parage aegeria* L. (Lepidoptera). *J. Comp. Physiol. A* 161: 891–898.

Schiff, H. and Candone, P. (1986) Superposition and scattering of visual fields in a compound, double eye. II. Stimulation sequences for different distances in a stomatopod from a bright habitat. *Comp. Biochem. Physiol.* 83A: 445–455.

Schikora, J., Spaethe, J., Brockmann, A., and Chittka, L. (2002) Colour vision and colour preference in *Bombus terrestris*—a population biological approach. *Zoology* 105: 28.

Schiller, C. (1957) *Instinctive Behavior*. New York: Hallmark Press.

Schiller, P. H. and Tehovnik, E. J. (2001) Look and see: How the brain moves your eyes about. *Prog. Brain Res.* 134: 127–142.

Schipperheyn, J. J. (1963) Respiratory eye movement and perception of stationary objects in the frog. *Acta Physiol. Pharmacol. Neerl.* 12: 157–159.

Schleidt, W. M. (1962) Die historische Entwicklung der Begriffe "Angeborenes auslösendes Schema" und "Angeborener Auslösemechanismus" in der Ethologie. *Z. Tierpsychol.* 19: 697–722.

Schmidtberg, H. (1999) Ultrastructural studies of the suckers of newly hatched *Eledone moschata* and *Octopus vulgaris* (Mollusca; Cephalopoda). In F. Olóriz and F. J. Rodríguez-Tovar (eds.), *Advancing Research on Living and Fossil Cephalopods*. New York: Kluwer Academic Plenum, pp. 203–222.

Schneider, D. (1954) Beitrag zu einer Analyse des Beute- und Fluchtverhaltens einheimischer Anuren. *Biol. Zbl.* 73: 225–282.

Schönenberger, N. (1977) The fine structure of the compound eye of *Squilla mantis* (Crustacea, Stomatopoda). *Cell Tiss. Res.* 176: 205–233.

Schulze Schencking, M. (1969) Untersuchungen zur visuellen Lerngeschwindigkeit und Lernkapazität bei Bienen, Hummeln und Ameisen. *Z. Tierpsychol.* 27: 513–552.

Schümperli, R. A. (1975) Monocular and binocular visual fields of butterfly interneurons in response to white- and coloured-light stimulation. *J. Comp. Physiol.* 103: 273–289.

Schümperli, R. A. and Swihart, S. (1978) Spatial properties of dark- and light-adapted visual fields of butterfly interneurones. *J. Insect Physiol.* 24: 777–784.

Schürg-Pfeiffer, E. (1989) Behavior-correlated properties of tectal neurons in freely moving toads. In J.-P. Ewert and M. A. Arbib (eds.), *Visuomotor Coordination: Amphibians, Comparisons, Models and Robots*. New York: Plenum, pp. 451–480.

Schürg-Pfeiffer, E., Spreckelsen, C., and Ewert, J.-P. (1993) Temporal discharge patterns of tectal and medullary neurons chronically recorded during snapping toward prey in toads *Bufo bufo* spinosus. *J. Comp. Physiol. A* 173: 363–376.

Schwerdtfeger, W. K. and Germroth, P. (eds.) (1990) *The Forebrain in Nonmammals.* Berlin: Springer-Verlag, pp. 57–65.

Schwind, R. P. S. (1991) Polarization vision in water insects and insects living on moist substrate. *J. Comp. Physiol. A* 169: 531–540.

Schwippert, W. W. and Ewert, J.-P. (1995) Effect of neuropeptide-Y on tectal field potentials in the toad. *Brain Res.* 669: 150–152.

Schwippert, W. W., Beneke, T. W., and Ewert, J.-P. (1995) Pretecto-tectal influences II. How retinal and pretectal inputs to the toad's tectum interact: A study of electrically evoked field potentials. *J. Comp. Physiol. A* 176: 181–192.

Schwippert, W. W., Röttgen, A., and Ewert, J.-P. (1998) Neuropeptide Y (NPY) or fragment NPY13-36, but not NPY18–36, inhibit retinotectal transfer in cane toads *Bufo marinus*. *Neurosci. Lett.* 253: 33–36.

Seah, W. K. and Li, D. (2001) Stabilimenta attract unwelcome predators to orb-webs. *Proc. Roy Soc. Lond. B* 268: 1553–1558.

Seeley, T. D. (1985) *Honeybee Ecology. A Study of Adaptation in Social Life.* Princeton, N.J.: Princeton Univ. Press.

Seidou, M., Sugahara, M., Uchiyama, H. Hiraki, K., Michinomae, M., Yoshihara, K., and Kito, Y. (1990) On the three visual pigments in the retina of the firefly squid, *Watasenia scintillans*. *J. Comp. Physiol. A* 166: 769–773.

Seidou, M., Narita, K., Michinomae, M., and Kito, Y. (1995) The firefly squid, *Watasenia scintillans*, has three visual pigments. In N. J. Abbott, R. Williamson, and L. Maddock (eds.), *Cephalopod Neurobiology. Neuroscience Studies in Squid, Octopus and Cuttlefish.* Oxford: Oxford Univ. Press, pp. 491–501.

Sekhar, V. and Reddy, R. (1988) Mechanosensory regulation of predatory evasion behavior in the cockroach, *Periplaneta americana*. *Curr. Sci.* 57(20): 1141–1142.

Seki T. and Vogt, K. (1998) Evolutionary aspects of the diversity of visual pigment chromophores in the class Insecta. *Comp. Biochem. Physiol.* 119B: 53–64.

Seki, T., Fujishita, S., Ito, M., Matsuoka, N., and Tsukida, K. (1987) Retinoid composition in the compound eyes of insects. *Exp. Biol.* 47: 95–103.

Seyfarth, E. A. (1985) Spider proprioception: Receptors, reflexes and control of locomotion. In F. G. Barth (ed.), *Neurobiology of Arachnids.* Berlin: Springer-Verlag, pp. 230–248.

Sharov, A. G. (1968) Phylogeny of the orthopteroidea. *Trans. Paleontol. Instit. Acad. Sci.* 118: 1–216.

Shashar, N. and Cronin, T. W. (1996) Polarization contrast vision in Octopus. *J. Exp. Biol.* 199: 999–1004.

Shashar, N. and Hanlon, R. T. (1997) Squids (*Loligo pealei* and *Euprymna scolopes*) can exhibit polarized light patterns produced by their skin. *Biol. Bull.* 193: 207–208.

Shashar, N., Addessi, L., and Cronin, T. W. (1995) Polarization vision as a mechanism for detection of transparent objects. In D. Gulko and L. Jokiel (eds.), *Ultraviolet Radiation and Coral Reefs*. HIMB Tech. Report 41, Kaneohe, Hawaii: Hawaii Institute of Marine Biology, pp. 207–211.

Shashar, N., Rutledge, P. S., and Cronin, T. W. (1996) Polarization vision in cutttlefish—a concealed communication channel? *J. Exp. Biol.* 199: 2077–2084.

Shashar, N., Hanlon, R. T., and Petz, A. D. (1998) Polarization vision helps detect transparent prey. *Nature* 393: 222–223.

Shashar, N., Hagan, R., Boal, J. G., and Hanlon, R. T. (2000) Cuttlefish use polarization sensitivity in predation on silvery fish. *Vison Res.* 40: 71–75.

Shashar, N., Borst, D. T., Ament, S. A., Saidel, W. M., Smolowitz, R. M., and Hanlon, R. T. (2001) Polarization reflecting iridophores in the arms of the squid *Loligo pealeii. Biol. Bull.* 201: 267–268.

Shaw, S. R. (1975) Retinal resistance barriers and electrical lateral inhibition. *Nature* 255: 480–482.

Shelton, P. M. J., Stephen, R. O., Scott, J. J. A., and Tindall, A. R. (1992) The apodeme complex of the femoral chordotonal organ in the metathoracic leg of the locust *Schistocerca gregaria. J. Exp. Biol.* 163: 345–358.

Sherry, D. F. (1998) Neural mechanisms of spatial representation. In S. Healy (ed.), *Spatial Representation in Animals*. Oxford: Oxford University Press, pp. 131–157.

Shimohigashi, M. and Tominaga, Y. (1991) Identification of UV, green and red receptors and their projection to lamina in the cabbage butterfly, *Pieris rapae. Cell Tiss. Res.* 263: 49–59.

Shimozawa, T. and Kanou, M. (1984) Varieties of filiform hairs: Range fractionation by sensory afferents and cercal interneurons of a cricket. *J. Comp. Physiol.* A 155: 485–493.

Shinn, E. A. and Dole, J. W. (1979a) Evidence for a role for olfactory cues in the feeding response of Western toads (*Bufo boreas*). *Copeia* 1979: 163–165.

Shinn, E. A. and Dole, J. W. (1979b) Lipid components of prey odors elicit feeding responses in western toads Bufo boreas. *Copeia* 1979: 275–278.

Silberglied, R. E. (1984) Visual communication and sexual selection among butterflies. In R. I. Vane-Wright and P. R. Ackery (eds.), *The Biology of Butterflies*. London: Academic Press, pp. 207–223.

Silver, S. C., Patterson, J. A., and Mobbs, P. G. (1983) Biogenic amines in cephalopod retina. *Brain Res.* 273: 366–368.

Simmons, P. J. and Rind, F. C. (1992) Orthopteran DCMD neuron: A reevaluation of responses to moving objects. II. Critical cues for detecting approaching objects. *J. Neurophysiol.* 68: 1667–1682.

Sivak, J. G. (1991) Shape and focal properties of the cephalopod ocular lens. *Can. J. Zool.* 69: 2501–2506.

Sivak, J. G., West, J. A., and Campbell, M. C. (1994) Growth and optical development of the ocular lens of the squid (*Sepioteuthis lessoniana*). *Vision Res.* 34: 2177–2187.

Sklansky, J. and Wassel, G. N. (1981) *Pattern Classifiers and Trainable Machines*. New York: Springer-Verlag.

Smith, S. R., Wheeler, B. C., Dowd, J. P., and Comer, C. M. (1991) Investigation of a multicellular neural code for directed movement. Proc. 13th Int. Conf. *IEEE Engr. Med. Biol. Soc.* 1: 457–458.

Snyder, A. S. and Laughlin, S. B. (1975) Dichroism and absorption by photoreceptors. *J. Comp. Physiol.* 100: 101–116.

Snyder, A. W. (1973) Polarization sensitivity of individual retinula cells. *J. Comp. Physiol. A* 83: 331–360.

Snyder, A. W. (1979) Physics of vision in compound eyes. In H. J. Autrum (ed.), *Handbook of Sensory Physiology. Vol. VII/6A Vision in Invertebrates*. Berlin: Springer-Verlag, pp. 225–313.

Snyder, A. W. and Miller, W. H. (1978) Telephoto lens system of falconiform eyes. *Nature* 275: 127–129.

Snyder, A. W., Menzel, R., and Laughlin, S. B. (1973) Structure and function of the fused rhabdom. *J. Comp. Physiol. A* 87: 99–135.

Sobel, E. C. (1990) The locust's use of motion parallax to measure distance. *J. Comp. Physiol. A* 167: 579–588.

Spaethe, J., Tautz, J., and Chittka, L. (2001) Visual constraints in foraging bumblebees: Flower size and color affect search time and flight behavior. *Proc. Nat. Acad. Sci. U.S.A.* 98: 3898–3903.

Sparks, D. L. (1999) Conceptual issues related to the role of the superior colliculus in the control of gaze. *Curr. Opin. Neurobiol.* 9: 698–707.

Sparks, D. L. and Nelson, J. (1987) Sensory and motor maps in the mammalian superior colliculus. *Trends Neurosci.* 10: 312–317.

Spreckelsen, C., Schürg-Pfeiffer, E., and Ewert J.-P. (1995) Responses of retinal and tectal neurons in non-paralyzed toads *Bufo bufo* and *B. marinus* to the real size versus angular size of objects moved at variable distance. *Neurosci. Lett.* 184: 105–108.

Srinivasan, M. V. (1992) Distance perception in insects. *Curr. Direct. Psychol. Sci.* 1: 22–25.

Srinivasan, M. V. (1993) Even insects experience visual illusions. *Curr. Sci.* 64: 649–654.

Srinivasan, M. V. (1994) Pattern recognition in the honeybee: Recent progress. *J. Insect Physiol.* 40: 183–194.

Srinivasan, M. V. and Bernard, G. D. (1975) The effect of motion on visual acuity of the compound eye: A theoretical analyis. *Vison Res.* 15: 515–525.

Srinivasan, M. V. and Zhang, S. W. (1998) Probing perception in a miniature brain: Pattern recognition and maze navigation in honeybees. *Zoology* 101: 246–259.

Srinivasan, M. V., Zhang, S. W., and Rolfe, B. (1993) Is pattern vision in insects mediated by "cortical" processing? *Nature* 362(8): 539–540.

Srinivasan, M. V., Zhang, S. W., and Witney, K. (1994) Visual discrimination of pattern orientation by honeybees: Performance and implications for "cortical" processing. *Phil. Trans. Roy. Soc. Lond. B.* 343: 199–210.

Srinivasan, M. V., Zhang, S. W., and Bidwell, N. (1997) Visually mediated odometry in honeybees. *J. Exp. Biol.* 200: 2513–1522.

Srinivasan, M. V., Zhang, S. W., and Zhu, H. (1998) Honeybees link sights to smells. *Nature (London)* 396: 637–638.

Srinivasan, M. V., Poteser, M., and Kral, K. (1999) Motion detection in insect orientation and navigation. *Vison Res.* 39: 2749–2766.

Srinivasan, M. V., Zhang, S. W., Altwein, M., and Tautz, J. (2000) Honeybee navigation: Nature and calibration of the "odometer." *Science* 287: 851–853.

Staudacher, E. (1998) Distribution and morphology of descending brain neurons in the cricket *Gryllus bimaculatus. Cell Tiss. Res.* 294: 187–202.

Stavenga, D. G. (1979) Pseudopupils of compound eyes. In H. Autrum (ed.), *Handbook of Sensory Physiology.* Vol. VII/6C Comparative Physiology and Evolution of Vision in Invertebrates. Berlin: Springer-Verlag, pp. 357–439.

Stavenga, D. G. (1989) Pigments in compound eyes. In D. G. Stavenga and R. C. Hardie (eds.), *Facets of Vision.* Berlin: Springer-Verlag, pp. 152–172.

Stavenga, D. G. (1992) Eye regionalization and spectral tuning of retinal pigments in insects. *Trends Neurosci.* 15: 213–218.

Stavenga, D. G. (2002a) Colour in the eyes of insects. *J. Comp. Physiol. A* 188: 337–348.

Stavenga, D. G. (2002b) Reflections on colourful ommatidia of butterfly eyes. *J. Exp. Biol.* 205: 1077–1085.

Stavenga, D. G., Smits, R. P., and Hoenders, B. J. (1993) Simple exponential functions describing the absorbance bands of visual pigment spectra. *Vison Res.* 33: 1011–1017.

Stavenga, D. G., Kimoshita, M., Yang, E.-C., and Arikawa, K. (2001) Retinal regionalization and heterogeneity of butterfly eyes. *Naturwissenschaften* 88: 477–481.

Steiner, A., Paul, R., and Gemperlein, R. (1987) Retinal receptor types in *Aglais urticae* and *Pieris brassicae* (Lepidoptera), revealed by analysis of the electroretinogram obtained with Fourier interferometric stimulation (FIS). *J. Comp. Physiol. A* 160: 247–258.

Stephens, D. W. (1991) Change, regularity and value in the evolution of animal learning. *Behav. Ecol.* 2: 77–89.

Sternthal, D. E. (1974) Olfactory and visual cues in the feeding behaviour of the leopard frog (*Rana pipiens*). *Z. Tierpsychol.* 34: 239–246.

Stevens, K. H. (1987) Implicit versus explicit computation. *Behav. Brain Sci.* 10: 387–388.

Stierle, I. E., Getman, M., and Comer, C. M. (1994) Multisensory control of escape in the cockroach *Periplaneta americana* I. Initial evidence from patterns of wind-evoked behavior. *J. Comp. Physiol. A* 174: 1–11.

Stowe, S. (1977) The retina-lamina projection in the crab *Leptograpsus variegatus*. *Cell Tiss. Res.* 185: 515–525.

Stowe, S. (1983) A theoretical explanation of intensity independent variation of polarization sensitivity in crustacean retinula cells. *J. Comp. Physiol. A* 153: 435–441.

Strausfeld, N. J. and Blest, A. D. (1970) Golgi studies on insects. Part I. The optic lobes of Lepidoptera. *Phil. Trans. Roy. Soc. Lond. B* 258: 81–134.

Strausfeld, N. J. and Nassel, D. R. (1981) Neuroarchitecture of brain regions that subserve the compound eyes of crustacea and insects. In H. Autrum (ed.), *Handbook of Sensory Physiology*. vol. VII/6B, Comparative Physiology and Evolution of Vision in Invertebrates. Berlin: Springer-Verlag, pp. 1–132.

Straznicky, K. and Gaze, R. M. (1972) The development of the tectum in *Xenopus laevis*: An autoradiographic study. *J. Embryol. Exp. Morphol.* 28: 87–115.

Sugawara, K., Katagiri, Y., and Tomita, T. (1971) Polarized light responses from octopus single retinular cells. *J. Fac. Sci., Hokkaido Univ.*, 6 Zoology 17: 581–586.

Suko, T. (1958) Studies on the development of the crayfish. VI. The reproductive cycle. *Sci. Rept. Saitama Univ.* 13(1) 79–91.

Suzuki, T. and Makino-Tasaka, M. (1983) Analysis of retinal and 3-dehydroretinal in the retina by high-pressure liquid chromatography. *Anal. Biochem.* 129: 111–119.

Suzuki, H. and Tasaki, K. (1983) Inhibitory retinal efferents from dopaminergic cells in the optic lobe of the octopus. *Vison Res.* 23: 451–457.

Suzuki, T., Makino-Tasaka, M., and Eguchi, E. (1984) 3-Dehydroretinal (vitamin A2 aldehyde) in crayfish eye. *Vison Res.* 24: 783–787.

Suzuki, T., Arikawa, K., and Eguchi, E. (1985) The effects of light and temperature on the rhodopsin-porphyropsin visual system of the crayfish, *Procambarus clarkia. Zool. Sci.* 2: 455–461.

Svenson, G. J. and Whiting, M. F. (2004) Phylogeny of Mantodea based on molecular data: evolution of a charismatic predator. *Syst. Entomol.*, in press.

Swihart, C. A. and Swihart, S. L. (1970) Colour selection and learned feeding preferences in the butterfly, *Heliconius charitonius* Linn. *Anim. Behav.* 18: 60–64.

Swihart, S. L. (1970) The neural basis of colour vision in the butterfly, *Papilio troilus*. *J. Insect Physiol.* 16: 1623–1636.

Swihart, S. L. and Gordon, W. C. (1971) Red photoreceptor in butterflies. *Nature* 231: 126–127.

Switkes, E. and Crognale, M. A. (1999) Comparison of color and luminance contrast: Apples versus oranges? *Vison Res.* 39: 1823–1831.

Syrkin, G. and Gur, M. (1997) Colour and luminance interact to improve pattern recognition. *Perception* 26: 127–140.

Székely, G. and Lázár, G. (1976) Cellular and synaptic architecture of the optic tectum. In R. Llinás and W. Precht (eds.), *Frog Neurobiology*. Berlin: Springer-Verlag, pp. 407–434.

Tarsitano, M. S. and Andrew, R. (1999) Scanning and route selection in the jumping spider *Portia labiata*. *Anim. Behav.* 58: 255–265.

Tarsitano, M. S. and Jackson, R. R. (1992) Influence of prey movement on the performance of simple detours by jumping spiders. *Behaviour* 123: 106–120.

Tarsitano, M. S. and Jackson, R. R. (1994) Jumping spiders make predatory detours requiring movement away from prey. *Behaviour* 131: 65–73.

Tarsitano, M. S. and Jackson, R. R. (1997) Araneophagic jumping spiders discriminate between detour routes that do and do not lead to prey. *Anim. Behav.* 53: 257–266.

Tarsitano, M. S., Jackson, R. R., and Kirchner, W. (2000) Signals and signal choices made by araneophagic jumping spiders while hunting the orb-weaving spiders *Zygiella x-notata* and *Zosis genicularis*. *Ethology* 106: 595–615.

Tasaki, I. and Nakaye, T. (1984) Rapid mechanical responses of the dark-adapted squid retina to light pulses. *Science* 223: 411–413.

Tasaki, K. and Karita, K. (1966a) Intraretinal discrimination of horizontal and vertical planes of polarized light by octopus. *Nature* 209: 934–935.

Tasaki, K. and Karita, K. (1966b) Discrimination of horizontal and vertical planes of polarized light by the cephalopod retina. *Jpm. J. Physiol.* 16: 205–216.

Tasaki, K., Norton, A. C., and Fukada, Y. (1963) Regional and directional differences in the lateral spread of retinal potentials in the octopus. *Nature* 198: 1206–1208.

Tasaki, K., Tsukahara, Y., Suzuki, H., and Nakaye, T. (1982) Two types of inhibition in the octopus retina. In A. Kaneko, N. Tsukahara, and K. Uchizono (eds.), *Neurotransmitters in the Retina and the Visual Centers*. Biomedical Research Supplement, Dec. 1982, Tokyo: Biomedical Research Foundation, pp. 41–44.

Tauber, E. and Camhi, J. M. (1995) The wind-evoked escape behavior of the cricket *Gryllus bimaculatus*: Integration of behavioral elements. *J. Exp. Biol.* 198: 1895–1907.

Taylor, P. W. and Jackson, R. R. (1999) Habitat-adapted communication in *Trite planiceps*, a New Zealand jumping spider (Araneae, Salticidae). *NZ J. Zool.* 26: 127–154.

Taylor, P. W., Jackson, R. R., and Robertson, M. B. (1998) A case of blind spider's bluff?: Prey-capture by jumping spiders (Araneae, Salticidae) in the absence of visual cues. *J. Arachnol.* 26: 369–381.

Teller, D. Y. and Bornstein, M. H. (1987) Infant color vision and color perception. In P. Salapatek and L. Cohen (eds.), *Handbook of Infant Perception. From Sensation to Perception*. Orlando, Fla.: Academic Press, pp. 185–236.

Terrace, H. S. (1985) Animal cognition: Thinking without language. *Phil. Trans. Roy. Soc. Lond. B* 308: 113–128.

Thomson, J. D. (1981) Field measures of flower constancy in bumblebees. *Am. Midl. Nat.* 105: 377–380.

Thorndike, E. L. (1911) *Animal Intelligence*. New York: Macmillan.

Tinbergen, L. (1960) The natural control of insects in pinewoods. Factors influencing the intensity of predation by songbirds. *Archs. Neer. Zool.* 13: 265–343.

Tinbergen, N. (1951) *The Study of Instinct*. Reprinted 1989. Oxford: Oxford Univ. Press/Clarendon Press.

Toates, F. (1988) Motivation and emotion from a biological perspective. In V. Hamilton, G. H. Bower, and N. H. Frijda (eds.), *Cognitive Perspectives on Emotion and Motivation*. Dordrecht, Netherlands: Kluwer, pp. 3–35.

Toates, F. (1996) Cognition and evolution—an organization of actions perspective. *Behav. Process.* 35: 239–250.

Toh, Y. (1977) Fine structure of antennal sense organs of the male cockroach, *Periplaneta americana*. *J. Ultrastruct. Res.* 60(3): 373–394.

Toh, Y. (1981) Fine structure of sense organs on the antennal pedicel and scape of the male cockroach, *Periplaneta americana*. *J. Ultrastruct. Res.* 77(2): 119–132.

Toh, Y. and Yokohari, F. (1985) Structure of the antennal chordotonal sensilla of the American cockroach. *J. Ultrastruct. Res.* 90: 124–134.

Tomarev, S. I., Zinovieva, R. D., and Piatigorsky, J. (1991) Crystallins of the octopus lens. Recruitment from detoxification enzymes. *J. Biol. Chem.* 266: 24226–24231.

Tonosaki, A. (1965) The fine structure of the retinal plexus in *Octopus vulgaris*. *Z. Zellforsch.* 67: 521–532.

Tóth, P., Csank, G., and Lázár, G. (1985) Morphology of the cells of origin of descending pathways to the spinal cord in *Rana esculenta*. A tracing study using cobalt-lysine complex. *J. Hirnforsch.* 26: 365–383.

Townson, S. M., Chang, B. S. W., Salcedo, E., Chadwell, L. V., Pierce, N. E., and Britt, S. G. (1998) Honeybee blue- and ultraviolet-sensitive opsins: Cloning, heterologous expression in *Drosophila* and physiological characterization. *J. Neurosci.* 18: 2412–2422.

Trachtenberg, M. C. and Ingle, D. (1974) Thalamo-tectal projections in the frog. *Brain Res.* 79: 419–430.

Trevino, D. L. and Larimer, J. L. (1970) The responses of one class of neurons in the optic tract of crayfish (*Procambarus*) to monochromatic light. *Vis. Res.* 25: 149–154.

Troje, N. (1993) Spectral categories in the learning behaviour of blowflies. *Z. Naturforsch. C* 48: 96–104.

Trueman, E. R. (1980) Swimming by jet propulsion. *Soc. Exp. Biol. Sem. Ser.* 5: 93–105.

Tsai, H.-J. (1991) Neuronal motion after-response induced in the tectal neurons of toads by moving textured background. *Brain, Behav. Evol.* 37: 161–167.

Tsai, H.-J. and Ewert, J.-P. (1987) Edge preference of retinal and tectal neurons in common toads (*Bufo bufo*) in response to worm-like moving stripes: The question of behaviorally relevant "position indicators." *J. Comp. Physiol. A* 161: 295–304.

Tsai, H.-J. and Ewert, J.-P. (1988) Influence of stationary and moving textured backgrounds on the response of visual neurons in toads (*Bufo bufo* L.). *Brain, Behav. Evol.* 32: 27–38.

Tsin, A. T. C. and Beatty, D. D. (1979) Scotopic visual pigment composition in the retinas and vitamin A in the pigment epithelium of the goldfish. *Exp. Eye Res.* 29: 15–26.

Tsukahara, Y. (1989) Shikaku masshou soku yokusei kikou (Mechanisms of peripheral lateral inhibition in vision). *Doubutsu Seiri* (Animal Physiology) *Tokyo* 6: 58–65 (in Japanese).

Tsukahara, Y. and Tasaki, K. (1972) Dark recovery of ERP in isolated octopus retina. *Tohoku J. Exp. Med.* 108: 97–98.

Tulk, A. (1844) Habits of the mantis. *Ann. Mag. Nat. Hist.* 14: 78.

Tyo, J. S., Rowe, M. P., Pugh, E. N., Jr., and Engheta, N. (1996) Target detection in optically scattering media by polarization-difference imaging. *Appl. Opt.* 35: 1855–1870.

Valdez, C. M. and Nishikawa, K. C. (1997) Sensory modulation and behavioral choice during feeding in the Australian frog, *Cyclorana novaehollandiae*. *J. Comp. Physiol. A* 180: 187–202.

van Hateren, J. H., Srinivasan, M. V., and Wait, P. B. (1990) Pattern recognition in bees: Orientation discrimination. *J. Comp. Physiol. A* 167: 649–654.

van Staaden, M. J. and Römer, H. (1997) Sexual signalling in bladder grasshoppers: Tactical design for maximizing calling range. *J. Exp. Biol.* 200: 2597–2608.

van Staaden, M. J. and Römer, H. (1998) Evolutionary transition from stretch to hearing organs in ancient grasshoppers. *Nature* 394: 773–776.

van Staaden, M. J., Reiser, M., Ott, S., Papst, M. A., and Römer, H. (2003) Serial hearing organs in the atympanate grasshopper *Bullacris membracioides* (Orthoptera, Pneumoridae). *J. Comp. Neurol.* 465: 579–592.

van Staaden, M. J., Rieser M., Ott, S. R., Papst, M. A., and Römer, H. (2003) Serial hearing organs in the atympanate grasshopper *Bullacris membracioides* (Orthoptera, Pneumoridae). *J. Comp. Neurol.* 465: 579–592.

Vanegas, H. (ed.) (1984) *Comparative Neurology of the Optic Tectum.* New York: Plenum.

Vanhoutte, K. A. J., Eggen, B. J. L., Janssen, J. J. M., and Stavenga, D. G. (2002) Opsin cDNA sequences of a UV and green rhodopsin of the satyrine butterfly *Bicyclus anynana*. *Insect Biochem. Mol. Biol.* B32: 1383–1390.

Varju, D. (1989) Prey attack in crayfish: Conditions for success and kinematics of body motion. *J. Comp. Physiol. A* 165: 99–107.

Ventura, D. F., Zana, Y., Souza, J. Md., and DeVoe, R. D. (2001) Ultraviolet colour opponency in the turtle retina. *J. Exp. Biol.* 204: 2527–2596.

Vogel, S., Westerkamp, C., Thiel, B., and Gessner, K. (1984) Ornithophilie auf den Canarischen Inseln. *Plant. Syst. Evol.* 146: 225–248.

Vogt, K. (1983) Is the fly visual pigment a rhodopsin? *Z. Naturforsch.* 38c: 329–333.

Vogt, K. (1989) Distribution of insect visual chromophores: Functional and phylogenetic aspects. In D. G. Stavenga and R. C. Hardie (eds.), *Facets of Vision*. Berlin: Springer-Verlag, pp. 134–151.

von der Heydt, R. and Peterhans, E. (1989) Cortical contour mechanisms and geometrical illusion. In D. M. Lam and C. D. Gilbert (eds.), *Neural Mechanisms of Visual Perception*. Houston, Tex.: Gulf Publishing, pp. 157–170.

von der Heydt, R., Peterhans, E., and Baumgartner, G. (1984) Illusory contours and cortical neuron responses. *Science* 224: 1260–1262.

von Frisch, K. (1914) Der Farbensinn und Formensinn der Biene. *Zool. J. Physiol.* 37: 1–238.

von Frisch, K. (1949) Die Polarisation des Himmels licht als orien terender Factor bei den Tanzend der Bienen. *Experimentia* 5: 142–148.

von Frisch, K. (1967) *The Dance Language and Orientation of Bees*. Reprinted 1993. Cambridge, Mass.: Harvard Univ. Press.

von Frisch, K. (1971) *Bees: Their Vision, Chemical Senses and Language*. Ithaca, N.Y.: Cornell Univ. Press.

von Frisch, O. (1962) Zur Biologie des Zwergchamäleons (*Microsaurus pumilus*). *Z. Tierpsychol.* 19(3): 276–289.

von Holst, E. and Mittelstaedt, H. (1950) Das Reafferenzprinzip. *Naturwissenschaften* 37: 464–476.

von Kries, J. A. (1905) Influence of adaptation on the effects produced by luminous stimuli. In *Handbuch der Physiologie des Menschens*, vol. 3. Braunschweig, Germany: Viehweg, pp. 109–282.

von Uexküll, J. (1909) *Umwelt und Innenwelt der Tiere*. Berlin: Springer-Verlag.

von Uexküll, J. (1934) A stroll through the worlds of animals and men: A picture book of invisible worlds. Reprinted 1957 in C. H. Schiller (ed.), *Instinctive Behavior: The Development of a Modern Concept*. New York: International Universities Press, pp. 5–80.

von Wietersheim, A. and Ewert, J.-P. (1978) Neurons of the toad's (*Bufo bufo* L.) visual system sensitive to moving configurational stimuli: A statistical analysis. *J. Comp. Physiol.* 126: 35–42.

Vorobyev, M. and Brandt, R. (1997) How do insect pollinators discriminate colors? *Isr. J. Plant. Sci.* 45: 103–113.

Vorobyev, M. and Menzel, R. (1999) Flower advertisement for insects: Bees, a case study. In S. N. Archer, M. B. A. Djamgoz, E. R. Loew, J. C. Partridge, and S. Vallerga (eds.), *Adaptive Mechanisms in the Ecology of Vision*. Dordrecht, Netherlands: Kluwer, pp. 537–553.

Vorobyev, M., Osorio, D., Bennett, A. T. D., and Cuthill, I. C. (1998) Tetrachromacy, oil droplets and bird plumage colours. *J. Comp. Physiol. A* 183: 621–633.

Wachowitz, S. and Ewert, J.-P. (1996) A key by which the toad's visual system gets access to the domain of prey. *Physiol. Behav.* 60: 877–887.

Waddington, K. D. (2001) Subjective evaluation and choice behavior by nectar- and pollen-collecting bees. In L. Chittka and J. D. Thomson (eds.), *Cognitive Ecology of Pollination*. Cambridge: Cambridge Univ. Press, pp. 41–60.

Waddington, K. D. and Holden, L. R. (1979) Optimal foraging: On flower selection by bees. *Am. Nat.* 114: 179–196.

Walcher, F. (1994) Der Einfluss visueller Deprivation auf die Entfernungsmessung bei *Tenodera sinensis* während der frühen postembryonalen Entwicklung. Masteri thesis, Univ. of Graz, Graz, Austria.

Walcher, F. and Kral, K. (1994) Visual deprivation and distance estimation in the praying mantis larva. *Physiol. Entomol.* 19: 230–240.

Wald, G. (1953) The biochemistry of vision. *Ann. Rev. Biochem.* 22: 497–526.

Wald, G. (1967) Visual pigment of crayfish. *Nature* 215: 1131–1133.

Wald, G. (1968) Single and multiple visual system in arthropods. *J. Gen. Physiol.* 51: 125–156.

Wallace, G. K. (1959) Visual scanning in the desert locust *Schistocerca Gregaria* (Forskal). *J. Exp. Biol.* 36: 512–525.

Wang, D. L. and Ewert, J.-P. (1992) Configurational pattern discrimination responsible for dishabituation in common toads *Bufo bufo* (L.): Behavioral tests of the predictions of a neural model. *J. Comp. Physiol. A* 170: 317–325.

Wang, D. L., Arbib, M. A., and Ewert, J.-P. (1991) Dishabituation hierarchies for visual pattern discrimination in toads: A dialogue between modeling and experimentation. In M. A. Arbib and J.-P. Ewert (eds.), *Visual Structures and Integrated Functions*. Berlin: Springer-Verlag, pp. 427–441.

Wanless, F. R. (1978) A revision of the spider genus *Portia* (Araneae: Saltcidae). *Bull. Brit. Mus. Nat. Hist. Zool. Lond.* 34: 83–124.

Wanless, F. R. (1984) A review of the spider subfamily Spartaeinae nom. n. (Araneae: Salticidae). *Bull. Brit. Mus. Nat. Hist. Zool. Lond.* 9: 213–257.

Warrant, E., Porombka, T., and Kirchner, W. H. (1996) Neural image enhancement allows honeybees to see at night. *Proc. Roy. Soc. Lond. B* 263: 1521–1526.

Waser, N. M. (1986) Flower constancy: Definition, cause and measurement. *Am. Nat.* 127: 593–603.

Waterman, T. H. (1981) Polarization sensitivity. In H. Autrum (ed.), *Handbook of Sensory Physiology*. vol. VII/6B, Comparative Physiology and Evolution of Vision in Invertetrates Berlin: Springer-Verlag, pp. 283–469.

Waterman, T. H. (1984) Natural polarized light and vision. In M. Ali (ed.), *Photoreception and Vision in Invertetrates*. NATO Advanced Science Series A, vol. 74, New York: Plenum, pp. 63–114.

Waterman, T. H. and Fernandez, H. R. (1970) E-vector and wavelength discrimination by retinular cells of the crayfish *Procambarus*. *Z. verg. Physiol.* 68: 154–174.

Waterman, T. H., Fernandez, H. R., and Goldsmith, T. H. (1969) Dichroism of photosensitive pigment in rhabdoms of the crayfish *Orconectes*. *J. Gen. Physiol.* 54: 415–432.

Weerasuriya, A. (1989) In search of the motor pattern generator for snapping in toads. In J.-P. Ewert and M. A. Arbib (eds.), *Visuomotor Coordination: Amphibians, Comparisons, Models and Robots*. New York: Plenum, pp. 589–614.

Weerasuriya, A. and Ewert, J.-P. (1981) Prey-selective neurons in the toad's optic tectum and sensorimotor interfacing: HRP studies and recording experiments. *J. Comp. Physiol.* 144: 429–434.

Weerasuriya, A. and Ewert, J.-P. (1983) Afferents of some dorsal retino-recipient areas of the brain of *Bufo bufo*. *Soc. Neurosci. Abstr.* 9: 536.

Weerasuriya, A., Baker, C. R., and Ball, N. A. (1994) How do small frogs capture long earthworms? *Soc. Neurosci. Abstr.* 20(1): 168.

Wehner, R. (1971) The generalization of directional visual stimuli in the honey bee, *Apis mellifera*. *J. Insect Physiol.* 17: 1579–1591.

Wehner, R. (1981) Spatial vision in arthropods. In H. Autrum (ed.), *Handbook of Sensory Physiology*. vol. 7/6C, *Vision in Invertebrates*. Berlin: Springer-Verlag, pp. 287–616.

Wehner, R. (1987) "Matched filters"—neural models of the external world. *J. Comp. Physiol. A* 161: 511–531.

Wehner, R. (1989a) Neurobiology of polarization vision. *Trends Neurosci.* 12: 353–359.

Wehner, R. (1989b) The hymenopteran skylight compass: Matched filtering and parallel coding. *J. Exp. Biol.* 146: 63–85.

Wehner, R. (2001) Polarization vision—a uniform sensory capacity? *J. Exp. Biol.* 204: 2589–2596.

Wehner, R. and Bernard, G. D. (1993) Photoreceptor twist: A solution to the false-color problem. *Proc. Nat. Acad. Sci.* USA 90: 4132–4135.

Wehner, R. and Lanfranconi, B. (1981) What do ants know about the rotation of the sky? *Nature* 293: 731–733.

Wehner, R., Bleuler, S., and Shah, D. (1990) Bees navigate using vectors and routes rather than maps. *Naturwissenschaften.* 77: 479–482.

Wehner, R., Michel, B., and Antonsen, P. (1996) Visual navigation in insects: Coupling of egocentric and geocentric information. *J. Exp. Biol.* 199: 129–140.

Weiss, R. M. (2001) Vision and learning in some neglected pollinators: Beetles, flies moths and butterflies. In L. Chittka and J. D. Thomson (eds.), *Cognitive Ecology of Pollination—Animal Behavior and Floral Evolution.* Cambridge: Cambridge Univ. Press, pp. 171–190.

Wells, H. and Wells, P. H. (1986) Optimal diet, minimal uncertainty and individual constancy in the foraging of honey bees, *Apis mellifera. J. Anim. Ecol.* 55: 881–891.

Wells, H., Wells, P., and Contreras, D. (1986) Effects of flower-morph frequency and distribution on recruitment and behaviour of honeybees. *J. Apic. Res.* 25: 139–145.

Wells, M. J. (1978) *Octopus: Physiology and Behaviour of an Advanced Invertebrate.* London: Chapman and Hall.

Wells, M. J. and O'Dor, R. K. (1991) Jet propulsion and the evolution of the cephalopods. *Bull. Mar. Sci.* 49: 419–432.

Wells, M. J. and Wells, J. (1959) Hormonal control of sexual maturity in *Octopus. J. Exp. Biol.* 36: 1–33.

Wells, M. J., Freeman, N. H., and Ashburner, M. (1965) Some experiments on the chemo-tactile sense of octopuses. *J. Exp. Biol.* 43: 553–563.

Wells, P. H. and Wells, H. (1985) Ethological isolation of plants 2. Odour selection by honeybees. *J. Apic. Res.* 24: 86–92.

Werbos, P. J. (1995) Backpropagation: Basis and new developments. In M. A. Arbib (ed.), *The Handbook of Brain Theory and Neural Networks.* Cambridge, Mass.: MIT Press, pp. 134–139.

Werner, A., Menzel, R., and Wehrhahn, C. (1988) Color constancy in the honeybee. *J. Neurosci.* 8: 156–159.

Westby, G. W., Keay, K. A., Redgrave, P. L., Dean, P., and Bannister, M. (1990) Output pathways from rat superior colliculus mediating approach and avoidance have different sensory properties. *Exp. Brain Res.* 81: 626–638.

Westin, J., Langberg, J. J., and Camhi, J. M. (1977) Responses of giant interneurons of the cockroach *Periplaneta americana* to wind puffs of different directions and velocities. *J. Comp. Physiol.* 121: 307–324.

White, R. H., Xu, H., Munch, T., Bennett, R. R., and Grable, E. A. (2003) The retina of *Manduca sexta*: Rhodopsin-expression, the mosaic of green-, blue- and UV-sensitive photoreceptors and regional specialization. *J. Exp. Biol.* 206: 3337–3348.

Widder, E. A. (1999) Bioluminescence. In S. N. Archer, M. B. A. Djamgoz, E. R. Loew, J. C. Partrige, and S. Vallerga (eds.), *Adaptive Mechanisms in the Ecology of Vision*. Dordrecht, Netherlands: Kluwer, pp. 555–581.

Widmer, A., Schmid-Hempel, P., Estoup, A., and Scholl, A. (1998) Population genetic structure and colonization history of *Bombus terrestris* s. I. (Hymenoptera: Apidae) from the Canary Islands and Madeira. *Heredity* 81: 563–572.

Wiens, J. A. (1970) Effects of early experience on substrate pattern selection in *Rana aurora* tadpoles. *Copeia* 3: 543–548.

Wiens, J. A. (1972) Anuran habitat selection: Early experience and substrate selection in *Rana cascade* tadpoles. *Anim. Behav.* 20: 218–220.

Wiersma, C. A. G. (1938) Function of the giant fibers of the central nervous system of the crayfish. *Proc. Soc. Exp. Biol. Med. U.S.A.* 38: 661–662.

Wiggers, W. and Roth, G. (1994) Depth perception in salamanders: The wiring of visual maps. *Eur. J. Morphol.* 32: 311–314.

Wilcox, R. S., Jackson, R. R., and Gentile, K. (1996) Spiderweb smokescreens: Spider trickster uses background noise to mask stalking movements. *Anim. Behav.* 51: 313–326.

Wilczynski, W. and Northcutt, R. G. (1977) Afferents to the optic tectum of the leopard frog: An HRP study. *J. Comp. Neurol.* 173: 219–229.

Wilczynski, W. and Northcutt, R. G. (1983a) Connections of the bullfrog striatum: Afferent organization. *J. Comp. Neurol.* 214: 321–332.

Wilczynski, W. and Northcutt, R. G. (1983b) Connections of the bullfrog striatum: Efferent projections. *J. Comp. Neurol.* 214: 333–343.

Wiley, R. H. (1991) Associations of song properties with habitats for territorial oscine birds of eastern North America. *Am. Nat.* 138: 973–993.

Wiley, R. H. and Richards, D. G. (1978) Physical constraints on sound communication in the atmosphere: Implications for the evolution of animal vocalizations. *Behav. Ecol. Sociobiol.* 3: 69–94.

Willey, M. B. and Jackson, R. R. (1993) Olfactory cues from conspecifics inhibit the web-invasion behaviour of *Portia*, a web-invading, araneophagic jumping spider (Araneae, Salticidae). *Can. J. Zool.* 71: 1415–1420.

Williams, D. S. (1983) Changes of photoreceptor performance associated with the daily turnover of photoreceptor membrane in the locust. *J. Comp. Physiol. A* 150: 509–519.

Williams, D. S. and McIntyre, P. (1980) The principal eyes of a jumping spider have a telephoto component. *Nature* 228: 578–580.

Williams, P. H. (1994) Phylogenetic relationships among bumble bees (*Bombus* Latr.): A reappraisal of morphological evidence. *Syst. Entomol.* 19: 327–344.

Williamson, R. (1995a) A sensory basis for orientation in cephalopods. *J. Mar. Biol. Assoc. UK* 75: 83–92.

Williamson, R. (1995b) The statocysts of cephalopods. In N. J. Abbott, R. Williamson, and L. Maddock (eds.), *Cephalopod Neurobiology. Neuroscience Studies in Squid, Octopus and Cuttlefish.* Oxford: Oxford Univ. Press, pp. 503–520.

Williamson, R. and Budelmann, B. U. (1985) The response of the *Octopus* angular acceleration receptor system to sinusoidal stimulation. *J. Comp. Physiol. A* 156: 403–412.

Williamson, R. and Budelmann, B. U. (1991) Convergent inputs to *Octopus* oculomotor neurones demonstrated in a brain slice preparation. *Neurosci. Lett.* 121: 215–218.

Williamson, R., Ichikawa, M., and Matsumoto, G. (1994) Neuronal circuits in cephalopod vision. *Netherlands J. Zool.* 44: 272–283.

Winston, M. L. (1991) *The Biology of the Honey Bee.* Cambridge, Mass.: Harvard Univ. Press.

Withers, G. S., Fahrbach, S. E., and Robinson, G. E. (1993) Selective neuro-anatomical plasticity and division of labour in the honeybee. *Nature* 364: 238–240.

Witt, P. N. (1975) The web as a means of communication. *Biosci. Comm.* 1: 7–23.

Wittmann, D., Radtke, R., Cure, J., and Schifino-Wittmann, M. T. (1990) Coevolved reproductive strategies in the oligolectic bee *Callonychium petuniae* (Apoidea andrenidae) and three purple flowered *Petunia* species (Solanaceae) in southern Brazil. *Z. Zool. Syst. Evolutionsforsch.* 28: 157–165.

Woodcock, A. E. R. and Goldsmith, T. H. (1970) Spectral responses of sustaining fibers in the optic tracts of crayfish (*Procambarus*). *Z. Vergl. Physiol.* 69: 117–133.

Woodhams, P. L. and Messenger, J. B. (1974) A note on the ultrastructure of the *Octopus* olfactory organ. *Cell Tiss. Res.* 152: 253–258.

Wyszecki, G. and Stiles, W. S. (1982) *Color Science: Concepts and Methods, Quantitative Data and Formulae*, vol. 2. New York: Wiley.

Yager, D. D. (1990) Sexual dimorphism of auditory function and structure in praying mantises (Mantodea; Dictyoptera). *J. Zool. Lond.* 221: 517–537.

Yamaguchi, T., Katagiri, Y., and Ochi, K. (1976) Polarized light responses from retinular cells and sustaining fibers of the mantis shrimp. *Biol. J. Okayama Univ.* 17: 61–66.

Yamamoto, M. (1984) Photoreceptor collaterals in the cuttlefish retina. *Zool. Sci.* 1: 501–503.

Yamamoto, M. and Takasu, N. (1984) Membrane particles and gap junctions in the retinas of two species of cephalopods, *Octopus ocellatus* and *Sepiella japonica. Cell Tiss. Res.* 237: 209–218.

Yamamoto, T., Tasaki, K., Sugawara, Y., and Tonosaki, A. (1965) Fine structure of the octopus retina. *J. Cell Biol.* 25: 345–359.

Yamamoto, T. Y., Tonosaki, A., Kataoka, S., Tasaki, K., and Tsukahara, Y. (1976) Synaptic interconnections of visual cells in some molluscan retinas. In E. Yamada and S. Mishima (eds.), *Structure of the Eye*, vol. III. Tokyo: Japanese Journal of Opthalmology, pp. 193–202.

Yamashita, S. and Tateda, H. (1976) Spectral sensitivities of jumping spiders' eyes. *J. Comp. Physiol. A* 105: 29–41.

Yang, E. C. and Maddess, T. (1997) Orientaion-sensitive neurons in the brain of the honeybee (*Apis mellifera*). *J. Insect Physiol.* 43: 329–336.

Yang, E. C. and Osorio, D. (1991) Spectral sensitivities of photoreceptors and lamina monopolar cells in the dragonfly, *Hemicordulia tau. J. Comp. Physiol. A* 169: 663–669.

Yang, X. L. and Wu, S. M. (1991) Feedforward lateral inhibition in retinal bipolar cells: Input-output relation of the horizontal cell-depolarizing bipolar cell synapse. *Proc. Natl. Acad. Sci. U.S.A.* 88: 3310–3313.

Ye, S. and Comer, C. M. (1996) Correspondence of escape-turning behavior with activity of descending mechanosensory interneurons in the cockroach, *Periplaneta americana. J. Neurosci.* 16: 5844–5853.

Ye, S., Leung, V., Khan, A., Baba, Y., and Comer, C. M. (2003) The antennal system and cockroach evasive behavior I: Roles for visual and mechanosensory cues in the response. *J. Comp. Physiol. A* 189: 89–96.

Yoerg, S. I. (1991) Ecological frames of mind: The role of cognition in behavioral ecology. *Quart. Rev. Biol.* 66: 287–301.

Young, J. Z. (1960a) The statocysts of *Octopus vulgaris. Proc. Roy. Soc. Lond.* 152: 3–29.

Young, J. Z. (1960b) The visual system of *Octopus*. (1) Regularities in the retina and optic lobes of *Octopus* in relation to form discrimination. *Nature* 186: 836–839.

Young, J. Z. (1963) Dark- and light-adaptation in the eyes of some cephalopods. *Proc. Zool. Soc. Lond.* 140: 255–272.

Young, J. Z. (1971) *The Anatomy of the Nervous System of Octopus vulgaris*. Oxford: Oxford Univ. Press.

Young, J. Z. (1973) Receptive fields of the visual system of the squid. *Nature* 241: 469–471.

Young, J. Z. (1988) Octopus brain. In L. N. Irwin (ed.), *Comparative Neuroscience and Neurobiology. Readings from the Encyclopedia of Neuroscience*. Boston: Birkhauser, pp. 97–99.

Young, J. Z. (1989a) The angular acceleration receptor system of diverse cephalopods. *Phil. Trans. Roy. Soc. Lond. B* 325: 189–238.

Young, J. Z. (1989b) The Bayliss-Starling Lecture. Some special senses in the sea. *J. Physiol. Lond.* 411: 1–25.

Young, J. Z. (1991) Light has many meanings for cephalopods. *Vis. Neurosci.* 7: 1–12.

Young, J. Z. (1995) Multiple matrices in the memory system of *Octopus*. In N. J. Abbott, R. Williamson, and L. Maddock (eds.), *Cephalopod Neurobiology. Neuroscience Studies in Squid, Octopus and Cuttlefish.* Oxford: Oxford Univ. Press, pp.

Young, R. E. (1972) Function of extra-ocular photoreceptors in bathypelagic cephalopods. *Deep-Sea Res.* 19: 651–660.

Young, R. E. and Roper, C. F. E. (1976) Bioluminescent countershading in midwater animals: Evidence from living squid. *Science* 191: 1286–1288.

Young, R. E., Roper, C. F. E., and Walters, J. F. (1979) Eyes and extraocular photoreceptors in midwater cephalopods and fishes: Their role in detecting downwelling light or coun-terillumination. *Mar. Biol.* 51: 371–380.

Zeil, J. (1989) Substrate slope and the alignment of acute zones in semi-terrestial crabs *Ocypode ceratophthalmus. J. Exp. Biol.* 152: 573–576.

Zeil, J. and Hofmann, M. (2001) Signals from 'crabworld': Cuticular reflections in a fiddler crab colony. *J. Exp. Biol.* 204: 2501–2569.

Zentall, T. R. and Hogan, D. E. (1978) Same/different concept learning in the pigeon: The effect of negative instances and prior adaptation to transfer stimuli. *J. Exp. Analysis Behav.* 30: 177–186.

Zhang, S. W. and Srinivasan, M. V. (1994) Prior experience enhances pattern discrimina-tion in insect vision. *Nature* 368: 330–333.

Zhang, S. W., Bartsch, K., and Srinivasan, M. V. (1996) Maze learning by honeybee. *Neurobiol. Learn. Mem.* 66(3): 267–282.

Zhang, S. W., Lehrer, M., and Srinivasan, M. V. (1998) Eye-specific route-learning and interocular transfer in walking honeybees. *J. Comp. Physiol. A* 182(6): 745–754.

Zhang, S. W., Lehrer, M., and Srinivasan, M. V. (1999) Honeybee memory: Navigation by associative grouping and recall of visual stimuli. *Neurobiol. Learn. Mem.* 72: 180–201.

Zhang, S. W., Mizutani, A., and Srinivasan, M. V. (2000) Maze navigation by honeybees: Learning path regularity. *Learn. Mem.* 7: 364–374.

Zollinger, H. (1988) Biological aspects of color naming. In I. Rentschler, B. Herzberger, and D. Epstein (eds.), *Beauty and the Brain. Biological Aspects of Aesthetics.* Basel, Switzerland: Birkhauser Verlag, pp. 149–164.

Zuker, C. S., Cowan, A. F., and Rubin, G. M. (1985) Isolation and structure of a rhodopsin gene from *Drosophila. Cell* 40: 851–858.

Taxonomic Index

General Subject Index